A Colour Atlas of
Otorhinolaryngology

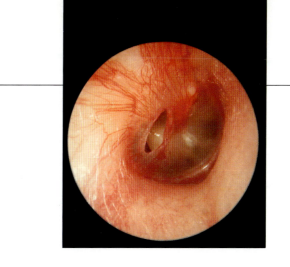

A Colour
Atlas of
Otorhinolaryngology

Bruce Benjamin
OBE, DLO, FRACS, FAAP
Clinical Professor of Otorhinolaryngology
Sydney University, Australia

Brian Bingham
MB ChB, FRCS
Honorary Senior Lecturer in Otolaryngology, University of Glasgow
Consultant ENT Surgeon, Victoria Infirmary, Glasgow, UK

Michael Hawke
MD, FRCS(C)
Professor of Otolaryngology, University of Toronto
Chief of Otolaryngology, St Joseph's Hospital, Toronto, Canada

Heinz Stammberger
MD
Professor of Otorhinolaryngology, University of Graz, Austria

Edited by Michael Hawke

With a contribution from

Kees Buiter, MD
Associate Professor of Otorhinolaryngology
University of Groningen, The Netherlands

Allen W Tarro, DMD
Merrimack Valley Oral Surgeons Inc., Lowell, Massachusetts, USA

MARTIN DUNITZ

Text © Martin Dunitz Ltd 1995
Artwork © Bruce Benjamin, Brian Bingham, Michael Hawke and Heinz Stammberger 1995,
except as otherwise acknowledged

First published in the United Kingdom in 1995 by
Martin Dunitz Ltd, 7–9 Pratt Street, London NW1 0AE

Reprinted 1997

A CIP record for this book is available from the British Library

ISBN 1-85317-122-0

A 35-mm colour slide collection in four volumes, based on
600 images in this book, is also available.

Composition by Scribe Design, Gillingham, Kent,
United Kingdom

Printed and bound in Spain
by Grafos, S.A. Arte Sobre papel

Contents

**This Atlas is dedicated to
Dr Karl Storz
Instrument maker**

Preface

Although the clinical features of a patient's history may suggest a possible diagnosis, definitive determination of disease is ultimately dependent on signs elicited by visual inspection; nowhere is this more important than in the field of otorhinolaryngology. Examination of the ear, nasal cavities, nasopharynx, oral cavity, larynx, tracheobronchial tree and oesophagus have been dependent in the past on naked-eye examination but with modern technology the search for diagnostic information now relies on sophisticated optical systems including the operating microscope, flexible fibreoptic nasopharyngolaryngoscope and rigid rod lens telescopes.

Photography for documentation has fascinated physicians since the larynx was first successfully photographed over 100 years ago by French, of New York, who utilized sunlight reflected from a headmirror, a laryngeal mirror and a primitive photographic device. Since then methods that have been acclaimed for demonstration of disease include artists' illustrations such as Netter's beautifully coloured, anatomically accurate works and Kleinsasser's modern photography utilizing the beam splitter of the operating microscope. In 1969 the first edition of *Atlas of Ear, Nose and Throat Diseases, including Bronchoesophagology* was published by Georg Thieme, edited by Walter Becker of Bonn, Germany. The other distinguished contributing authors were Richard Buckingham (Chicago), Paul Holinger (Chicago), Wolfgang Steiner and Michael Jaumann (Erlangen) and Walter Messerklinger (Graz). This atlas was a great milestone in the depiction of disease: the photographs demonstrated otorhinlaryngologic and bronchoesophagolic pathology as a foundation upon which rational therapy could be developed. Becker's conception was that an atlas should point out the salient visual features of a disorder to assist the physician in recognition and understanding of the disease, leading to correct management.

Since Becker's Atlas technology for photographic documentation has improved. There have been many successful methods but the most reliable and versatile modern system employs a 35 mm single frame, single lens reflex camera with Hopkins telescopes and a synchronized, computer-controlled, automatic exposure remote electronic flash generator. Routine photographic documentation of any area accessible to a telescope is now a practical reality, utilizing either black-and-white or colour film, although the latter provides better depth, warmth and added reality. Colour reproduction from the original 35 mm transparencies must be painstakingly and accurately achieved, not only to retain the information in the original photograph but to maintain consistency from one colour separation to the other throughout the book. Martin Dunitz publishers have been most cooperative and patient in this endeavour and have earned the respect and appreciation of the authors.

In the field of ear, nose and throat/head and neck surgery, photographic documentation is of supreme importance. It provides an objective, natural colour record with accurate detail eminently suitable for teaching. The rigid glass lens rod system in the Hopkins telescopes permits the use of miniature endoscopes which provide magnified clear full-colour wide-angled images with unlimited photographic capabilities.

The authors of this new text, *A Colour Atlas of Otorhinolaryngology*, have used the Karl Storz photographic equipment and wish to pay tribute to Dr Karl Storz. The young Karl Storz, born in 1911, served an apprenticeship in his father's firm where he learned to appreciate the need for high-quality surgical instruments. In 1945 Karl Storz, with his father's assistance, founded the present firm of Karl Storz GmbH in Tuttlingen, southern Germany. At first, the firm made specialized instruments in collaboration with Kleinsasser, Messerklinger and Maassen and expanded the field of bronchoscopy which was then primarily applied to the removal of inhaled foreign bodies. By the end of the 1940s, Karl Storz had designed his own optical system and produced optical and flexible forceps for use with rigid bronchoscopes. By the early 1950s, a new system with a flash tube for photo-documentation was made and by 1960 Karl Storz recognized that glass fibres could be used not only for the transmission of illumination but also for reflecting the image to the eye of the examiner. The era of cold light had begun. The value of the principle of the rod lens system designed by Professor H. H. Hopkins was recognized by Karl

Storz, leading to a sustained period of rapid growth. Production now embraced every specialized medical field for adults, children and infants. In addition, the Karl Storz endoscopes and fibreoptic telescopes were applied in the technology of engine construction, air and space travel, architecture and archaeology. Dr Storz has been awarded a Doctorate of Medicine at the University of Marburg and numerous other honours from many countries. He has guided his world-famous firm for many years and is now supported by his daughters, Sybill Storz-Reling and Gudrun Koller-Storz, while looking forward to his grandson, Karl-Christian, becoming an able successor.

The majority of the photographs in this Atlas were taken with the Karl Storz state-of-the-art photographic equipment developed by the brilliant application of fine instrument making, optics, electronics, photographic technique and a practical knowledge of the needs of the clinician. The Atlas is dedicated to Dr Karl Storz.

Bruce Benjamin

Acknowledgements

The authors are grateful to the following for permission to reproduce figures:

Dr Kees Buiter, Department of Otorhinolaryngology, University of Groningen, for 2.87, 2.93, 2.96, 2.97, 2.101, 2.116, 2.117, 2.173, 2.195, 2.197, 2.267, 2.268, 2.272, 2.290, 2.291, 2.292, 2.293, 2.294, 2.295 and 2.296;

John Cowpe, Department of Oral Surgery, University of Wales College of Medicine, Cardiff, for 3.11, 3.37, 3.42, 3.46, 3.49, 3.52, 3.55, 3.56, 3.67, 3.68, 3.70, 3.71, 3.72, 3.75, 3.76, 3.77, 3.79, 3.80, 3.106, 3.107, 3.119, 3.121 and 3.127;

John Crowther, Department of Otolaryngology, Victoria Infirmary, Glasgow, for 6.37 and 6.38;

Dr Benjamin Fisher, The Wellsley Hospital, Toronto, for 1.60 and 3.133;

Liam Flood, Department of Otolaryngology, North Riding Infirmary, Middlesbrough, for 3.108, 6.8, 6.9, 6.17, 6.24, 6.25, 6.56;

Dr Jeremy Freeman, Department of Otolaryngology, University of Toronto, for 6.10;

Dr Michael Hawke and Dr Anthony F. Jahn, *Diseases of the Ear: Clinical and Pathological Aspects* (Gower: London 1987), for 1.4 and 1.86;

Dr U. Joshi, Department of Genitourinary Medicine, Glasgow Royal Infirmary, for 3.24 and 3.74;

Robin Kell, Department of Otolaryngology, Victoria Infirmary, Glasgow for 3.208, 6.30 and 6.50;

Dr M. A. Knowling and the Editor of the *Canadian Medical Association Journal* for 1.24;

Dr Mark May, The Sinus Surgery Center, Shadyside Hospital, Pittsburgh, for 2.22 and 2.24;

Dr David P. Mitchell, Staff Otolaryngologist, The Hospital for Sick Children, Toronto, for 1.17, 1.79 and 1.80;

Laura Mitchell, Department of Orthodontics, Middlesbrough General Hospital, for 3.26, 3.27, 3.33, 3.35, 3.36 and 3.39;

The Mouth Clinic, Sunnybrook Medical Centre, Toronto, for 3.150;

Dr Colin Munro, Department of Dermatology, Southern General Hospital, Glasgow, for 3.8, 3.9, 3.17, 3.18, 3.22, 3.23, 3.25, 3.81, 3.82, 3.89, 3.91, 3.93, 3.94, 3.95 and 3.96;

Ahmes L. Pahor, Department of Otolaryngology, Sandwell District General Hospital, for 3.168;

David Ritchie, Accident and Emergency Department, Victoria Infirmary, Glasgow, for 6.58;

Derek Russell, Department of Oral Surgery, Victoria Infirmary, Glasgow, for 3.6, 3.43, 3.45, 3.47, 3.48, 3.50, 3.51, 3.54, 3.56, 3.58, 3.59, 3.65, 3.66, 3.73, 3.83, 3.92, 3.110, 3.112, 3.125, 3.126, 3.147, 3.153, 3.154, 3.156, 3.162, 3.171 and 3.177;

Dr Sandy Sharp, Department of Haematology, Victoria Infirmary, Glasgow, for 3.20, 3.21, 3.53, 3.102–3.105, 3.159 and 3.160;

Dr Allen W. Tarro, Merrimack Valley Oral Surgeons Inc., Lowell, Massachusetts, for 6.63–6.71;

Dr Ian Witterick, Mount Sinai Hospital, Toronto, for 6.28.

The authors would particularly like to thank Dr Buiter for his contribution to Chapter 2; Dr Tarro for his contribution to Chapter 6; and Paul Rodgers of Hartlepool Medical Illustration Department and the staff of the Department of Medical Illustration in the Victoria Infirmary, Glasgow, for their help with Chapters 3 and 6.

1
The ear

Introduction

The ear is traditionally divided into four anatomical areas: the pinna or external ear, the external auditory canal, the middle ear and the inner ear. In this Atlas the first three of these areas will be covered in detail. Each of these areas plays its own distinct role in the auditory process and is affected by its own distinct group of diseases.

The pinna

The outermost portion of the ear, the external ear, is a flattened, funnel-shaped appendage composed of a fibroelastic cartilaginous skeleton covered by skin, which is located on the side of the head. The external ear is also called the pinna or auricle.

The funnel shape of the pinna has a role to play in sound localization and sound amplification. Both sound localization and sound amplification also depend upon the ability to move the pinna for maximal reception. These two acoustic functions are more highly developed in some other mammals (such as the horse, dog and bat), as is demonstrated by the relatively greater size, projection and musculature of the auricle in these species. In humans the pinna plays only a minor, but still significant, role in sound localization and, to a lesser extent, amplification. The folds and convolutions of the pinna are also thought to provide some protection to the external auditory canal from insects and foreign objects.

By virtue of its external location, the pinna is exposed to the effects of the elements (especially to solar irradiation) as well as to those of wind, cold and local trauma. The majority of disorders affecting the pinna involve the skin which covers its surface; in this area, therefore, the otorhinolaryngologist must have a sound knowledge of dermatology. In any examination of the pinna all areas must be inspected, and the examiner must never forget to 'look behind the ear'.

The external auditory canal

The second area is the external auditory canal. The external canal provides a conduit through which the airborne sound waves collected by the pinna are transmitted to the tympanic membrane. Because of its length and slightly convoluted shape, the external canal also provides a great deal of protection for the tympanic membrane.

The external auditory canal originates at the medial end of the conchal bowl and extends medially to the tympanic membrane. For anatomical purposes, the lateral surface of the tympanic membrane is considered to be part of the external auditory canal. Because of the oblique angulation of the tympanic membrane, the external canal measures approximately 25 mm in length along its posterior wall and 30 mm in length along its anterior wall.

The external auditory canal has developed a unique and highly efficient self-cleansing mechanism, in which there is a continuous migration of epithelium from the deep meatus to the outer portion of the canal where the keratin squames are shed.

Many of the disorders affecting the external auditory canal result from either a failure of the normal migratory self-cleansing mechanism or trauma to the epithelium lining the canal. The accumulation of moisture within the canal, and the unfortunate tendency of some individuals to insert foreign objects into the external canal, can break down the integrity of the epithelium lining the canal and thus predispose to the development of infections of the epithelium (otitis externa).

The middle ear

The third portion of the ear, the middle ear, is responsible for the transmission of sound waves from the tympanic membrane to the inner ear. The middle ear cleft or tubotympanic cavity originates in the nasopharynx at the nasopharyngeal opening of the Eustachian tube (the torus tubarius). The middle ear cleft consists of three major components: the middle ear cavity proper (which contains the three ossicles), the Eustachian tube (which provides a source of ventilation and pressure equalization) and the mastoid air cell system (whose exact function remains unclear). Proper functioning of the Eustachian tube is critical for the maintenance of aeration and the normal functioning of the middle ear; indeed, malfunction of the Eustachian tube is the prime cause of most disorders of the middle ear.

The anterior half of the middle ear cavity is lined by a respiratory ciliated type of epithelium which contains two types of mucus-producing cells: the goblet cells which are located in the epithelial layer and the seromucinous glands which are located in the subepithelial layer. The mucus produced by these glands serves as a protecting and lubricating mantle for the respiratory mucoperiosteum which is exposed to the air within the middle ear. Mucociliary flow is the major defence mechanism of respiratory epithelium and the role of the mucous blanket in this system is critical. In the absence of sufficient or normal mucus, the mucociliary clearance system fails.

Pinna

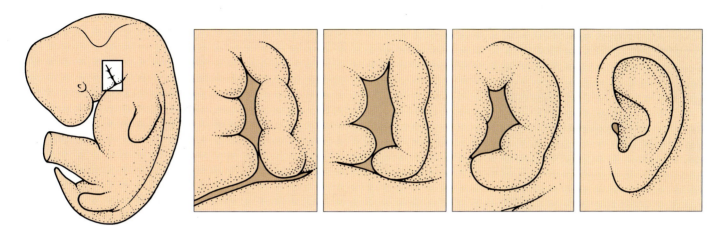

Figure 1.1
Embryology of the auricle

The pinna or external auricle is formed from six hillocks that arise around the dorsal extremity of the first branchial groove between 4 and 6 weeks of gestation. These hillocks are gradually transformed into the complex folds of the fully formed auricle.

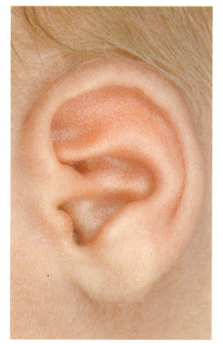

Figure 1.2
Normal newborn auricle

The newborn auricle demonstrates all the basic features of the adult pinna. By the age of 9 years, the auricle has usually reached its adult size.

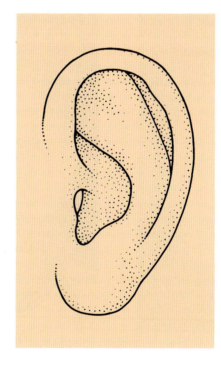

Figure 1.3
Surface anatomy of the external ear

The common surface landmarks of the pinna are illustrated. While the relative proportion of the structures varies from individual to individual, their presence is relatively constant.

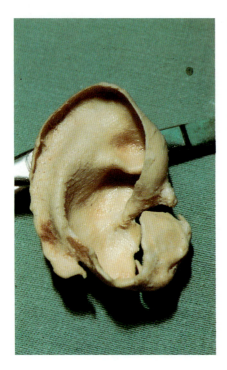

Figure 1.4
Cartilaginous skeleton of the pinna

The shape of the external auricle is determined by its underlying fibroelastic cartilaginous 'skeleton'.

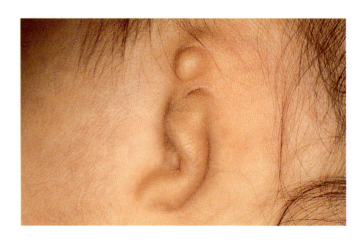

Figure 1.5
Microtia

The term 'microtia' is used when there is gross under-development of the pinna with a blind or absent external auditory canal. Congenital malformations of the external ear are frequently associated with malformations of other portions of the ear or face.

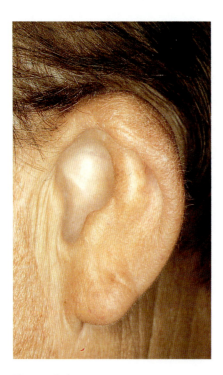

Figure 1.6
Atresia

In this patient there is a partial atresia of the pinna and a complete atresia of the external auditory canal.

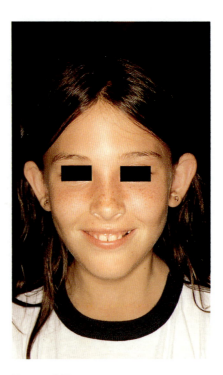

Figure 1.7
Outstanding ear

Minor deformities of the helix and antihelix are the most common malformations of the external ear. Outstanding ears are inherited by means of an autosomal dominant gene with complete penetrance and variable expressivity. When the angle between the auricle and the side of the head is greater than normal, the result is an outstanding ear.

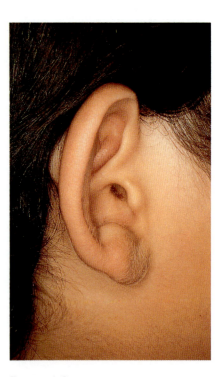

Figure 1.8
Cupped ear

The redundant and overhanging helical fold in this patient has produced a 'cupped ear'.

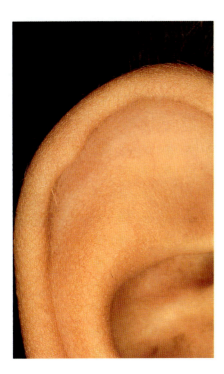

Figure 1.9
Darwin's tubercle

Darwin's tubercle is a small cartilaginous protuberance most commonly situated along the concave edge of the posterosuperior helix. A Darwin's tubercle is inherited by means of an autosomal dominant gene with variable expressivity. Darwin's tubercle usually projects anteriorly from the concave edge of the posterosuperior helix.

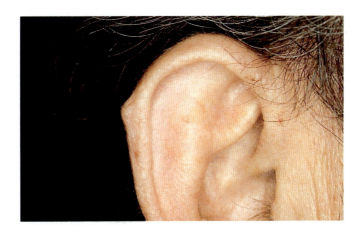

Figure 1.10
Occasionally, a Darwin's tubercle will project posteriorly from the convex border of the helix.

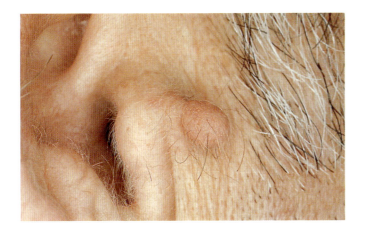

Figure 1.11
Preauricular tag

Preauricular tags are small congenital pedunculated projections arising from the skin along the anterior border of the external ear. The most common location for a preauricular tag is just anterior to the upper border of the tragus.

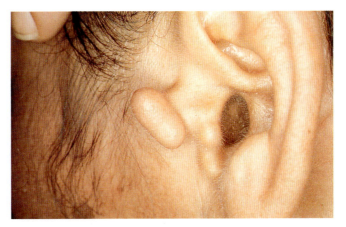

Figure 1.12
Accessory auricle

A preauricular appendage that contains a cartilaginous core is called an 'accessory auricle'. Accessory auricles represent a small ectopic remnant of one of the embryological hillocks.

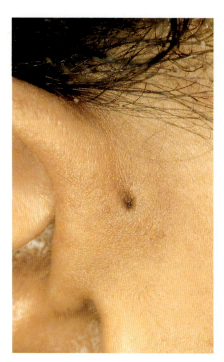

Figure 1.13

Preauricular pit

Preauricular pits are relatively shallow pits that result either from a failure in the fusion of the primitive ear hillocks or from the defective closure of the first branchial cleft. Preauricular pits are most characteristically located in, or just in front of, the anterior crus of the helix. Preauricular pits are inherited through an autosomal dominant gene with incomplete penetrance.

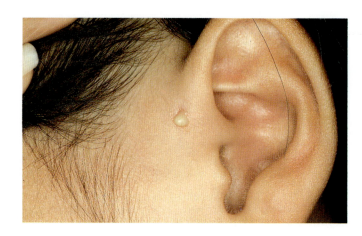

Figure 1.14

Infected preauricular sinus

A preauricular sinus is deeper than a preauricular pit, and the sinus tract is lined with a stratified squamous or columnar epithelium. The tract of a preauricular sinus may become chronically infected and emit a painless, foul-smelling, milky discharge.

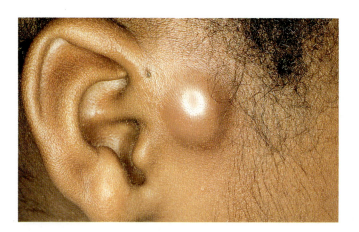

Figure 1.15

Preauricular cyst

If the external opening of the tract of a preauricular sinus becomes closed, the epithelium lining of the tract will continue to shed epithelial squames into the tract, thereby producing a preauricular cyst.

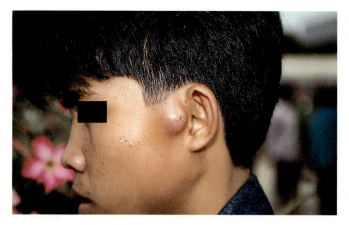

Figure 1.16

Infected preauricular cyst

When an infection develops in a preauricular sinus, it is usually more acute and associated with pain and swelling in the area of predilection for preauricular pits and sinuses. As there is no external connection in a preauricular sinus, a mini-abscess usually forms, which, if left untreated, will eventually drain from the sinus through the skin.

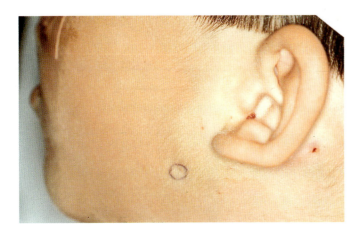

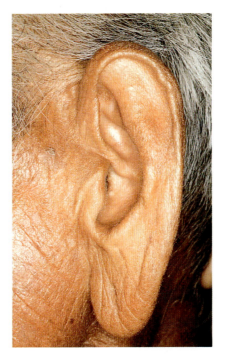

Figure 1.18

Elongated lobule

This elongated and large lobule produces an external ear that is Buddha-like in appearance. Elongated lobules are inherited by means of an autosomal dominant gene.

Figure 1.17

Collaural fistula

A collaural fistula is a rare fistula which has two openings. The lower opening is usually located in the neck between the angle of the mandible and the sternomastoid muscle. The epithelial-lined tract runs upwards to its superior opening, which is usually located in the floor of the external auditory canal or in the intertragal notch.

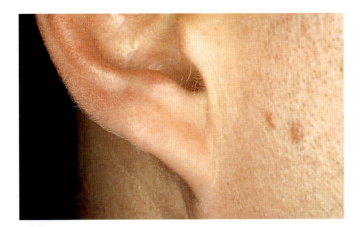

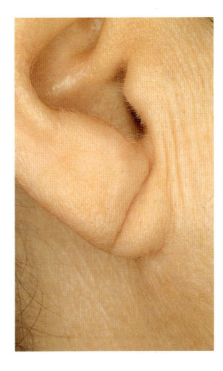

Figure 1.20

Creased lobule

With increasing age an oblique crease may appear in the lobule. This is known as a creased lobule and appears to indicate a predisposition to obstructive coronary artery disease.

Figure 1.19

Attached lobule

The insertion of the lobule into the side of the head varies from fully attached (the outer edge of the lobule forming a straight line, as seen in this photograph) to fully detached (a separate lobule that curves up to the side of the head). Attached lobules appear to be genetically recessive to detached lobules.

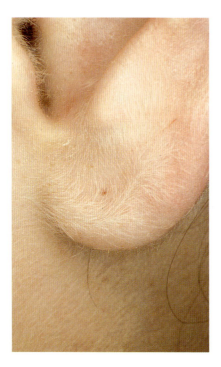

Figure 1.21
Hairy lobule

The fine hair covering this patient's lobule resulted from a persistence of the vellus hair.

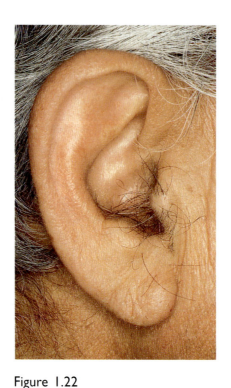

Figure 1.22
Hairy tragus

With age, coarse hairs may appear on the male tragus. This secondary sex characteristic is known as 'hairy tragus'. It is interesting to note that the word 'tragus' is derived from the Greek 'tragos' (goat), which alludes to the resemblance of these hairs to a goat's beard.

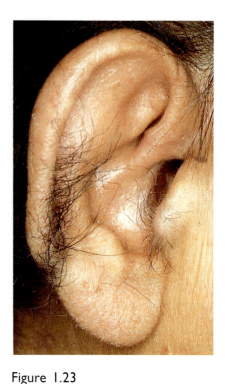

Figure 1.23
Hairy pinna

The development of coarse hairs over the pinna is called a 'hairy pinna'. These coarse hairs most commonly appear over the lower portion of the helix. Hairy pinna occurs only in males and is a Y-linked trait. The expression of hairy pinna increases with age.

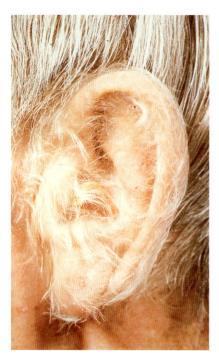

Figure 1.24
Hypertrichosis lanuginosa acquisita

Hypertrichosis lanuginosa acquisita is the term applied to the excessive growth of fine hair of the lanugus or vellus type. Hypertrichosis lanuginosa acquisita is associated with the use of certain medicines such as phenytoin, streptomycin, penicillamine and minoxidil. Certain metabolic conditions, including porphyria, pregnancy, hyperthyroidism, malnutrition and occasionally the presence of malignant disease, have also been associated with this condition.

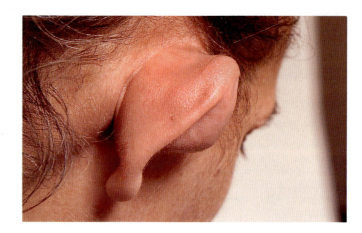

Figure 1.25
Haematoma

Haematoma of the auricle is usually the result of blunt trauma sustained during such activities as boxing or wrestling. If the trauma tears one of the small vessels that lie between the perichondrium and the underlying auricular cartilage, then blood will collect in the subperichondrial plane, thereby elevating the perichondrium from the underlying cartilage. The loose subcutaneous tissue between the skin and the perichondrium on the medial aspect of the auricle usually provides considerable mobility, and as a result a haematoma forms less commonly on the medial surface of the auricle unless the auricular cartilage has been fractured.

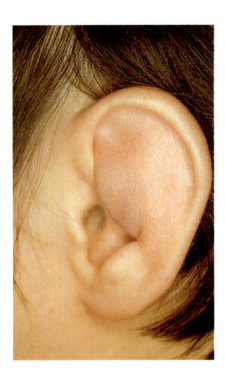

Figure 1.26
Traumatic seroma

Chronic trauma from friction may irritate the perichondrium and produce a subperichondrial serous or serosanguineous seroma. A seroma will usually persist for several days after the original injury.

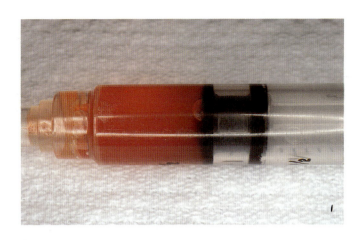

Figure 1.27
Traumatic seroma

When a seroma fails to resolve spontaneously, aspiration of the subperichondrial blood-tinged serous transudate may be necessary.

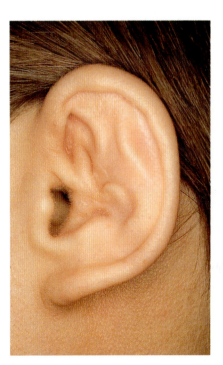

Figure 1.28
Cauliflower ear

Severe or repeated trauma to the auricle may produce areas of subperichondrial separation, shearing and localized haemorrhage, which result in devitalization of the underlying cartilage. This devitalization and its associated healing process may produce excessive subcutaneous fibrous tissue and scar formation, which deform the surface of the pinna.

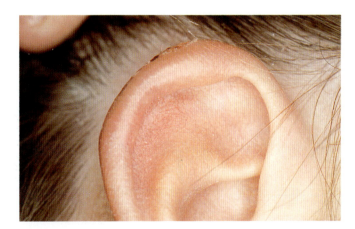

Figure 1.29
solar dermatitis

The superior portion of the pinna is susceptible to acute solar damage (sunburn). The superior portion of this pinna shows erythema, oedema and blistering, which are the result of a 'second-degree sunburn'. As will be seen later, repeated solar damage predisposes an individual to premalignant and malignant cutaneous changes.

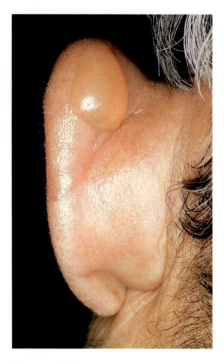

Figure 1.30
Frostbite

Tissue damage from extreme cold is similar in appearance to that sustained from heat injuries. Note the large serous-filled bulla with oedema of the surrounding skin. This is a second-degree frostbite.

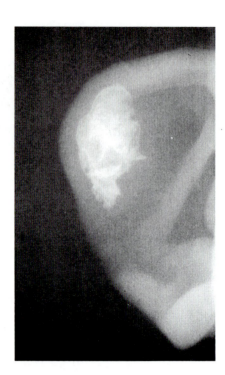

Figure 1.31
Frostbite-induced ossification of the auricular cartilage

The soft-tissue radiograph of the pinna of this patient who had severe frostbite many years previously revealed extensive calcification throughout the posterior superior portion of the auricular cartilage. This was clinically manifest as a rocky hard pinna.

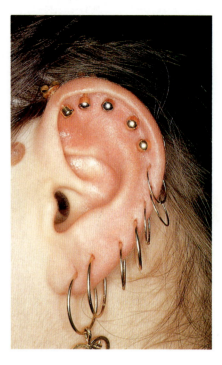

Figure 1.32
Multiple earrings

'Beauty is in the eye of the beholder'. Some individuals favour wearing more than one earring in each ear. The upper five earrings in this patient have penetrated through the auricular cartilage and thus predispose the patient to perichondritis.

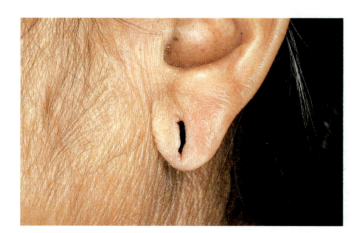

Figure 1.33
Elongated earring hole

Years of traction from a heavy earring have gradually elongated the hole in this lobule.

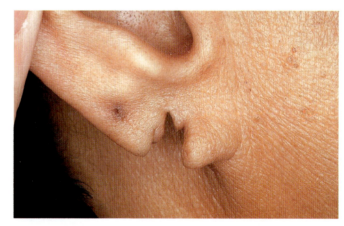

Figure 1.34
Traumatic split lobule

The irregular cut-out deformity in this lobule was the result of the traumatic avulsion of an earring. Such injuries usually occur when a large hoop type of earring is accidentally grasped and pulled by an infant or young child.

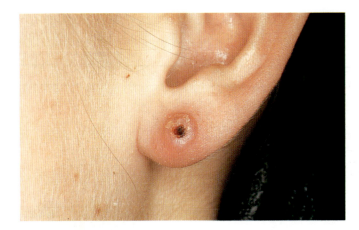

Figure 1.35
Foreign body, lobule

This hypertrophic swelling around the earring tract was the result of a chronic foreign body reaction to the metal keeper of an earring that had become embedded within the lobule.

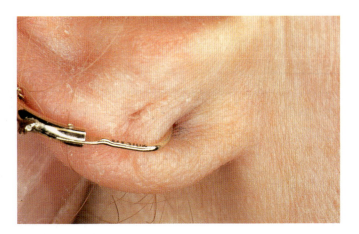

Figure 1.36
Black dermatography

The black discolouration seen around the entrance of the earring hole in this patient is the result of a phenomenon called black dermatography. Black dermatography results from the use of powdered cosmetics that contain zinc oxide or titanium dioxide. These two products are harder than the metal of the jewellery worn and gradually abrade tiny metallic particles which are so small that they do not reflect light and thus appear black. These patients mistakenly blame the black discolouration on the jewellery rather than on the cosmetic.

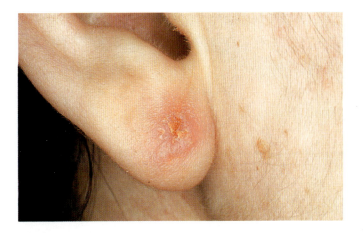

Figure 1.37
Infected earring tract

Localized infections within the earring tract are usually the result of poor hygiene. In these patients pressure on the lobule will frequently expel a tiny drop of pus.

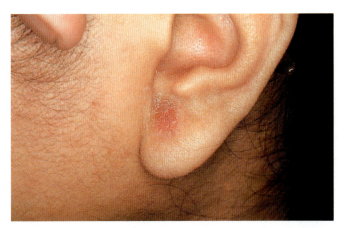

Figure 1.38
Contact dermatitis

The red and excoriated area around the earring tract in the lobule of this patient was the result of a nickel contact dermatitis.

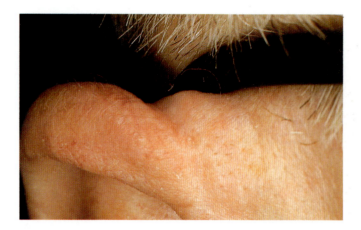

Figure 1.39
Pressure atrophy

Long-standing pressure on the skin may cause absorption or atrophy of the underlying subcutaneous tissue. The grooved area running across the helical rim in this patient is the result of long-standing pressure from the horn of a behind-the-ear hearing aid.

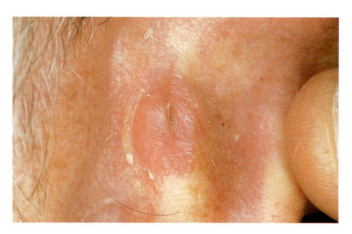

Figure 1.40
Pressure ulceration

Pressure from the overly tight temple bar of this patient's eye glasses has caused a pressure or 'decubitus' ulcer on the posterior surface of the pinna.

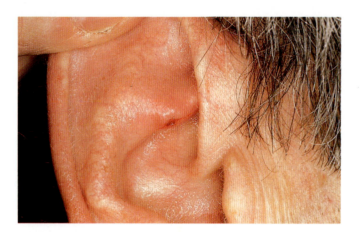

Figure 1.41
Ear mould ulceration

Long-standing pressure from a poorly fitting ear mould has caused ulceration of the upper portion of the antitragus.

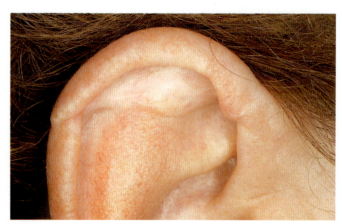

Figure 1.42
Traumatic partial avulsion

As the blood supply to the auricle is excellent and its metabolic demands relatively low, primary reattachment of an auricle is frequently successful, even when there is only a tenuous pedicle present.

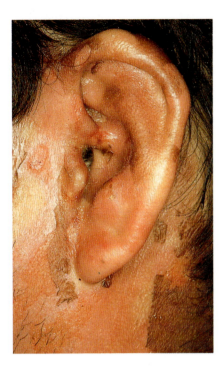

Figure 1.43
Second-degree burn

The second-degree burn affecting this patient's pinna and the side of his head was the result of an accidental spillage of hot soup. Unfortunately, the hot liquid ran into the meatus causing second-degree burn in the external canal and thermal perforation of the tympanic membrane.

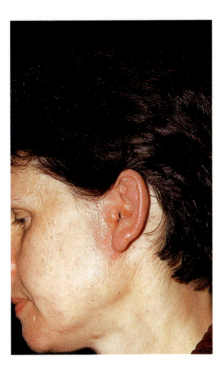

Figure 1.44
Contact dermatitis

Contact dermatitis of the external ear is relatively common and may be confused with infectious otitis externa. Patients with contact dermatitis complain primarily of itching rather than pain. Note the acute erythema and oedema of the skin and subcutaneous tissue, and the telltale extension of the cutaneous reaction onto the skin in front of the lobule where the offending medication has tracked.

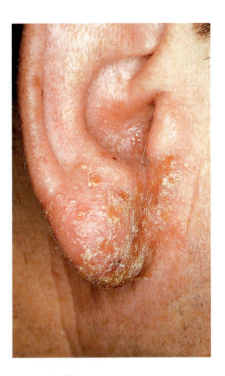

Figure 1.45
Contact dermatitis of lobule

A neomycin-containing ointment has produced in this patient an erythematous, weeping allergic reaction which has tracked inferiorly along the path of the secretions.

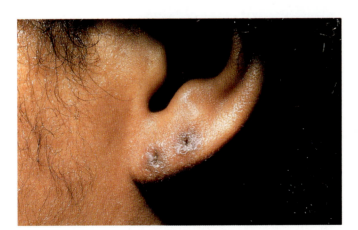

Figure 1.46
Metal contact dermatitis

The two hyperpigmented circles around the earring tracts in this patient's lobule were the result of a nickel contact dermatitis.

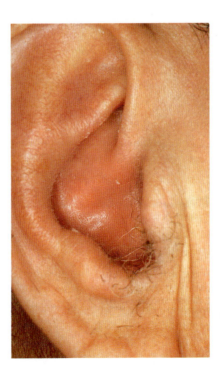

Figure 1.47
Ear mould contact dermatitis

The shiny, atrophic and itchy erythematous area located on the conchal bowl of this patient was the result of an allergy to the material used to make his ear mould.

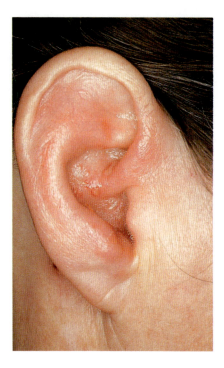

Figure 1.48

Herpes zoster (shingles)

Herpes zoster is an acute localized viral infection of the skin caused by the varicella zoster virus. This large DNA-containing virus of the herpes virus groups causes, in the early stage, scattered pustules in the skin of the involved sensory dermatome.

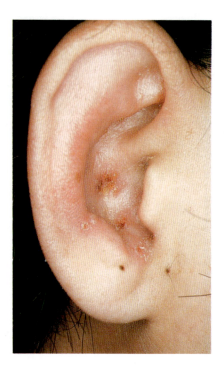

Figure 1.49

Herpes zoster (shingles)

Over time the pustules rupture, dry out and become crusted. When herpes zoster involves the sensory portion of the geniculate ganglion of the facial nerve, it may produce a lower motor neuron facial paralysis and associated herpetic eruption over the affected dermatomes. This is called the Ramsay Hunt syndrome (herpes zoster oticus).

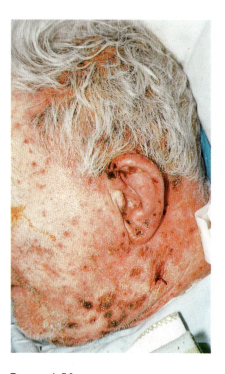

Figure 1.50

Disseminated herpes zoster

In patients with a deficient immune defence system, such as this patient with leukaemia, herpes zoster infection may spread dramatically.

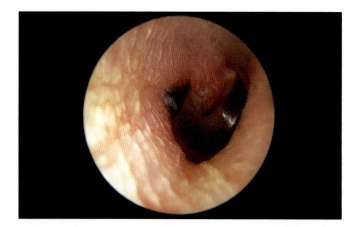

Figure 1.51

Herpes zoster of the tympanic membrane

Herpes zoster may involve the skin lining the external auditory canal. The haemorrhagic bleb over the anterosuperior portion of this patient's left tympanic membrane was a result of herpes zoster.

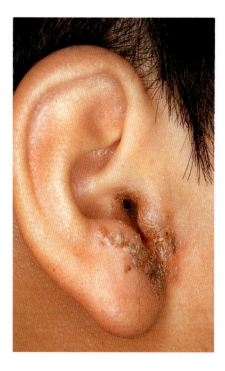

Figure 1.52

Impetigo contagiosa

The *Staphylococcus aureus*-laden discharge from the middle ear of this patient has caused a localized superficial infective dermatitis (impetigo) over the upper portion of the lobule. Ulcerative impetigo is a result of a deeper bacterial skin infection most commonly the result of group A streptococci, staphylococci or a mixture of these bacteria. Note the ulceration in the postauricular crease of this patient.

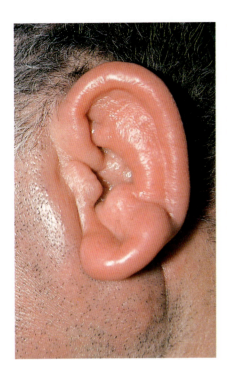

Figure 1.53

Erysipelas

Erysipelas is an acute, localized but spreading superficial cellulitis usually caused by group A beta haemolytic streptococci and characterized by involvement of the lymphatics. The cutaneous lesions are bright red, well demarcated and tender, with an elevated and distinct advancing peripheral margin.

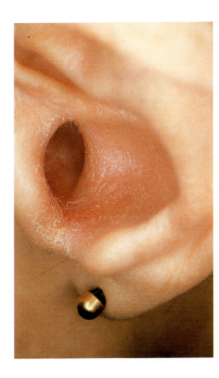

Figure 1.54

Chronic dermatitis

While healthy skin normally provides an effective physical and chemical barrier against the numerous bacteria and fungi to which it is constantly exposed, under conditions of trauma, moisture or maceration this effective antimicrobial barrier may break down. The result may be a chronic infective dermatitis caused by bacteria, fungi or a mixture of both. The diffuse dermatitis throughout this patient's conchal bowl is the result of infection by *Staph. aureus* and *Candida albicans* secondary to the wearing of a hearing aid ear mould.

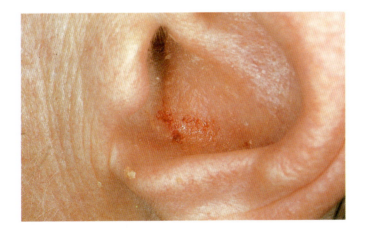

Figure 1.55

Neurodermatitis

Itching is a common feature in patients with chronic dermatitis and repeated scratching of the pruritic area may break down the skin barrier, allowing dermatitis to develop. The term 'neurodermatitis' has been applied to these patients in whom telltale areas of excoriation or bleeding are frequently seen.

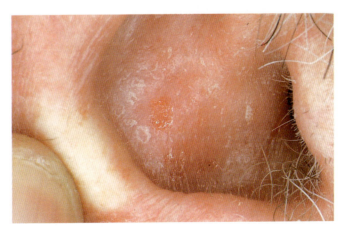

Figure 1.56

Fungal dermatitis

In this patient the increased moisture and trauma of wearing a hearing aid mould was responsible for a local fungal dermatitis caused by *Candida albicans*. As it is impossible to differentiate clinically a bacterial dermatitis from a fungal infection, culture of the involved area is of great value.

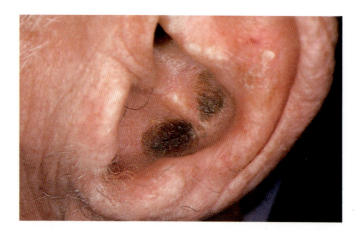

Figure 1.57

Neglect keratosis

Sheets of keratin squames are constantly pushed up to the surface of the skin and shed during normal epidermal maintenance. The outermost layer of squames (the stratum corneum) is normally rubbed away by contact with clothing or as a result of personal toilet. Neglected areas of skin may accumulate patches of thick keratin debris, resulting in a pigmented, greasy, raised lesion that at first glance resembles an area of seborrhoeic keratosis. Unlike seborrhoeic keratosis, these areas of neglect keratosis are easily removed with a cotton-tipped applicator to reveal normal underlying skin.

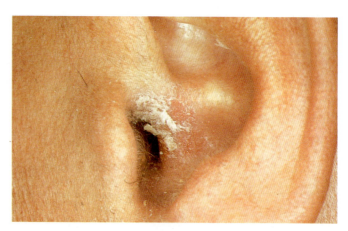

Figure 1.58

Psoriasis vulgaris

Psoriasis vulgaris is a hereditary disorder of skin characterized by an increased rate of epidermal cell replication. Note the sharply demarcated, salmon-coloured plaques of psoriasis just below the helical rim. The upper portion of the lesion is covered with the characteristic silvery scales.

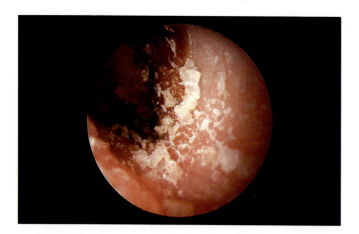

Figure 1.59

Psoriasis vulgaris of the external ear canal

Psoriatic dermatitis may extend into the external auditory canal. In this case the superficial external auditory canal will show a collection of white, silvery, scaly debris.

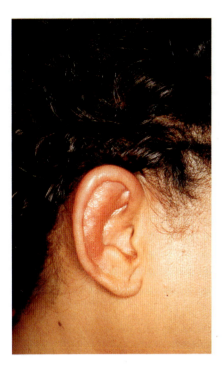

Figure 1.60
Relapsing polychondritis

Relapsing polychondritis is an episodic and generally progressive inflammation of the cartilaginous structures throughout the body. An autoimmune disorder is suspected since many of these patients have circulating antibodies to type II collagen (the collagen present in cartilage). Clinically, relapsing polychondritis is characterized by bilateral auricular chondritis, nasal chondritis, laryngeal chondritis, polyarthritis and respiratory tract chondritis. Ocular inflammation may also be present.

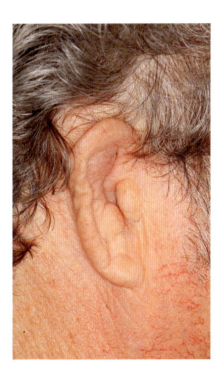

Figure 1.61
Relapsing polychondritis

This patient has relapsing polychondritis. There has previously been acute inflammation of the auricular cartilage. While the acute painful inflammatory stage has settled, the cartilage has degenerated, becoming soft and flabby and giving the pinna a crumpled appearance.

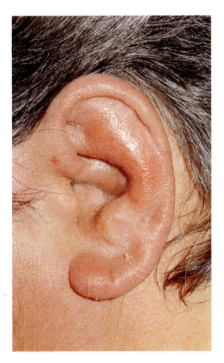

Figure 1.62
Perichondritis

Acute perichondritis is caused by a bacterial infection of the perichondrium, which is usually the result of trauma to the pinna. Acute perichondritis most commonly occurs following lacerations or incisions that extend through the perichondrium. Clinically, the skin of the pinna is diffusely swollen, painful and tender.

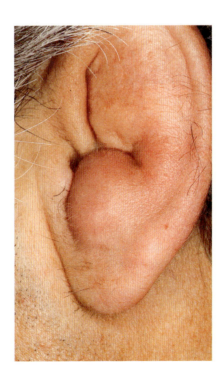

Figure 1.63
Idiopathic cystic chondromalacia of the external auricular cartilage

Benign idiopathic cystic chondromalacia (auricular pseudocyst) is a cystic degeneration of the auricular cartilage of unknown origin, which may be mistaken both clinically and histologically for relapsing polychondritis. Clinically, this disease presents as an isolated, unilateral, asymptomatic swelling, most commonly on the anterior surface of the pinna. These pseudocysts may be the result of repeated local minor trauma to the auricular cartilage.

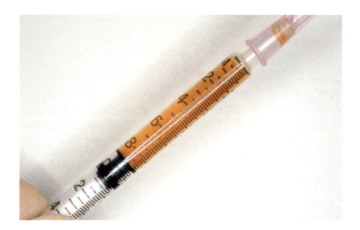

Figure 1.64

Idiopathic cystic chondromalacia (auricular pseudocyst)

Aspiration of the pseudocyst will produce a yellow or orange serous fluid. This syringe contains the contents of the area of idiopathic cystic chondromalacia affecting the pinna shown in Figure 1.63.

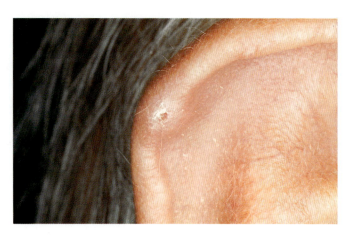

Figure 1.65

Chondrodermatitis nodularis helicis chronica (Winkler's nodule)

Chondrodermatitis nodularis helicis chronica is the formal name given to a discrete, firm, raised and frequently painful nodule, most commonly located on the apex of the helix of the ear. This disease appears to be the result of solar damage to the underlying cartilage, which undergoes degeneration and extrusion through the skin. These lesions are exquisitely tender to the touch. Local excision of the overlying skin and underlying auricular cartilage is curative.

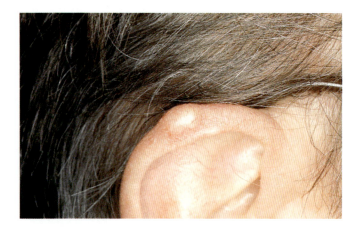

Figure 1.66

Gouty tophi

Gouty tophi are the result of the subcutaneous accumulation of deposits of monosodium urate crystals. These tophi present as painful, skin-covered nodules occurring most frequently on the helix. Tophi are gritty to palpation and the underlying yellow crystals may occasionally be seen through the skin.

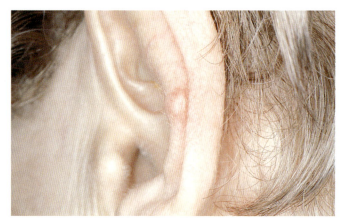

Figure 1.67

Rheumatoid nodule

Rheumatoid nodules may appear in the skin of the pinna.

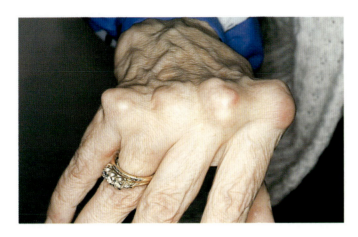

Figure 1.68
Rheumatoid arthritis

The diagnosis of the whitish raised lesion seen in the previous photograph was easily made by observation of severe rheumatoid arthritic changes affecting this patient's joints.

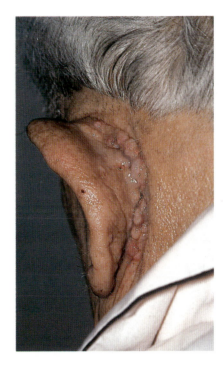

Figure 1.69
Primary cutaneous amyloid

The raised subcutaneous deposits in the postauricular crease of this patient's ear are the result of the deposition of amyloid. Amyloid is a complex fibrillar protein believed to originate from plasma cells.

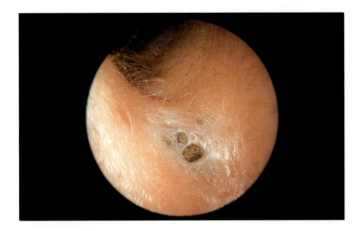

Figure 1.70
Comedones

A comedo consists of a collection of keratin debris and sebum trapped at the opening of a pilosebaceous follicle. If the follicle is closed this collection appears whitish and is referred to as a 'whitehead'. If the comedo is situated in an open follicle, the superficial contents darken with time and are called a ' blackhead'.

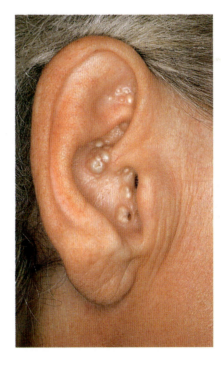

Figure 1.71
Milia

Milia are multiple, superficially located, small white cysts that arise from the lowest portion of the infundibulum in the region of the sebaceous duct. These tiny cysts differ from epidermal cysts only in size.

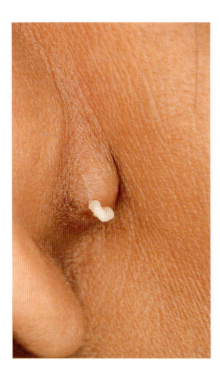

Figure 1.72
Epidermal cyst

Epidermal cysts are slow-growing, round, firm intradermal or subcutaneous cysts that arise most commonly from the infundibula of hair follicles.

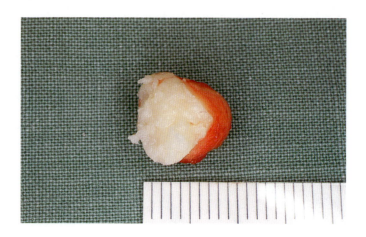

Figure 1.73
Epidermal cyst

Histologically, epidermal cysts are lined with a true epidermis, similar to that seen on the surface of the skin. The cyst itself is filled with laminated layers of keratin.

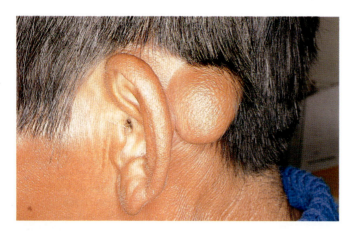

Figure 1.74
Trichilemmal (pilar) cyst

Trichilemmal cysts originate from the outer root sheath of the hair follicle (the trichilemma). Pilar cysts occur most commonly on the scalp where they are clinically indistinguishable from epidermal cysts. Histologically, a pilar cyst is lined with epithelial cells that lack visible intercellular bridges.

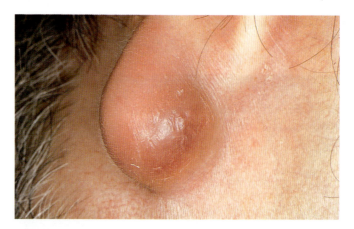

Figure 1.75
Epidermal inclusion cysts

The traumatic implantation of epidermis into the underlying soft tissue may produce a true epidermal inclusion cyst. The infected epidermal inclusion cyst in the lobule of this patient arose from the implantation of epidermal cells during ear piercing.

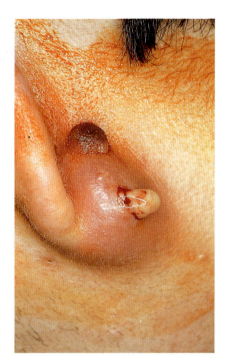

Figure 1.76

Infected epidermal cyst

An epidermal cyst may become infected. This is manifested by pain, tenderness and localized swelling. Incision and drainage of the cyst will release foul-smelling, purulent material containing necrotic keratin squames.

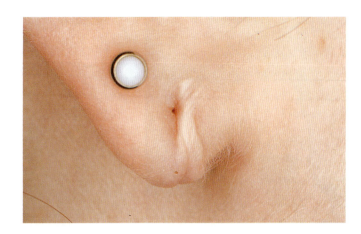

Figure 1.77

Hypertrophic ear

Hypertrophic scars are raised scars that remain within the confines of the wound and usually flatten spontaneously over 1–2 years.

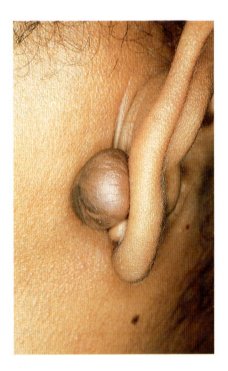

Figure 1.78

Keloid

Keloids not only persist but extend beyond the site of the original injury. Keloids occur more often in Blacks than in Whites and are more frequent in the second and third decades of life.

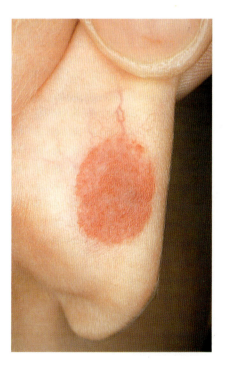

Figure 1.79

Capillary haemangioma

Capillary haemangioma or strawberry birthmark is a bright red, soft, lobulated, benign tumour consisting of numerous blood-filled, benign-looking capillaries. Seventy per cent of capillary haemangiomas undergo spontaneous resolution in the first decade of life.

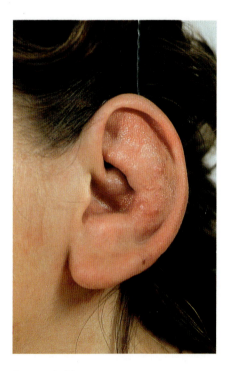

Figure 1.80

Arteriovenous malformation

Arteriovenous malformations may involve the blood vessels within the pinna. Clinically, an arteriovenous malformation will present with discolouration and distortion of the skin overlying the pinna. Palpation of the involved area will reveal pulsations, and auscultation will reveal a loud bruit.

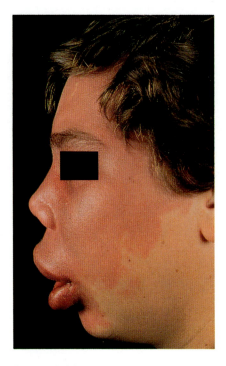

Figure 1.81

Naevus flammeus (port wine naevus)

In this patient with Sturge-Weber syndrome there is a large naevus flammeus involving the left side of the face.

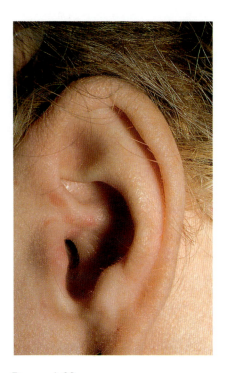

Figure 1.82

Venous lake

A venous lake is a small, raised, soft, blue lesion that may appear on the exposed surface of the pinna. These lesions may be caused by a localized venous capillary haemangioma or by a large venous lake. The diagnosis is readily apparent as these lesions empty when compressed by digital pressure.

Figure 1.83

Angiolymphoid hyperplasia with eosinophilia (Kimura's disease)

Kimura's disease or angiolymphoid hyperplasia with eosinophilia may present as raised angiomatous nodules arising on the pinna or superficial external auditory canal. These nodules usually persist, slowly increasing in number, and are associated with itching and bleeding after scratching.

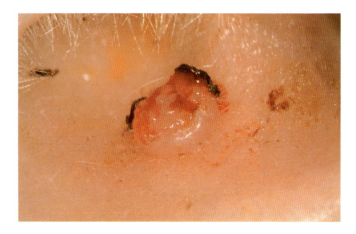

Figure 1.84

Keratoacanthoma

A keratoacanthoma is a benign, usually solitary, rapidly developing epithelial neoplasm that arises on the sun-exposed areas of fair-skinned, elderly individuals. The lesion is characterized by a firm, dome-shaped nodule with skin-coloured rolled edges and a central crater filled with keratin debris, which clinically and histologically resembles a squamous cell carcinoma. Because of its resemblance to squamous cell carcinoma, a biopsy is indicated.

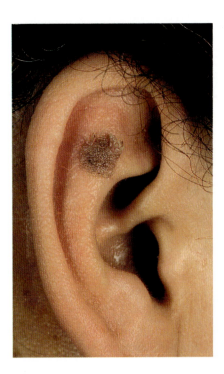

Figure 1.85

Seborrhoeic keratosis

Seborrhoeic keratoses are benign tumours that appear after the third decade of life. Clinically, they appear as raised, greasy, 'stuck-on' lesions with visible keratotic plugs filling a central irregular crypt. Seborrhoeic keratosis may vary in colour from light yellow through brown to black with the intensity of the colour varying with the amount of melanin pigment present in the lesion. When examined with a magnifying glass, keratin or horn cysts can be seen on the surface of the lesion.

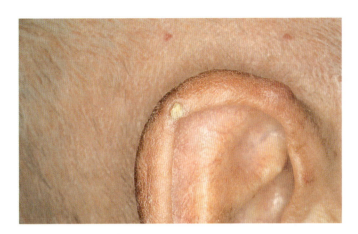

Figure 1.86

Solar keratosis (actinic keratosis or senile keratosis)

Solar keratoses are premalignant lesions that arise on sun-exposed areas of the skin. Clinically, solar keratoses appear as dry, rough and adherent scaly lesions. Occasionally, solar keratoses produce a circumscribed, conical, hyperkeratotic excrescence, which is known as a cutaneous horn. A solar keratosis is considered to be premalignant as it may develop into a squamous cell carcinoma.

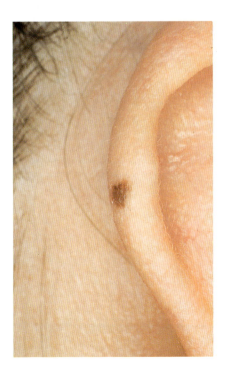

Figure 1.87

Junctional naevus

The flat, circumscribed, dark brown macule present on the posterior helical rim of this young child is a junctional naevus.

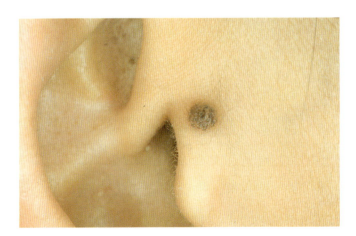

Figure 1.88

Compound naevus

This raised, pigmented lesion present on the superior border of the tragus is a compound naevus.

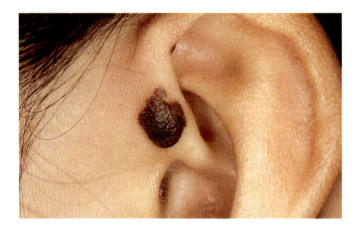

Figure 1.89

Intradermal naevus

This larger and more extensively raised, pigmented, dome-shaped lesion on the upper border of the tragus is an intradermal naevus.

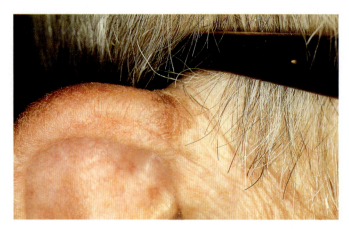

Figure 1.90

Solar lentigo

Solar lentigo is another lesion that develops from repeated exposure to the sun. These lesions rarely occur before the fourth decade of life, slowly increasing in both size and number. Clinically, solar lentigo appears as multiple, uniformly pigmented, dark brown, flat lesions with an irregular outline.

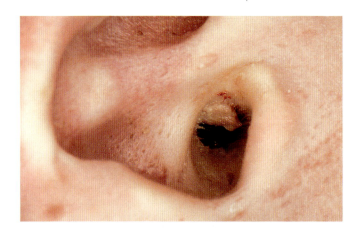

Figure 1.91

Verruca vulgaris

Verruca vulgaris or the common wart is a benign, localized area of epithelial hyperplasia caused by the human wart virus of the papova virus group. Verrucae appear as firm, circumscribed elevated papules with a filiform or papillomatous and hyperkeratotic surface.

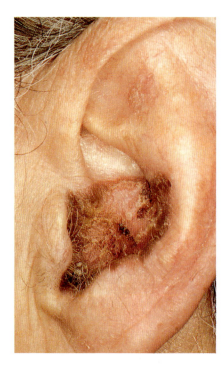

Figure 1.92

Basal cell carcinoma

Basal cell carcinoma is the most common cutaneous malignancy. These tumours usually develop in skin that has been subject to actinic damage, and it is therefore not surprising that basal cell carcinomas are the most common malignant tumour affecting the external ear. This area of 'chronic dermatitis' affecting the conchal bowl did not respond to appropriate topical antibiotic and anti-fungal preparations, and was diagnosed on biopsy as a basal cell carcinoma.

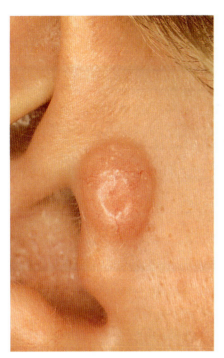

Figure 1.93
Basal cell carcinoma

Basal cell carcinomas may present with many different clinical appearances. Any chronically ulcerated or raised lesion that persists should be biopsied.

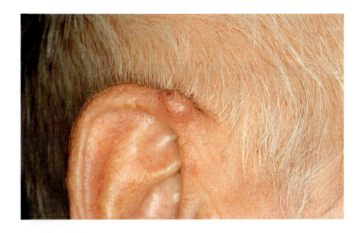

Figure 1.94
Squamous cell carcinoma

Squamous cell carcinoma of the auricle is a relatively uncommon malignant tumour that arises from keratinocytes damaged by exposure to sunlight. The diagnosis of a squamous cell carcinoma is made by biopsy. As with basal cell carcinoma, any lesion that does not heal or shows any suggestion of invasion of the underlying tissues should be biopsied.

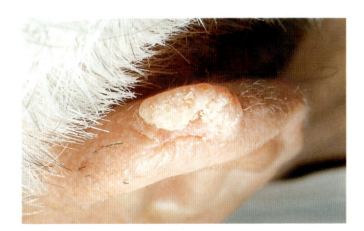

Figure 1.95
Verrucous carcinoma

Verrucous carcinoma is a low-grade squamous cell carcinoma that is slow growing and initially exophytic and wart-like in appearance. Verrucous carcinoma is characterized by slow and continual advancement with a special predisposition for destruction of adjacent bony structures.

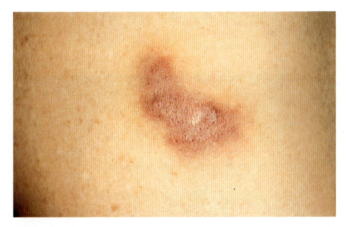

Figure 1.96
Kaposi's sarcoma

Kaposi's sarcoma is a sarcoma of vascular cell origin whose incidence has increased dramatically as a result of the worldwide epidemic of acquired immune deficiency syndrome (AIDS). Kaposi's sarcoma usually presents as a raised purplish-red nodule that continues to expand and enlarge. The diagnosis is made by biopsy. Diagnosis of Kaposi's sarcoma strongly raises the possibility of HIV-positive status.

External auditory canal

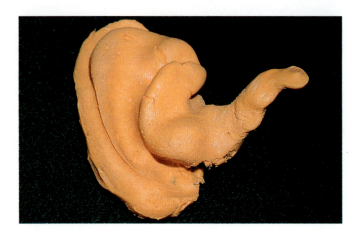

Figure 1.97

Normal superficial external auditory canal

The external auditory canal is divided into three distinct sections: the external or cartilaginous section, the medial or bony section and the lateral surface of the tympanic membrane. The relationship of the conchal bowl of the pinna to the external auditory canal is shown.

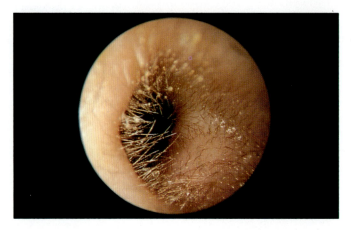

Figure 1.98

Cartilaginous portion of the external auditory canal

The skin lining the outer or cartilaginous portion of the external auditory canal is thick, hair-bearing skin containing numerous sebaceous and ceruminous glands. The cartilaginous portion of the external canal is relatively strong, mobile and is supported within a surrounding cartilaginous framework. (The right ear is shown.)

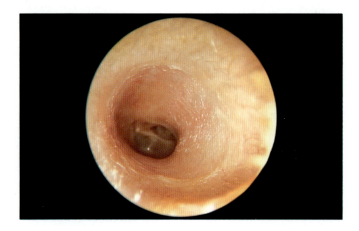

Figure 1.99

Isthmus

The lumen of the external auditory canal is narrowest at the junction between the outer cartilaginous and inner bony portions. This area is known as the 'isthmus'. (The left ear is shown.)

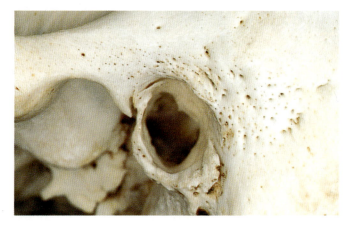

Figure 1.100

Bony external auditory canal

The medial (deep) or bony portion of the external auditory canal is surrounded by a bony framework, which consists primarily of the U-shaped tympanic bone. (The left ear is shown.)

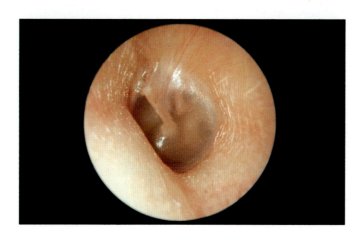

Figure 1.101
Bony external auditory canal

The skin lining the bony portion of the external auditory canal is thin and lacks adnexal structures, i.e. hairs and glands. (The left ear is shown.)

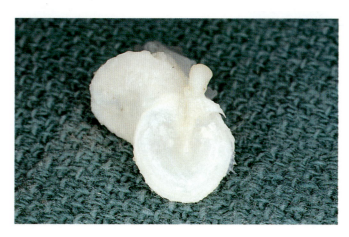

Figure 1.102
Tympanic portion of the external auditory canal

The external auditory canal ends at the tympanic membrane. The epithelium covering the lateral surface of the tympanic membrane is considered to be the tympanic portion of the external auditory canal. Note the oblique angle of the tympanic membrane in this dissection of the epithelium lining the bony external canal and the adjacent lateral portion of the tympanic membrane. (The left ear is shown.)

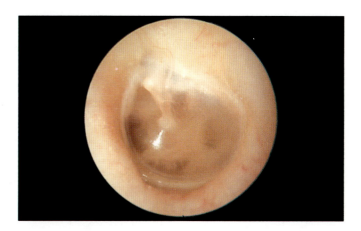

Figure 1.103
Tympanic membrane

The tympanic membrane appears as a pale grey, semi-transparent membrane positioned obliquely at the medial end of the external auditory canal. (The left ear is shown.)

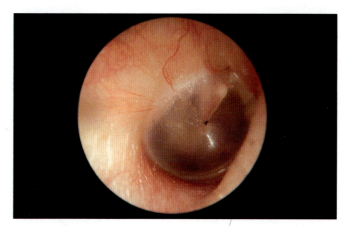

Figure 1.104
Epithelial migration I

The normal self-cleansing of the external auditory canal is the result of the miraculous ability of the epithelium lining the canal to migrate in an outward direction. In this volunteer (right ear) an ink dot has been applied to the surface of the tympanic membrane in the region of the umbo.

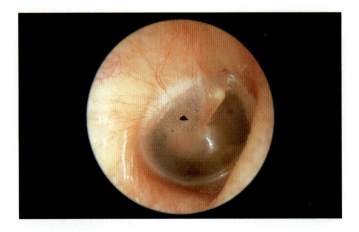

Figure 1.105

Epithelial migration 2

Two months later the ink dot has migrated in a radial or centrifugal direction over the surface of the tympanic membrane to a position overlying the area of the incudostapedial joint.

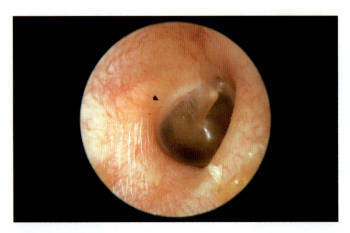

Figure 1.106

Epithelial migration 3

Two months later the ink dot has migrated onto the bony external auditory canal in the 10 o'clock position.

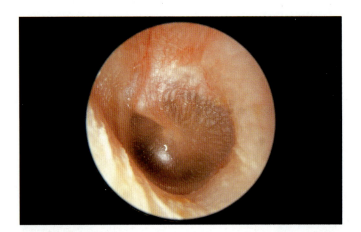

Figure 1.107

Keratin patches on the tympanic membrane

Small, radially oriented patches of thickened keratin squames can often be seen on the surface of the tympanic membrane. These patches consist of older and thicker keratin from the central portion of the tympanic membrane that has migrated centrifugally. (The left ear is shown.)

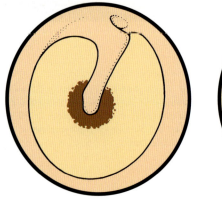

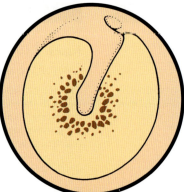

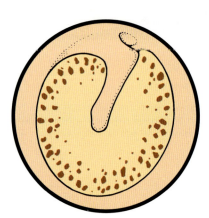

Figure 1.108

Keratin patches on the tympanic membrane

As the superficial keratin layer of the central portion of the tympanic membrane migrates centrifugally, it must also spread laterally to cover the widened peripheral areas of the drum, resulting in the development of separation lines.

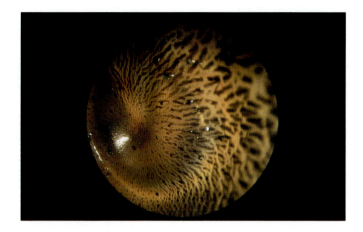

Figure 1.109

Keratin patches on the tympanic membrane: osmium staining

The shape, size and number of keratin patches can be clearly seen in this cadaveric specimen (left ear) in which the keratin patches have been emphasized by staining with osmium tetroxide.

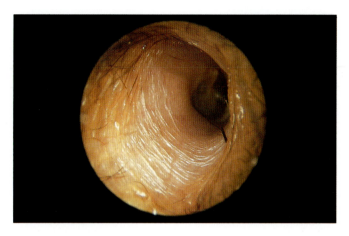

Figure 1.110

Transverse epithelial wrinkles

Transverse wrinkles are superficial waves or corrugations that lie at right angles to the long axis of the external auditory canal. These wrinkles are present in most external canals and are most readily visible in the epithelium covering the posterior bony canal wall. These transverse wrinkles develop as the outwardly migrating stratum corneum of the deep canal becomes heaped up against the pressure of the stationary hairs of the superficial canal. (The right ear is shown.)

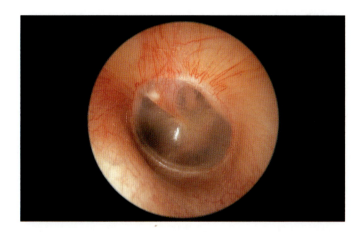

Figure 1.111

Vascular strip

The external surface of the tympanic is supplied by the deep auricular branch of the maxillary artery. This artery provides a leash of prominent vessels that pass down the superior canal wall. This area is called the 'vascular strip'. (The left ear is shown.)

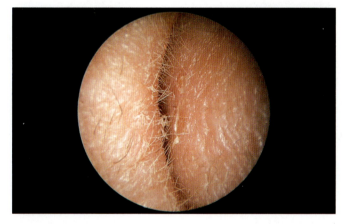

Figure 1.112

Collapsing external auditory canal

In some patients a structural deficiency in the surrounding and supporting fibroelastic cartilage allows the external portion of the auditory canal to collapse, leaving only a slit-like narrow lumen. Pressure against such an external auditory canal from a headphone may increase the amount of collapse to such an extent that the external canal becomes completely occluded. (The right ear is shown.)

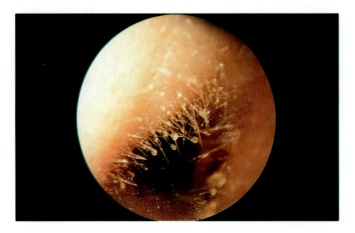

Figure 1.113

Cerumen

The openings of the ceruminous glands are located near the base of the hairs of the cartilaginous canal. The ceruminous glands produce a clear colourless secretion, which can be seen in this photograph (right ear) as tiny droplets along the hairs. While the secretions of the ceruminous glands are called 'cerumen', by tradition, this term is most commonly used to refer to ear wax (see Figure 1.116).

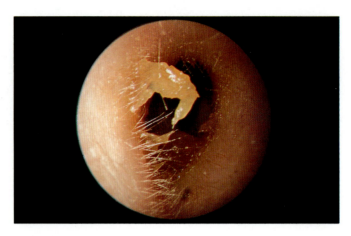

Figure 1.114

Cerumen

The normal outward migration of the epithelium lining the deep meatus will normally carry keratin debris and cerumen out into the cartilaginous portion of the external auditory canal. In this patient (right ear) a small collection of soft, light-brown cerumen is seen being elevated by the hairs of the cartilaginous canal.

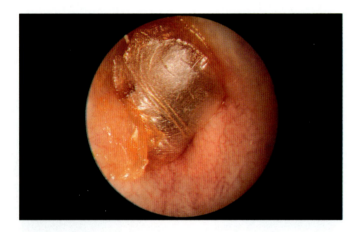

Figure 1.115

Veil of cerumen

In this patient (right ear) the superficial area of outwardly migrating keratin has become flipped across the external auditory canal where it lies like a drape or veil. This appearance most commonly results from the use of Q-tips, which elevate and rotate the superficial layer of the keratin lining the external auditory canal.

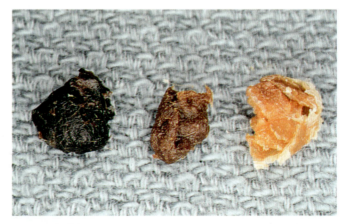

Figure 1.116

Colours of cerumen

Cerumen or ear wax is a complex mixture of desquamated keratin squames and hairs, combined with the secretions of the sebaceous and ceruminous glands. Cerumen varies in colour from golden yellow through brown to black.

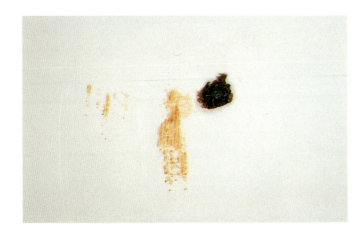

Figure 1.117

Colour of cerumen

The pigment(s) responsible for the colouration of cerumen has yet to be identified. Burnt ochre is the most common colour of cerumen, as seen in this smear made from a piece of dark-brown cerumen.

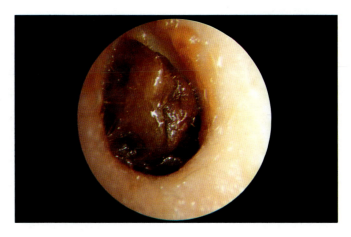

Figure 1.118

Cerumen accumulation

While cerumen is normally removed from the external auditory canal by the process of epithelial migration, in some patients it gradually collects along the floor of the external auditory canal. (The right ear is shown.)

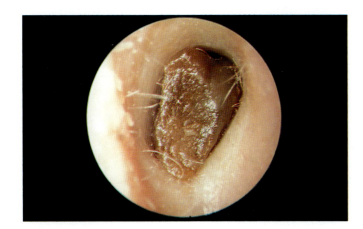

Figure 1.119

Cerumen accumulation

In some patients the plug of cerumen may accumulate to such an extent that it totally occludes the lumen of the external auditory canal. (The right ear is shown.)

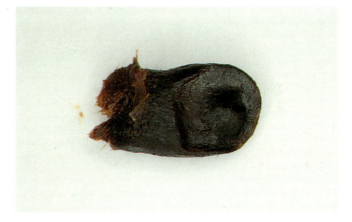

Figure 1.120

Massive cerumen plug

In some patients cerumen may accumulate to such an extent that it totally fills the external auditory canal and produces a mould or cast of the canal. Note the impression of the lateral surface of the tympanic membrane on the right side of this extensive cerumen plug.

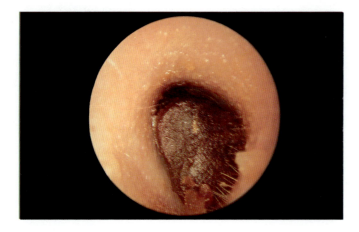

Figure 1.121
Inspissated hard cerumen

The external canal of this patient (left ear) is plugged with a bony-hard accumulation of cerumen. Black cerumen is more commonly encountered in the older age groups, and when it becomes dry and inspissated in consistency, it is more difficult to remove.

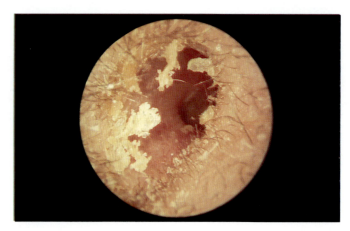

Figure 1.122
Oriental wax

Cerumen occurs in two forms: wet and dry. The usual type of cerumen found in Orientals is the dry type, commonly referred to as 'rice bran' wax, as it resembles particles of rice bran.

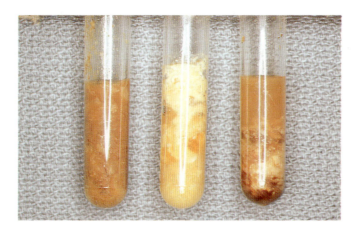

Figure 1.123
Ceruminolytics

The most effective ceruminolytics have an aqueous base. Note the swelling and dissolution of a cerumen plug caused by these aqueous solutions (from the left: sodium bicarbonate, hydrogen peroxide, and distilled water).

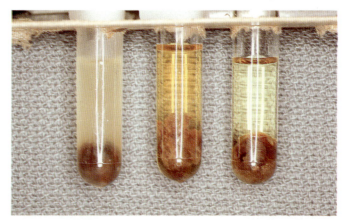

Figure 1.124
Ceruminolytics

In contrast, oily based solutions are not effective in breaking up a cerumen plug as seen in these organic solutions (from the left: Cerumol, Cerumenex, and olive oil).

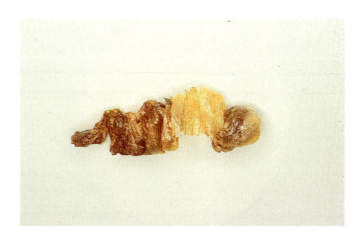

Figure 1.125

Keratin component of cerumen

The accumulation of cerumen is probably related to a deficiency in the separation and migration of the stratum corneum lining the epithelium of the external canal. Large unbroken keratin sheets are the single greatest constituent of cerumen, as seen in this cerumen plug that has been unrolled.

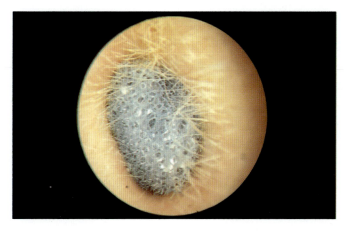

Figure 1.126

Foreign body

A wide variety of foreign bodies may become lodged in the external auditory canal whether by accident, neglect or deliberate insertion. The signs and symptoms of a foreign body depend on its size, location and composition of material. In this patient (left ear) a blue plug of sponge rubber can be seen filling the deep meatus.

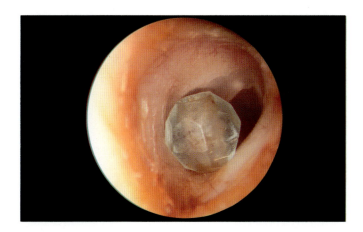

Figure 1.127

Foreign body

A purple plastic bead was inserted into the external auditory canal in this young child (right ear). A general anaesthetic was required for safe removal owing to the child's lack of cooperation.

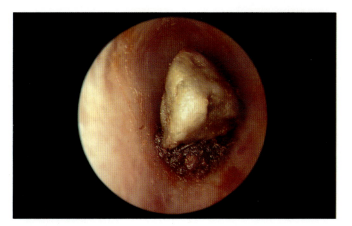

Figure 1.128

Foreign body

In this patient a small pebble has become lodged in the deep canal. This was easily removed by syringing.

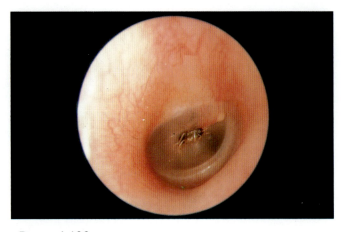

Figure 1.129

Foreign body

Animate foreign bodies, such as this tiny cockroach attached to the lateral surface of the tympanic membrane, may produce objective tinnitus, itching and severe pain.

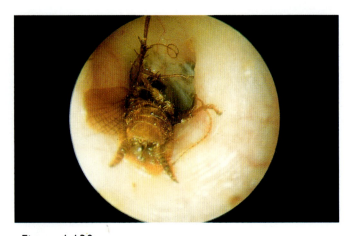

Figure 1.130

Foreign body

This larger cockroach produced severe pain and tinnitus. Injury to the epithelium from the sharp spurs on the insect's hind legs produced an acute otitis externa. It was not until the otitis externa had been treated successfully with topical antibiotics that the primary cause was observed.

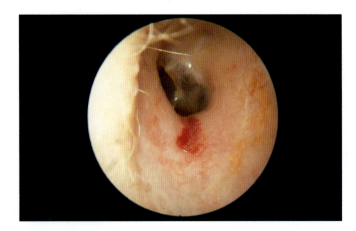

Figure 1.131

Haematoma, external auditory canal

The epithelium lining the bony or deep canal is extremely thin and easily traumatized. The use of a cotton-tipped applicator and aural cleansing has produced a haematoma in the skin overlying the floor of the bony external auditory canal. (The left ear is shown.)

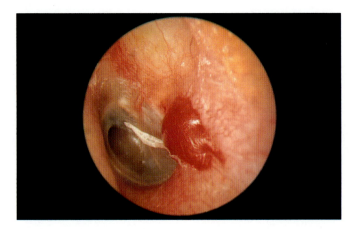

Figure 1.132

Extensive haematoma, external auditory canal

Following debridement of the external auditory canal, a more extensive subepithelial haematoma has formed. This haematoma (left ear) has elevated the superficial keratin layer.

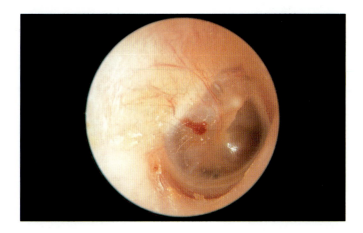

Figure 1.133

Haematoma, tympanic membrane

This asymptomatic haematoma located just behind the handle of the malleus resulted from the deep insertion of a cotton-tipped applicator during aural toilet. The friction of the cotton bud has produced a small superficial haematoma of the epithelium covering the tympanic membrane. (The right ear is shown.)

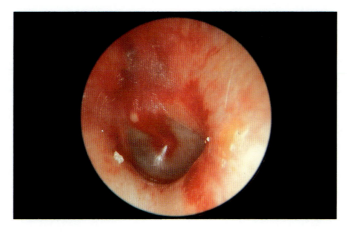

Figure 1.134

Haematoma, tympanic membrane

Following relatively traumatic wax curretage, a large haematoma has developed over the deep portion of the bony external auditory canal. The haematoma has tracked down on either side of the handle of the malleus. (The left ear is shown.)

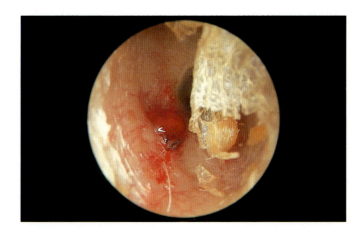

Figure 1.135

Laceration, external auditory canal

The delicate skin lining the bony external auditory canal has been lacerated during wax curettage. Active bleeding through the laceration can be seen. Because of the vascularity of the skin in this area, such bleeding may be troublesome and if not stopped may fill the deep canal with blood.

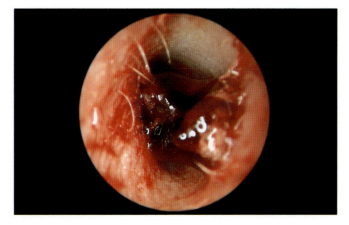

Figure 1.136

Fresh blood clot from external auditory canal

A blood clot in the external auditory canal should be removed when it is relatively fresh and still jelly-like in consistency.

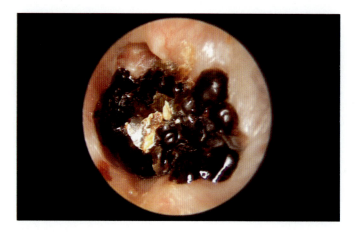

Figure 1.137

Old blood clot in external auditory canal

Once a blood clot is allowed to remain in the external auditory canal, it will become converted into a bony-hard, black, tar-like mixture, which is extremely difficult to remove.

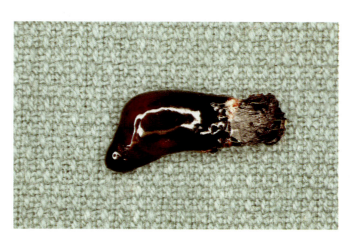

Figure 1.138

Blood clot from an external auditory canal

Bleeding from a traumatic laceration of an external auditory canal allowed this clot to fill the external auditory canal. Note how the outer (right) side of the clot has undergone dessication and hardening while the deeper (left) portion of the clot still has a jelly-like consistency.

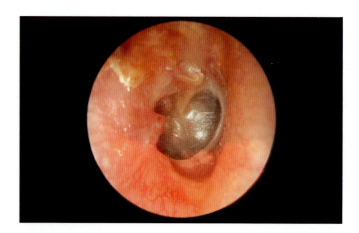

Figure 1.139

Keratin foreign body granuloma

Traumatic lacerations of the external auditory canal may allow the implantation of keratin squames into the subepithelial layers. These keratin squames act as powerful foreign bodies and elicit a foreign body granulation tissue response, as seen in this patient (right ear).

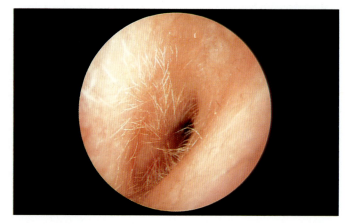

Figure 1.140

Early acute otitis externa

Acute diffuse otitis externa (swimmer's ear) is the most commonly encountered type of otitis externa. Exposure to moisture and local trauma are the most common predisposing factors. *Pseudomonas aeruginosa* is the usual pathogen. Initially the skin lining the external auditory canal becomes oedematous, has a shiny appearance, and is extremely tender. (The right ear is shown.)

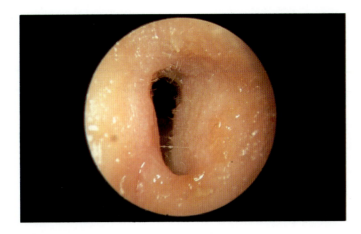

Figure 1.141
Acute otitis externa

As the acute otitis externa progresses, the swelling of the epithelial lining of the external canal increases and the infected epithelium exudes a watery or serous discharge. (The right ear is shown.)

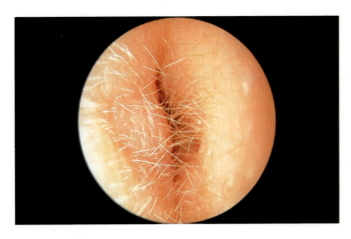

Figure 1.142
Severe acute otitis externa

As the acute otitis externa progresses, the swelling of the epithelium lining of the external canal may increase to such an extent that the lumen is totally occluded. Severe local pain and trismus is usually present. (The right ear is shown.)

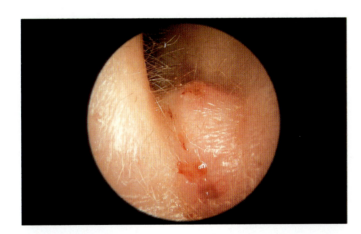

Figure 1.143
Acute localized otitis externa (furuncle)

A furuncle is a small staphylococcal abscess that arises at the base of a hair follicle. Furuncles only occur in the outer cartilaginous hair-bearing portion of the external canal. They appear as a red and extremely painful localized swelling.

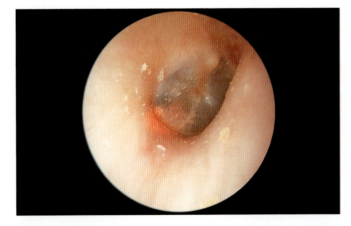

Figure 1.144
Chronic otitis externa

Chronic otitis externa, in contrast with acute otitis externa, is usually a painless condition in which itching, irritation and scanty otorrhoea are the predominant symptoms. The skin of the external auditory canal is thickened, shiny and usually erythematous. Normal cerumen is usually absent, as seen in this patient (right ear).

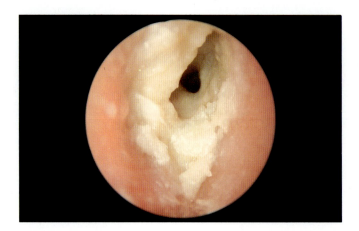

Figure 1.145
Chronic otitis externa

Chronic otitis externa may be the result of a bacterial, fungal or mixed infection. In this patient (right ear), the deep meatus is filled with a collection of moist, macerated keratin squames.

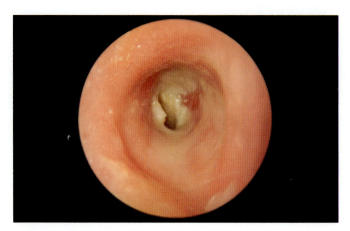

Figure 1.146
Chronic otitis externa

In this patient (left ear) the deep meatus is filled with a creamy yellow mixture of macerated keratin squames and purulent exudate. The offending organisms were micrococci and diphtheroids.

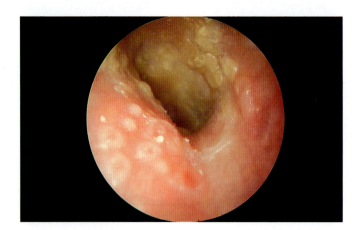

Figure 1.147
Chronic otitis externa

In this patient (right ear) the deep meatus contains a greenish exudate. The pustules seen on the skin of the external canal were the result of an unusual pustular form of *Pseudomonas* infection.

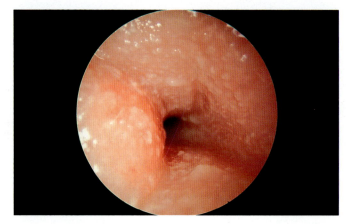

Figure 1.148
Hypertrophic otitis externa

In some patients, chronic infection in the skin lining the external auditory canal may result in diffuse fibrosis and thickening of the subepithelial layers, thereby narrowing the canal's lumen. This condition is referred to as chronic hypertrophic otitis externa. (The right ear is shown.)

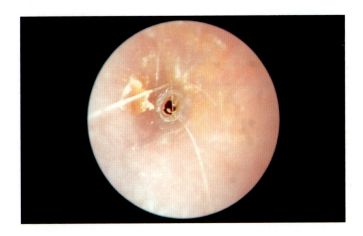

Figure 1.149

Acquired stenosis of the external auditory canal

In this patient (right ear) chronic trauma to the epithelium lining the bony canal and chronic otitis externa in this area have resulted in an acquired stricture and stenosis of the deep external auditory canal. The tiny pinhole-sized lumen that remains was, however, sufficient for normal hearing as long as the lumen was kept free from debris.

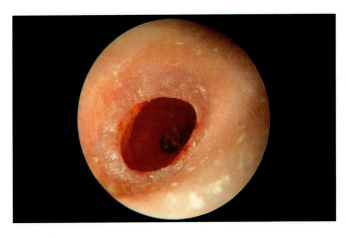

Figure 1.150

Acquired stenosis of the external auditory canal

Trauma from the continuing use of cotton-tipped applicators has caused circumferential ulceration, granulation tissue formation and the development of a web-like stenosis of the external auditory canal at the level of the isthmus.

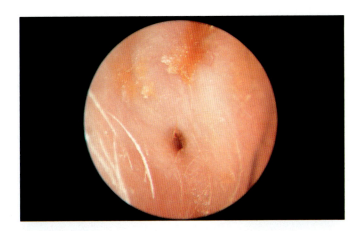

Figure 1.151

Acquired stenosis of the external auditory canal

In this patient (right ear) the lumen has been stenosed to such an extent that both sound conduction and migration are no longer possible.

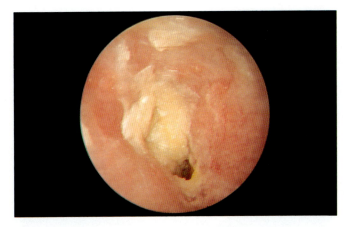

Figure 1.152

Otomycosis due to *Candida albicans*

Infection of the external auditory canal by fungal organisms is called otomycosis. The most common pathogenic fungi involved are *Aspergillus* and *Candida spp*. Infections with *Candida albicans* do not show any morphological evidence of fungi and as a result the diagnosis of otomycosis in these patients can only be made by culture. Patients with candidal otitis external frequently present with a creamy white exudate within the deep canal, as seen in this patient (left ear).

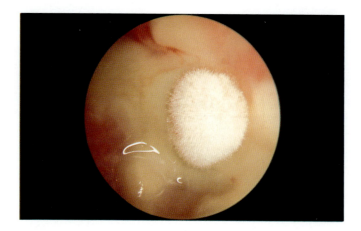

Figure 1.153

Aspergillus niger otomycosis

Otomycosis caused by *Aspergillus* can usually be diagnosed by the presence of a white, fluffy, cotton-like material, which represents the fungal hyphae. (The left ear is shown.)

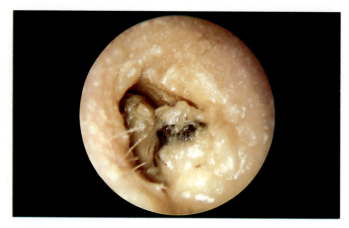

Figure 1.154

Aspergillus niger otomycosis

Another diagnostic feature of *Aspergillus* infections is the presence of coloured particles. The black debris represents the conidiophores of *Aspergillus niger*. (The left ear is shown.)

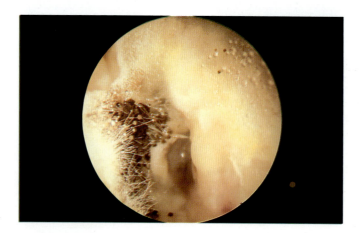

Figure 1.155

Aspergillus niger otomycosis

Note the collection of black debris and the fungal hyphae in this patient with *Aspergillus* otomycosis (right ear).

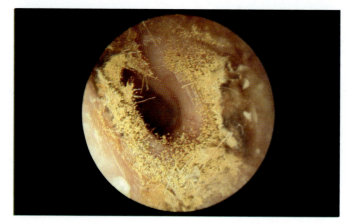

Figure 1.156

Otomycosis caused by *Aspergillus flavus*

In this patient (left ear) the multiple golden yellow dots are caused by the conidiophores of *Aspergillus flavus*.

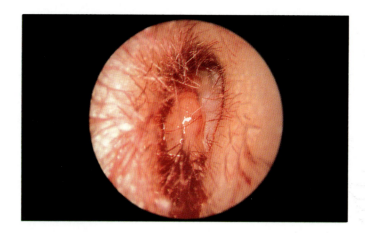

Figure 1.157

Malignant otitis externa

Malignant otitis externa is a severe and locally aggressive form of otitis externa that occurs in elderly diabetics and immunocompromised patients. The causative organism is usually *Pseudomonas aeruginosa*. Classically, malignant otitis externa presents as a severe pain in the ear associated with the appearance of exuberant granulation tissue arising from the floor of the external auditory canal at the junction of the bony and cartilaginous portions. (The right ear is shown.)

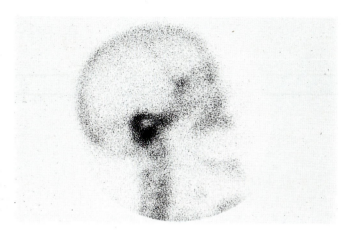

Figure 1.158

Malignant otitis externa: gallium scan

The spreading infection of malignant otitis externa can be seen in this gallium scan (right ear).

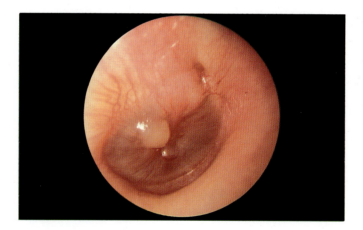

Figure 1.159

Myringitis bullosa (bullous myringitis)

Bullous myringitis is a specific form of viral otitis external, and is characterized by the appearance of blebs on the tympanic membrane and in the skin of the deep bony meatus associated with severe local pain. (The right ear is shown.)

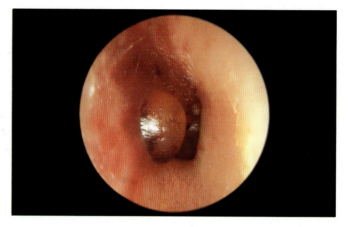

Figure 1.160

Severe myringitis bullosa (bullous myringitis)

The bleb present on the posterior bony canal wall and adjacent tympanic membrane contains a serous effusion with a small collection of blood in the more dependent portion. (The right ear is shown.)

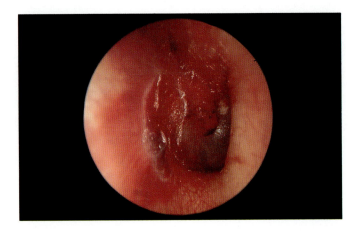

Figure 1.161

Severe myringitis bullosa (bullous myringitis)

Following rupture and aspiration of the contents of the large bulla seen in Figure 1.160, extensive subcutaneous and intracutaneous haemorrhage can be seen. Note the extensive haemorrhage along the handle of the malleus.

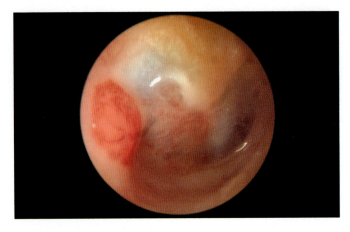

Figure 1.162

Localized granular myringitis

A chronic infection of the tympanic membrane associated with the appearance and persistence of painless, bright-red granulation tissue is termed 'granular myringitis'. Granular myringitis appears to be the result of chronic superficial infection of the thin epithelium covering the lateral surface of the tympanic membrane. Granular myringitis occurs in two distinct varieties: localized granulation tissue and diffuse granulation tissue. (The right ear is shown.)

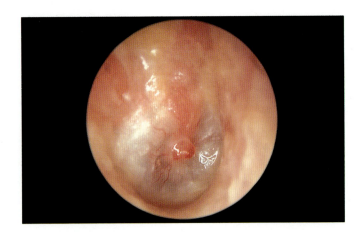

Figure 1.163

Localized granular myringitis

The pathogens responsible for granular myringitis may be either bacteria or fungi. In this patient (right ear) the chronic inflammation was the result of a candidal infection.

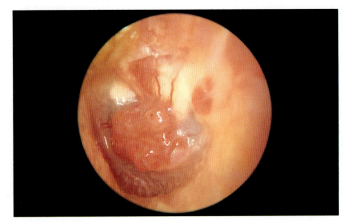

Figure 1.164

Diffuse granular myringitis

In this patient (left ear) a large portion of the tympanic membrane surface is covered with a diffuse granulation tissue.

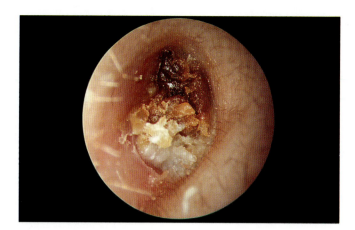

Figure 1.165

Keratosis obturans

Keratosis obturans is a condition in which the external auditory canal becomes occluded by an accumulation of keratin squamous debris. This condition appears to be the result of a defect in the normal self-cleansing migratory mechanism of the external auditory canal. (The right ear is shown.)

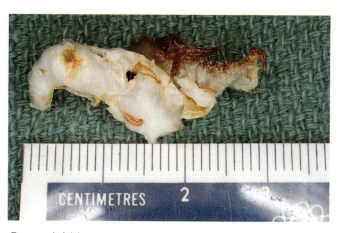

Figure 1.166

Keratin plug

The typical white plug which had occluded the external auditory canal is seen in this photograph. The lateral surface of the plug is covered with what appears to be relatively normal cerumen.

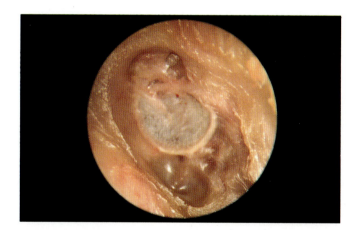

Figure 1.167

Widening of the bony canal secondary to keratosis obturans

The slowly enlarging plug of keratin squamous debris may exert enough pressure on the bone of the deep canal to cause substantial reabsorption. In these patients, following removal of the plug, an extremely wide, scooped-out external canal may be seen. The persistence of a keratin plug within the deep meatus in this patient (left ear, postmortem specimen) has caused gross resorption of the tympanic bone resulting in an extremely widened and deep canal.

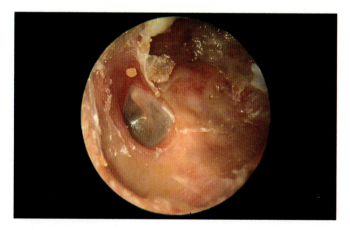

Figure 1.168

Automastoidectomy secondary to keratosis obturans

In this patient (left ear) the persistence of a keratin plug within the external auditory canal for a period of 5 years caused such pressure and resorption that the entire posterior bony canal wall and mastoid wall were resorbed, resulting in an automastoidectomy.

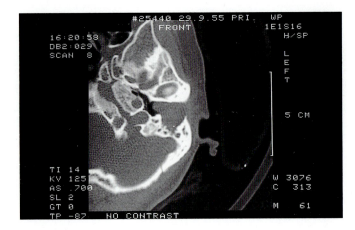

Figure 1.169

Automastoidectomy secondary to keratosis obturans

The massive keratin plug can be clearly seen in this axial CT scan of the left ear. Note how the plug has caused total resorption of the posterior bony canal wall and erosion of the mastoid process.

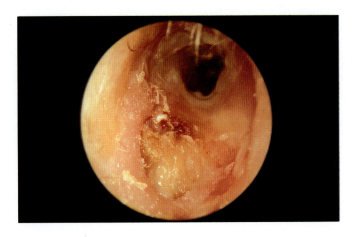

Figure 1.170

Osteitis of the tympanic bone (cholesteatoma of the external auditory canal)

Osteitis of the external auditory canal appears to result from local trauma, which disrupts the thin epithelium and underlying periosteum that overlies the tympanic bone. This allows the exposed tympanic bone to become infected, with the development of chronic osteitis. This results in an ulceration of the skin lining the floor of the external auditory canal with exposed devitalized bone. (The right ear is shown.)

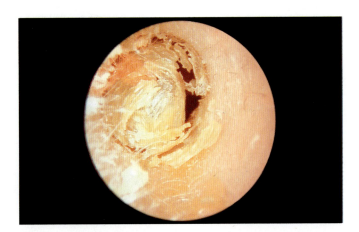

Figure 1.171

Irradiation changes in the external auditory canal

Irradiation of the external auditory canal may cause a secondary acute otitis externa as well as chronic changes such as those seen in this photograph (right ear). Radiation affects the sebaceous and ceruminous glands thereby interfering with the formation of normal cerumen. The result is an accumulation of keratin squamous debris in what is essentially a postirradiation acquired form of keratosis obturans.

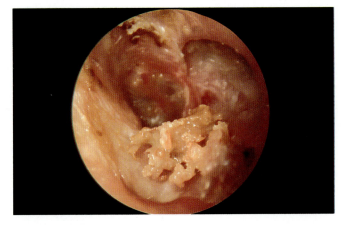

Figure 1.172

Irradiation osteitis

High levels of radiation may cause osteoradionecrosis of the tympanic bone with ulceration and sequestration similar to that seen in benign osteitis of tympanic bone. (The left ear is shown.)

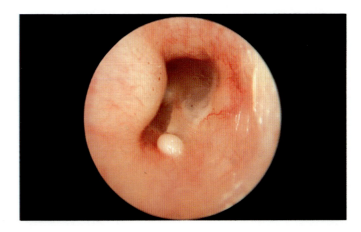

Figure 1.173
Exostosis

Exostoses of the bony ear canal are the result of localized areas of benign bony hypertrophy, which are thought to result from stimulation of the periosteum covering the medial surface of the tympanic bone by cold temperatures, e.g. swimming in cold water. Exostoses are usually multiple. Note the solitary white exostosis in the 12 o'clock position. (The right ear is shown.)

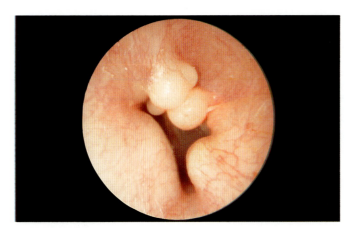

Figure 1.174
Multiple exostoses

This patient (left ear) has multiple exostoses. While the external canal has been significantly narrowed by multiple exostoses, the lumen is still of sufficient calibre for normal sound conduction and epithelial migration.

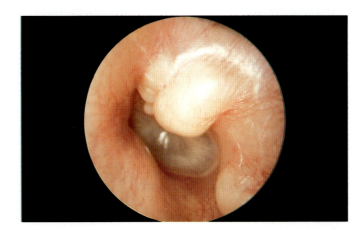

Figure 1.175
Multiple exostoses

The white colour of the exostoses is the result of thinning of the epithelium over the exostoses, allowing the ivory white colour of the underlying bone to be seen. (The left ear is shown.)

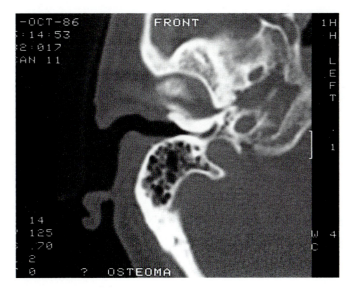

Figure 1.176
Multiple exostoses: CT scan

The dense ivory bone of exostoses arising from the anterior surface of the tympanic bone can be seen in this axial high-resolution CT scan.

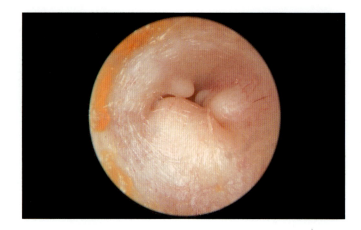

Figure 1.177

Severe multiple exostoses

In some patients the exostoses may grow to such an extent that the external auditory canal becomes almost totally occluded. (The left ear is shown.)

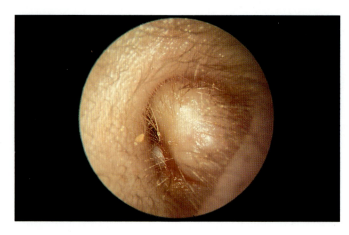

Figure 1.178

Osteoma of the tympanic bone

Osteomas of the deep ear canal are benign bony tumours that are relatively uncommon and usually solitary in occurrence. Osteomas appear as bony-hard pedunculated or sessile masses covered by normal canal skin. The large bony mass arising from the anterior canal wall was a pedunculated solitary osteoma.

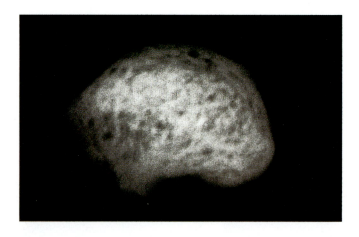

Figure 1.179

Osteoma of the tympanic bone: dental radiograph

Unlike exostoses, osteomas consist of a spongy or cancellous type of bone, as can be seen in this dental radiograph of a surgically removed osteoma.

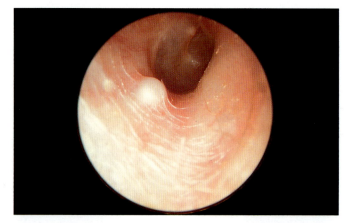

Figure 1.180

Epidermal inclusion cysts

Epidermal inclusion cysts in the skin of the external auditory canal usually result from trauma with implantation of epidermal cells into the dermis of the deep canal epithelium. Epidermal inclusion cysts have a pearly white colouration and are soft to palpation. (The right ear is shown.)

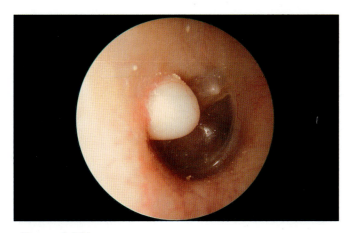

Figure 1.181

Epidermal inclusion cyst

The epidermal inclusion cyst seen in the 10 o'clock position in this patient (right ear) developed in the site of an endomeatal incision undertaken for access to the middle ear for stapedectomy.

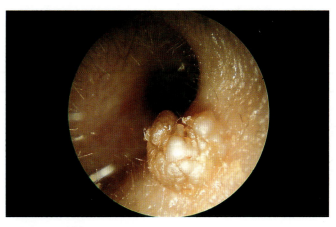

Figure 1.182

Papilloma of the external auditory canal

Squamous papillomas and viral papillomas not infrequently occur in the epithelium of the external auditory canal. Viral papillomas occur more commonly in the superficial canal skin. (The right ear is shown.)

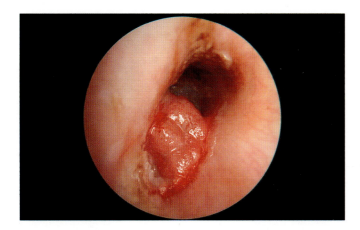

Figure 1.183

Aural polyp

Polyps encountered within the external auditory canal may arise from the skin lining the canal or from the mucosa of the middle ear, passing through a perforation of the tympanic membrane. Careful investigation needs to be undertaken to identify the origin of these benign granulation tissue polyps prior to excision. (The right ear is shown.)

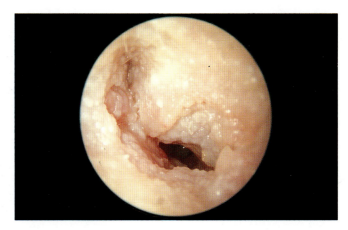

Figure 1.184

Carcinoma of the external auditory canal

Any unusual lesion arising from the skin of the external auditory canal should be carefully investigated and biopsied. This knobbly lesion (left ear) was a squamous cell carcinoma.

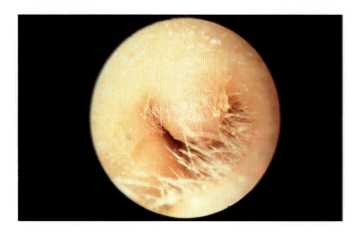

Figure 1.185
Adenocarcinoma of the external auditory canal

This innocuous dome-shaped subcutaneous mass (left ear) was diagnosed by excisional biopsy as an adenoid cystic adenocarcinoma.

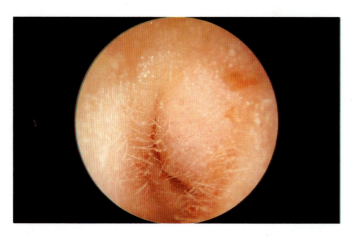

Figure 1.186
Ceruminoma of the external auditory canal

In contrast, this large subcutaneous lesion arising from the left anterior canal wall and narrowing the lumen of the external canal was a ceruminoma.

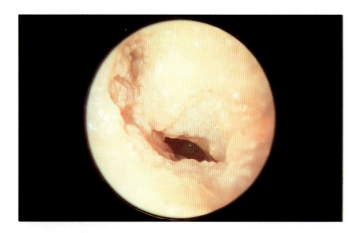

Figure 1.187
Carcinoma of the external auditory canal

Any unusual lesion of the external auditory canal should be biopsied. While the development of pain and bleeding have long been considered the hallmarks of malignancy in the ear, in our experience most cases lack these symptoms until very late in the course of the disease, The 'knobbly' lesion in this left external auditory canal is a well-differentiated squamous cell carcinoma.

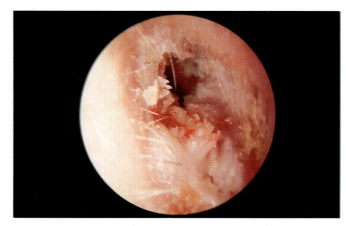

Figure 1.188
Verrucous carcinoma of the external auditory canal

The wart-like raised lesion arising from the floor of the cartilaginous external auditory canal was a verrucous carcinoma. (The left ear is shown.)

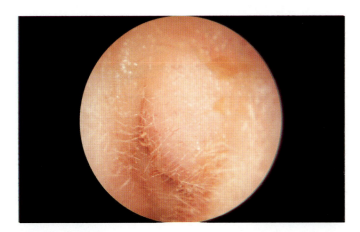

Figure 1.189

Ceruminoma of the external auditory canal

The smooth and 'benign' dome-shaped asymptomatic mass arising from the posterior cartilaginous canal wall is a ceruminoma.

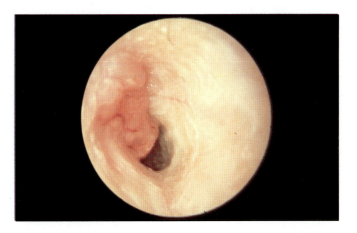

Figure 1.190

Secondary adenocystic adenocarcinoma of the external auditory canal

The irregular pink subcutaneous mass invading the skin lining the deep anterior canal wall of this left ear is adenoid cystic adenocarcinoma, which has spread posteriorly from the parotid gland.

Middle ear

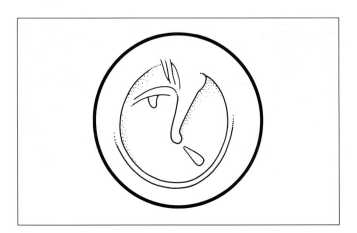

Figure 1.191
Normal right tympanic membrane

The normal tympanic membrane is a pale grey, ovoid, semi-transparent membrane, which sits at the medial end of the bony external auditory canal. This schematic diagram shows the anatomical landmarks that can be seen on and through a normal right tympanic membrane.

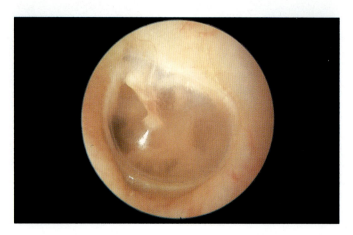

Figure 1.192
Normal tympanic membrane

The tympanic membrane provides a semi-transparent window through which the middle ear and some of its contents may frequently be visualized. Note in this photograph (left ear) the handle of the malleus with its short process superiorly and its cone of light anteroinferiorly. The long process of the incus can be seen in the posterosuperior quadrant, as can the chorda tympani nerve.

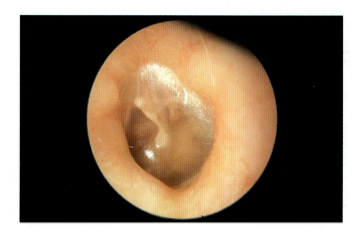

Figure 1.193
Prominent pars flaccida

The pars flaccida of this normal left tympanic membrane is very well developed. Note the slight outward bulging of the pars flaccida at the level of the head of the malleus.

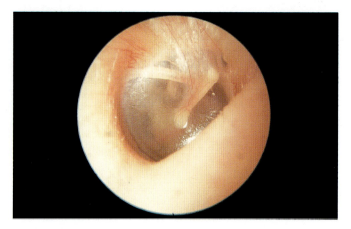

Figure 1.194
Prominent chorda tympani nerve

A very prominent chorda tympani nerve can been seen passing across the posterosuperior quadrant of this right tympanic membrane. Note the prominent posterior bulging of the anteroinferior bony canal wall, which hides the anterior sulcus of the tympanic membrane.

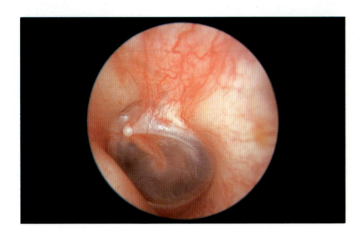

Figure 1.195
Vascular strip

The lateral surface of the tympanic membrane is supplied by the deep auricular branch of the maxillary artery, which sends a leash of prominent vessels down the superior canal wall. This area is called the 'vascular strip'. (The left ear is shown.)

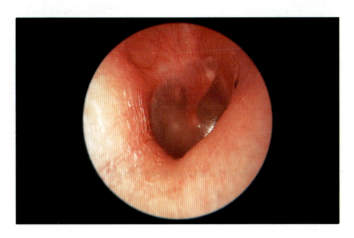

Figure 1.196
Prominent tympanic membrane vasculature

In some patients the blood supply of the vascular strip along the superior portion of the deep external auditory canal and the vessels that run from the vascular strip down either side of the handle of the malleus are unduly prominent. This is a variation of normal, which should not be interpreted as providing evidence of inflammation, i.e. an early acute otitis media. (The right ear is shown.)

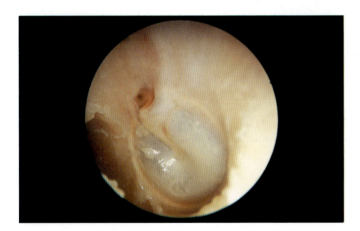

Figure 1.197
Shape of the tympanic membrane 1

The tympanic membrane is located obliquely to the central axis of the external auditory canal. This oblique angulation of the tympanic membrane gives the examiner a false impression that the tympanic membrane is flat and oval in shape, as seen in this cadaveric specimen of the left ear photographed through the external auditory canal.

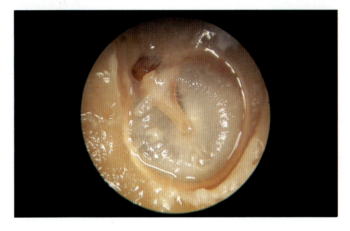

Figure 1.198
Shape of the tympanic membrane 2

In reality, the shape of the tympanic membrane is essentially circular and conical, as seen in this photograph of the previous specimen taken through a hole in the mastoid drilled at right angles to the actual axis of the tympanic membrane.

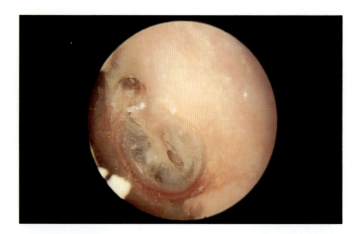

Figure 1.199

Optical illusions 1

This oblique angulation of the tympanic membrane is responsible for several optical illusions. Note the slit-like appearance of the myringotomy incision in this cadaveric specimen of the left ear photographed through the external auditory canal.

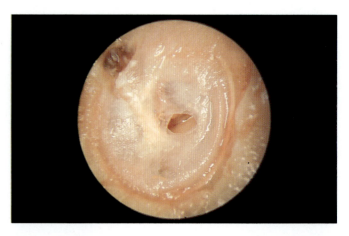

Figure 1.200

Optical illusion 2

The real size and shape of the defect in the tympanic membrane from the myringotomy can be seen in this photograph of the previous specimen (left ear) taken through a hole drilled in the mastoid in a plane at right angles to the true axis of the tympanic membrane.

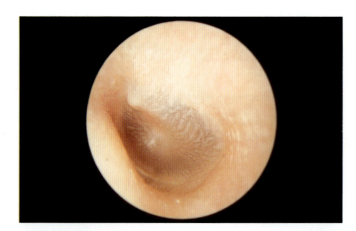

Figure 1.201

Keratin patches on the tympanic membrane

Small, radially oriented patches of thickened keratin squames are often seen on the surface of the tympanic membrane. These patches consist of older and thicker keratin from the central portion of the tympanic membrane, which has migrated centrifugally. These patches become more prominent when moistened and are consequently more easily seen after swimming. (The left ear is shown.)

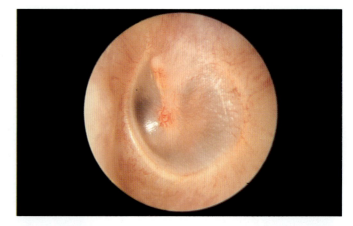

Figure 1.202

Keratin patches on the tympanic membrane

These small, radially oriented patches of thickened keratin squames are present on the surface of every tympanic membrane, although they cannot always be seen, as in this cadaveric tympanic membrane (left ear).

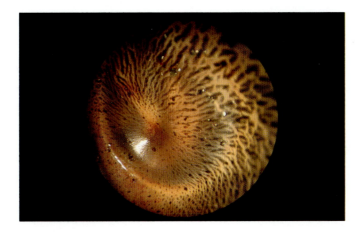

Figure 1.203

Keratin patches on the tympanic membrane: osmium staining

Osmium tetroxide stains keratin black, and can be used in the laboratory to demonstrate the presence of keratin patches. The shape, size and number of keratin patches can be clearly seen in this cadaveric specimen (left ear) in which the keratin patches have been emphasized by staining with osmium tetroxide.

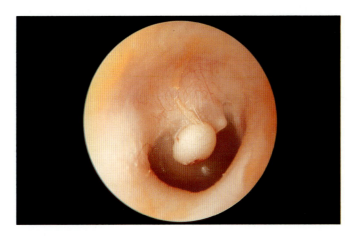

Figure 1.204

Congenital epidermal inclusion cyst of the tympanic membrane

The white cystic structure located in the central portion of the right tympanic membrane is a benign congenital epidermal cyst located lateral to the fibrous middle layer of the tympanic membrane.

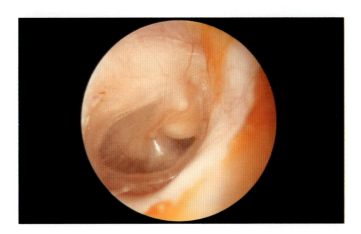

Figure 1.205

Small congenital epidermal cholesteatoma

The white cystic structure seen just behind the right tympanic membrane in the anterosuperior quadrant is a typical small congenital epidermal cholesteatoma.

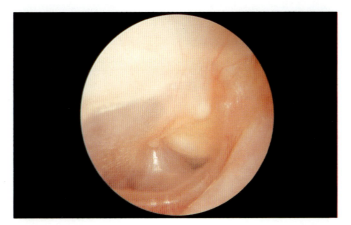

Figure 1.206

Small congenital epidermal cholesteatoma

A higher-power photograph of the right ear of the patient shown in Figure 1.205.

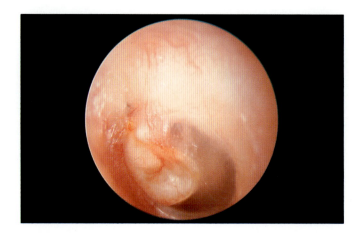

Figure 1.207

Congenital epidermal cholesteatoma, medium sized

The large white cystic structure seen deep to the tympanic membrane in this left ear is a medium-sized congenital epidermoid cholesteatoma of the middle ear.

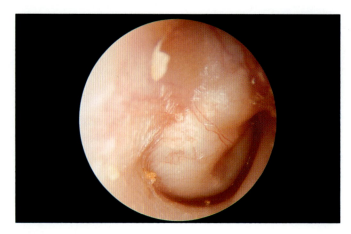

Figure 1.208

Extensive congenital epidermal cholesteatoma

The white bulging mass deep to the tympanic membrane in this right ear is a massive congenital epidermoid cholesteatoma of the middle ear.

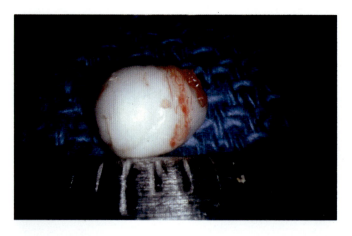

Figure 1.209

Congenital epidermal cholesteatoma: surgical specimen

The white, round, cyst-like structure is a small congenital cholesteatoma that was surgically removed.

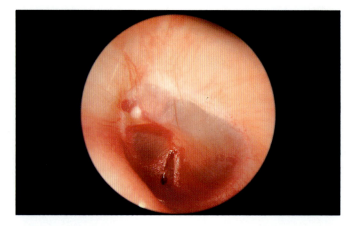

Figure 1.210

Traumatic perforation

Traumatic perforations of the tympanic membrane are the result of either sudden changes in pressure in the external auditory canal or direct trauma from an object inserted through the external auditory canal and into the tympanic membrane. The traumatic perforation seen in the anteroinferior quadrant of this young boy's left tympanic membrane resulted from a slap on the ear by his irate schoolmaster.

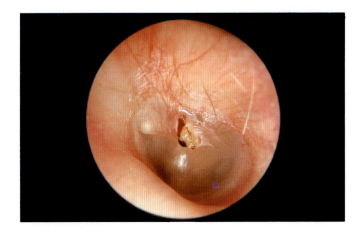

Figure 1.211

Healed traumatic perforation

Luckily this perforation healed completely and without complications 6 weeks later. Note the migrating scab which has moved to the posterosuperior quadrant of the tympanic membrane.

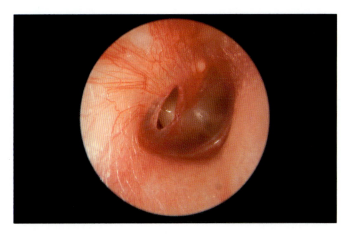

Figure 1.212

Traumatic perforation

The large linear perforation over the incudostapedial joint in the posterosuperior quadrant of this patient's right tympanic membrane resulted from the insertion of a cotton-tipped applicator too deeply into the external auditory canal.

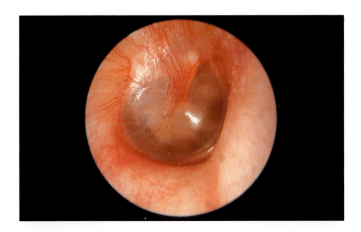

Figure 1.213

Healed traumatic perforation

Six weeks later the perforation had healed completely with no visible sequel.

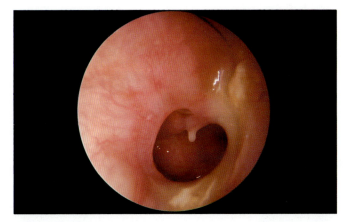

Figure 1.214

Thermal burn

The tympanic membrane may be perforated by welding sparks or hot liquids that are inadvertently poured down the external auditory canal. The large subtotal perforation in this right tympanic membrane resulted from an accidental spill of hot grease down the external auditory canal.

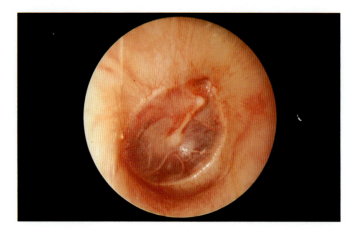

Figure 1.215
Barotrauma

The inability to equalize intratympanic with atmospheric pressure during descent in an aircraft or while diving in water may cause barotraumatic damage of the tympanic membrane or middle ear. This patient (right ear) shows the classic appearance of barotrauma following flying (6 hours earlier), namely a subepithelial haemorrhage along the handle of the malleus and over the posterosuperior annulus. Note the strands of fluid behind the lower half of the tympanic membrane.

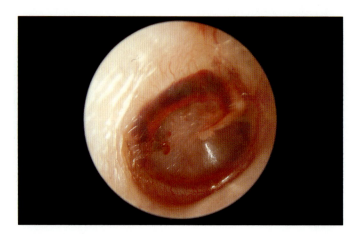

Figure 1.216
Barotrauma

Note the extensive area of subepithelial haematoma affecting the posterosuperior annulus and adjacent tympanic membrane. (The right ear is shown.)

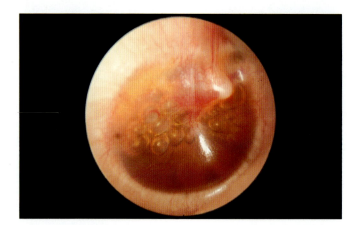

Figure 1.217
Barotrauma

This patient (right ear) developed a dark-orange serous effusion following barotrauma caused by travelling in an aircraft while having an upper respiratory infection.

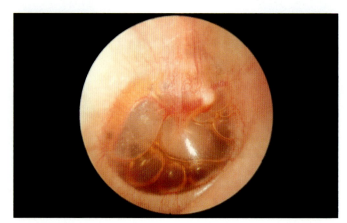

Figure 1.218
Barotrauma after autoinflation

Following a Valsalva manoeuvre, the patient shown in Figure 1.217 was able to clear most of the golden-yellow serous fluid from her middle ear.

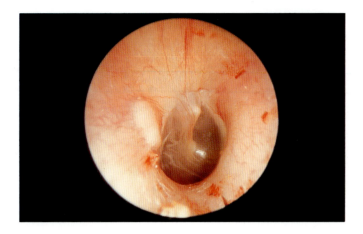

Figure 1.219

Temporal bone fracture

Temporal bone fractures may extend into the bony external auditory canal leaving telltale raised subepithelial bony fragments or subepithelial clefts along the fracture line. Note the displaced chip of bone beneath the epithelium of the posterior bony external canal in the 9 o'clock position (The right ear is shown.)

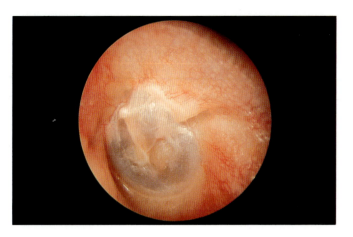

Figure 1.220

Temporal bone fracture

Note the diastasis of the posterosuperior bony canal wall in the 3 o'clock position. (The right ear is shown.)

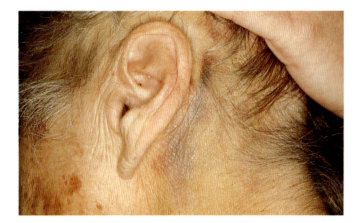

Figure 1.221

Battle's sign

Temporal bone fractures may be associated with bruising of the skin over the mastoid process, as seen in this patient. This is referred to as 'Battle's sign'.

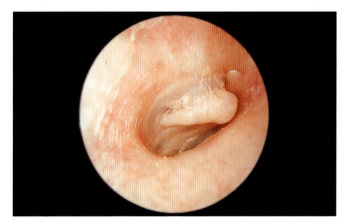

Figure 1.222

Temporal bone fracture with post-traumatic incus interposition

This patient (right ear) suffered a temporal bone fracture in childhood, when a truck ran over his head. During the injury, the incus was displaced onto the head of the stapes producing a post-traumatic incus interposition. Interestingly, the hearing was normal.

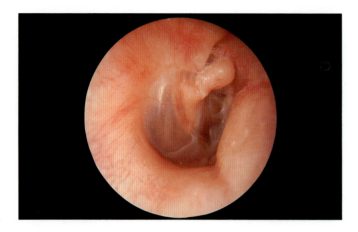

Figure 1.223

Temporal bone fracture with fracture of the malleus

In this patient (right ear) the head of the malleus has been fractured and rotated anteriorly. Note the fracture lines in the tympanic bone located at the 1, 2 and 5 o'clock positions.

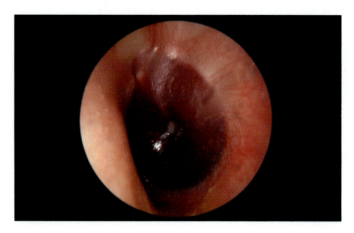

Figure 1.224

Haemotympanum

The presence of extravasated blood or blood-stained fluid in the middle ear is called a haemotympanum. A haemotympanum may develop following head injury with temporal bone fracture, barotrauma or in association with a severe otitis media. (The left ear is shown.)

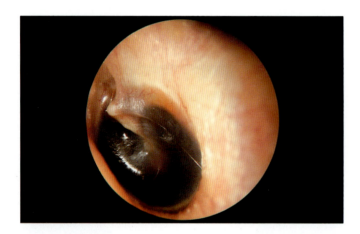

Figure 1.225

Haemotympanum

The older, dark-brown bloody fluid in this right middle ear has coloured the tympanic membrane black.

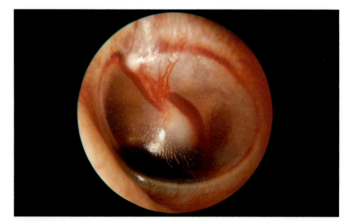

Figure 1.226

Partial haemotympanum

This patient has just had posterior nasal packing inserted for the control of severe epistaxis. The fresh blood seen behind the inferior portion of the tympanic membrane has entered the middle ear from the nasal cavity via the Eustachian tube.

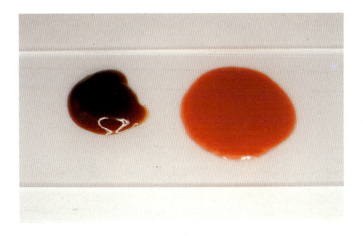

Figure 1.227

Haemotympanum fluid

The colour of fluid in the ear of a patient with a haemotympanum may vary from bright red, as seen on the right, to a chocolate brown colour, as seen on the left.

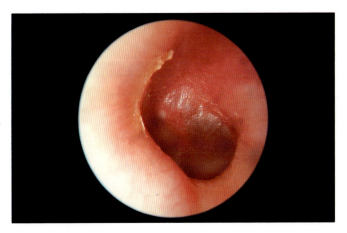

Figure 1.228

Early acute otitis media: stage of redness

The earliest changes in acute suppurative otitis media consist of redness, oedema and swelling in the pars flaccida (the upper fifth of the tympanic membrane). In this patient (left ear) the pars flaccida shows increased redness and slight outward bulging.

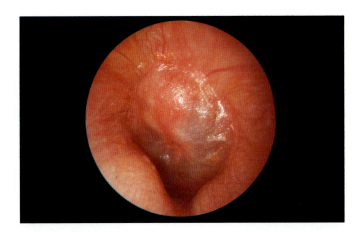

Figure 1.229

Early acute otitis media: stage of redness

In this patient (left ear) the pars flaccida shows redness, oedema and marked outward bulging.

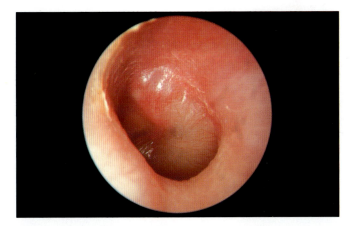

Figure 1.230

Otitis media: stage of suppuration

The stage of redness is shortly followed by the development of a mucopurulent exudate within the middle ear cleft. This creamy white fluid rapidly fills the middle ear and causes the tympanic membrane gradually to bulge outwards. This is the same patient as shown in Figure 1.228, 48 hours later.

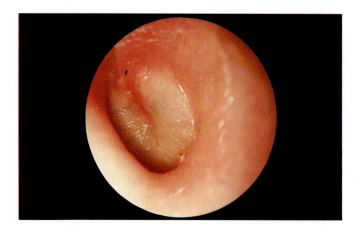

Figure 1.231

Severe acute otitis media

In this patient (left ear) the middle ear cleft is filled with creamy white mucopurulent material under pressure, which has caused the tympanic membrane to bulge laterally.

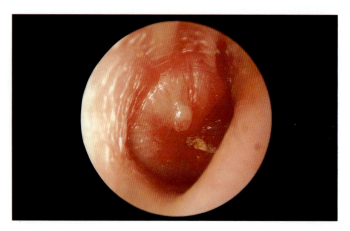

Figure 1.232

Severe acute otitis media

The small outward bulge in the centre of this right tympanic membrane is an area in which the fibrous middle layer has become necrotic and the thin epithelium is being herniated laterally by the pressure of the purulent fluid within the middle ear. It is through this area that a tiny perforation will shortly develop to allow the infected material within the middle ear to drain into the external auditory canal.

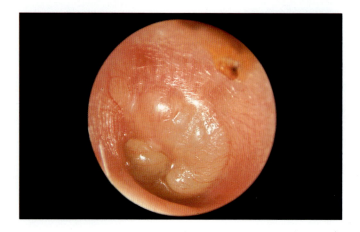

Figure 1.233

Severe acute otitis media

In this patient (left ear) the entire tympanic membrane is bulging laterally under the pressure of the infected purulent debris in the middle ear.

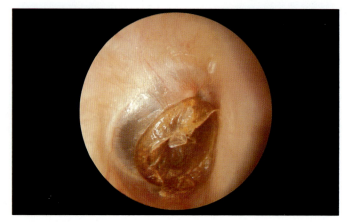

Figure 1.234

Serous and keratin casts of the tympanic membrane

In cases of severe otitis media the infection may spread through the tympanic membrane to such an extent that serous fluid weeps from the lateral surface of the tympanic membrane. The epithelium covering the tympanic membrane produces keratin squames at an increased rate. The end result is a golden-yellow brittle 'cast' covering the surface of the tympanic membrane. (The left ear is shown.)

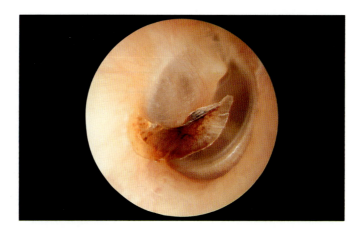

Figure 1.235

Cast of the tympanic membrane

Over time, following resolution of the infection, the cast covering the tympanic membrane will slowly separate and be carried out along the external auditory canal by normal migration. (The right ear is shown.)

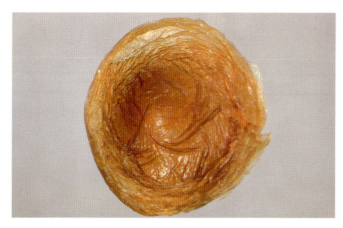

Figure 1.236

Serous and keratin cast

This circular cast was retrieved from the external canal of a young child. Initially the cast had covered the entire tympanic membrane.

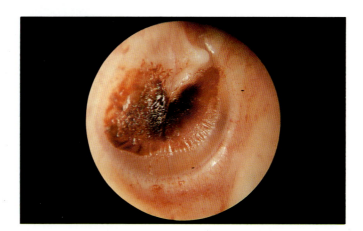

Figure 1.237

Tympanic membrane cast

A large blood-tinged dried cast can be seen covering most of this right tympanic membrane.

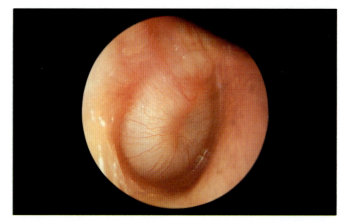

Figure 1.238

Mastoiditis

An incompletely treated or prolonged acute suppurative otitis media may extend from the middle ear into the mastoid air cell system, producing an acute mastoiditis. In this patient (right ear) the tympanic membrane is bulging out because of the presence of a chronic accumulation of purulent debris within the middle ear.

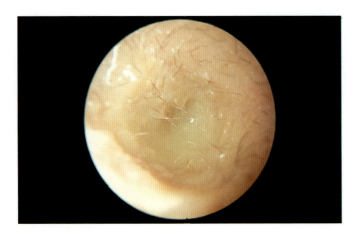

Figure 1.239

Mastoiditis

In this patient (right ear) the tympanic membrane has perforated as evidenced by the drainage of mucopurulent debris into the external auditory canal.

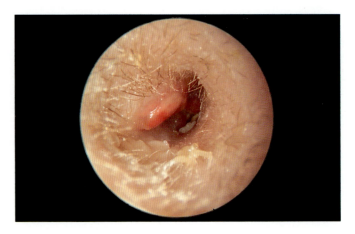

Figure 1.240

Mastoiditis

Following removal of the mucopurulent debris, a fistula through the canal into the mastoid process can be seen in the 9 o'clock position. (The right ear is shown.)

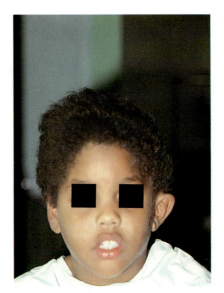

Figure 1.241

Subperiosteal abscess

A collection of pus under pressure beneath the periosteum over the left mastoid cortex will elevate the pinna, producing an outstanding ear, as seen in this patient.

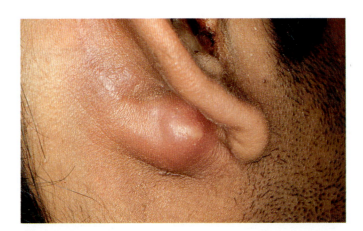

Figure 1.242

Subperiosteal abscess

In this patient the infection within the mastoid has perforated through the cortex laterally to produce a subcutaneous abscess over the mastoid tip. In the patient a large cholesteatoma was the predisposing factor.

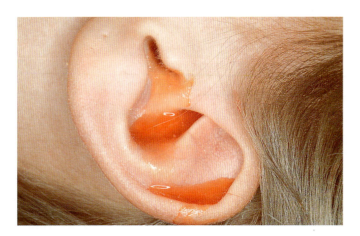

Figure 1.243
Cholesterol granuloma mastoiditis

In this patient chronic inflammation in the mastoid has resulted in the accumulation of cholesterol crystals together with a yellowy-brown fluid under pressure. Following myringotomy, copious quantities of fluid drained from the external canal.

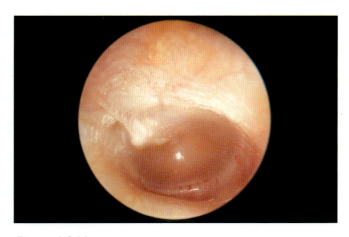

Figure 1.244
Mucoid otitis media

Mucoid otitis media is the most common cause of hearing loss in childhood. The mucoid fluid within this left middle ear has caused decreased translucency of the tympanic membrane. The inflammation that caused this mucoid otitis media to develop has caused vasodilatation of the radial vessels.

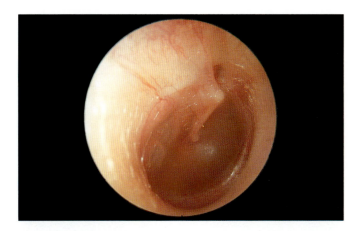

Figure 1.245
Mucoid otitis media

The mucoid fluid is opalescent in colour, as a result of which one cannot view through the tympanic membrane into the middle ear. The structures of the middle ear are obscured by this opalescent yellowish fluid. (The right ear is shown.)

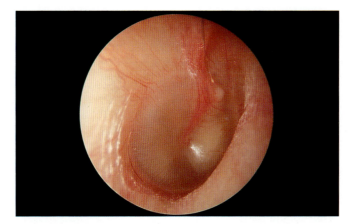

Figure 1.246
Mucoid otitis media

The differentiation between mild acute otitis media, mucoid otitis media and subacute otitis media can be quite subtle and is often a clinical judgement based on relatively indistinct findings. The creamy white mucoid effusion seen in this patient's left middle ear is an example of such a situation.

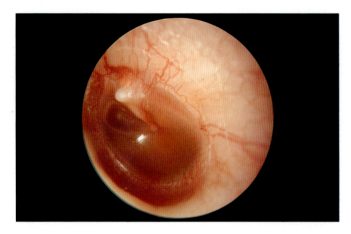

Figure 1.247

Mucoid otitis media

The mucoid fluid in this left middle ear has an orange tinge. Note the tiny air bubble anterior to the malleus handle.

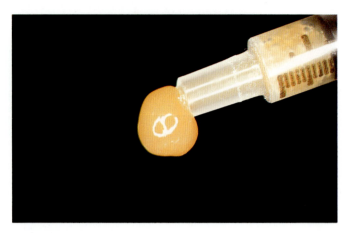

Figure 1.248

Mucoid otitis media

This fluid removed at myringotomy shows characteristic colouration and opacification of the middle ear exudate seen in patients with mucoid otitis media. Note the yellowish discolouration and thick tenacity.

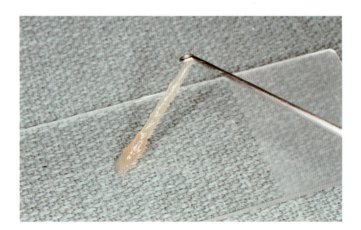

Figure 1.249

Mucoid otitis media

In this patient the fluid removed from the middle ear is opalescent and rubbery in consistency.

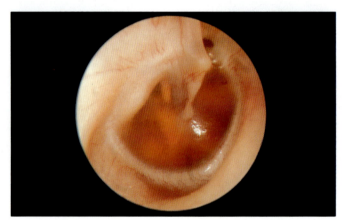

Figure 1.250

Serous otitis media

Serous otitis media results from persistent and complete eustachian tube obstruction. This condition is characterized by the accumulation of a golden-yellow or straw-coloured, thin, uninfected, watery serous fluid in the middle ear. The tympanic membrane shows a yellowish discolouration from the fluid within. (The right ear is shown.)

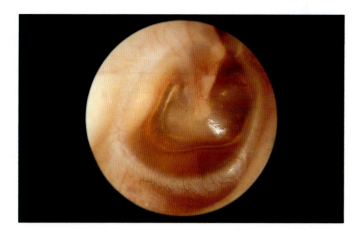

Figure 1.251
Serous otitis media post-Valsalva

This is the same patient as shown in Figure 1.250 following autoinflation by means of the Valsalva manoeuvre (attempting to exhale through the nose against pinched nostrils), which forces air up the Eustachian tube, reventilating the middle ear, as seen in this patient (right ear). Note how most of the golden-yellow watery fluid within the middle ear has been displaced by air.

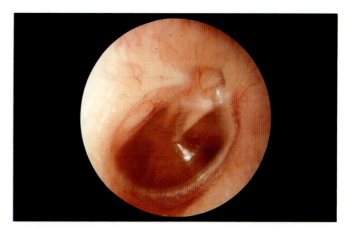

Figure 1.252
Serous otitis media

In many patients there is inward retraction of the tympanic membrane, which causes the short process of the malleus to become abnormally prominent and chalky white in colour. (The right ear is shown.)

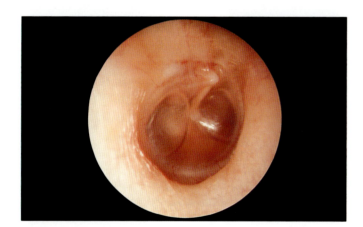

Figure 1.253
Serous otitis media: air–fluid level

When there is still air present within the middle ear, a well-defined air–fluid level may be seen.

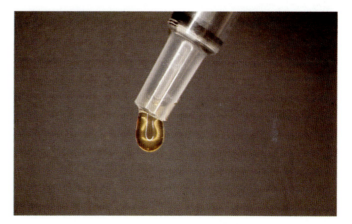

Figure 1.254
Serous fluid

The fluid obtained at myringotomy from patients with serous otitis media is clear, yellow or straw-coloured and watery.

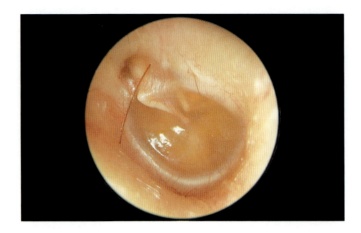

Figure 1.255

Myringotomy 1

The colour of the fluid within the middle ear gives the tympanic membrane a yellowish colour. (The left is shown.)

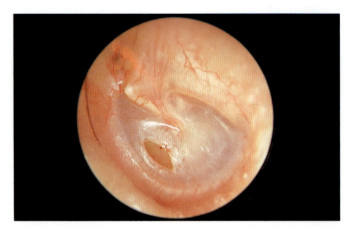

Figure 1.256

Myringotomy 2

Note the anteroinferior myringotomy incision in the patient shown in Figure 1.255, through which fluid in the middle ear has been aspirated. The myringotomy incision usually heals spontaneously within 7–14 days. Following removal of the fluid, the true colour of the tympanic membrane can be seen.

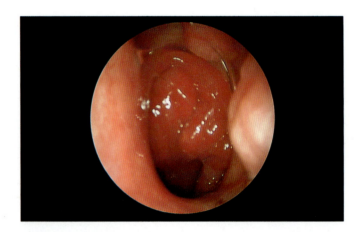

Figure 1.257

Carcinoma of the nasopharynx

A carcinoma of the nasopharynx must be suspected in any adult patient who presents with a persistent serous otitis media. In this patient the carcinoma arising from the posterior wall of the left nasopharynx was discovered with a Hopkin's rod nasopharyngeal endoscopic examination.

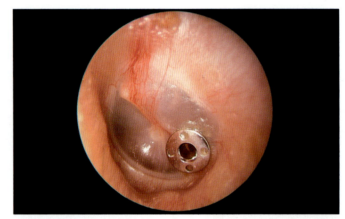

Figure 1.258

Ventilation tube

Ventilation tubes allow a more permanent aeration, ventilation and drainage of the middle ear. Note the stainless steel Reuter bobbin present in this patient's left tympanic membrane.

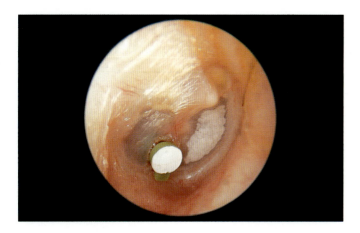

Figure 1.259

Castelli membrane ventilation tube

In this patient (right ear) the lumen of the green silastic ventilation tube is covered with a semi-permeable membrane to prevent the entrance of water into the tube during swimming.

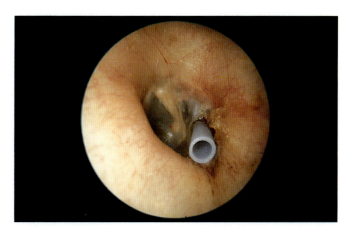

Figure 1.260

T-tube

In this patient (left ear) with chronic Eustachian tube insufficiency, a long purple silastic T-tube has been inserted in the inferior quadrant. T-tubes tend to stay in place for a relatively long period of time.

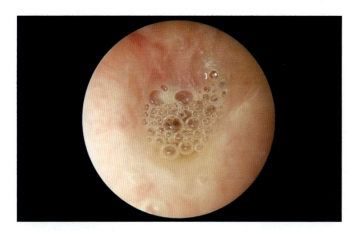

Figure 1.261

Otitis media in a patient with a ventilation tube 1

This patient with a ventilation tube in place developed an otitis media. The external auditory canal is filled with a mixture of air bubbles and purulent fluid, which has drained into the external auditory canal through the lumen of the tube. (The right ear is shown.)

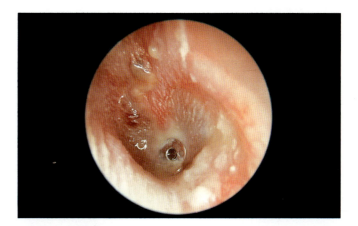

Figure 1.262

Otitis media in a patient with a ventilation tube 2

Following aspiration of the fluid seen in Figure 1.261, the stainless steel Reuter bobbin can be seen in place in the right tympanic membrane.

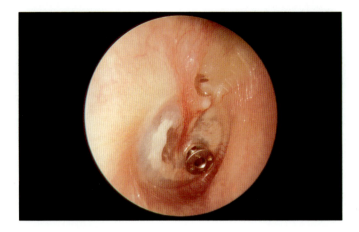

Figure 1.263
Extruding ventilation tube

Most ventilation tubes spontaneously extrude from 3 months to 2 years following insertion. The time interval between insertion and extrusion is a function of the individual patient and the type of tube inserted. Note the tiny collar of keratin accumulating behind the outer flange of this stainless steel Reuter bobbin tube. The action of the tympanic membrane and its accumulating collar of keratin will ultimately lever this tube out of the tympanic membrane. Note the patches of tympanosclerosis. (The right ear is shown.)

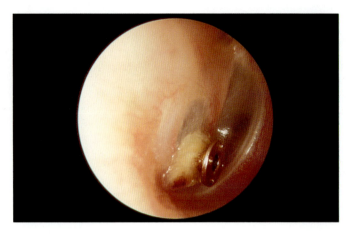

Figure 1.264
Extruding tube

A much larger collar of keratin has almost completely lifted this stainless steel Reuter bobbin out of its insertion site in the right tympanic membrane.

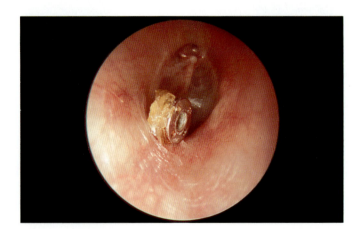

Figure 1.265
Extruded tube

Once a tube has extruded from the tympanic membrane, it will be carried outward by the normal migration of the epithelium lining the deep external auditory canal. (The right ear is shown.)

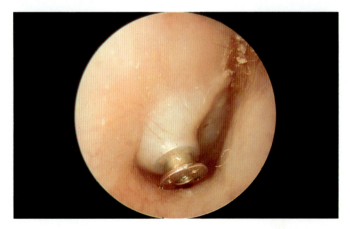

Figure 1.266
Acute otitis media with accelerated extrusion of a ventilation tube

This patient (right ear), whose ventilation tube had been inserted 1 week previously, developed an acute otitis media. The lumen of her ventilation tube has become plugged and the pressure of the purulent fluid accumulating within the middle ear is forcing the ventilation tube out of the tympanic membrane in an accelerated fashion.

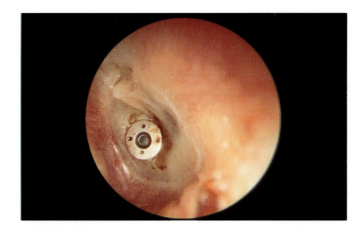

Figure 1.267
Blocked ventilation tube

The lumen of a ventilation tube must remain patent if the tube is to perform its intended functions: aeration, pressure equalization and, when necessary, drainage. The lumen of this stainless steel Reuter bobbin has become blocked by a small amount of clotted blood. (The left ear is shown.)

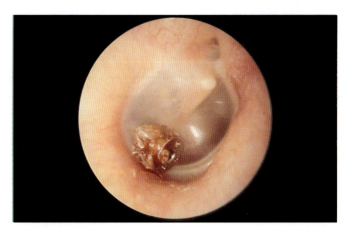

Figure 1.268
Blocked ventilation tube

The lumen of this tube has become blocked with a brittle, dry, orange crust, which formed when serous fluid leaking from the middle ear dried. Note how this crust has also collected under the outer flange of the tube. (The right ear is shown.)

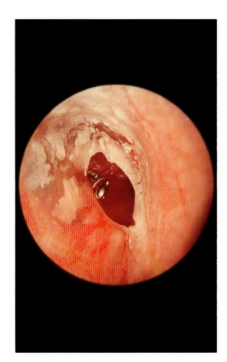

Figure 1.269
Ventilation tube in the middle ear

This patient (left ear) developed an acute otitis media shortly after the insertion of a stainless steel Reuter bobbin ventilation tube. The area of the tympanic membrane in which the ventilation tube was situated necrosed and the tube has fallen inwards.

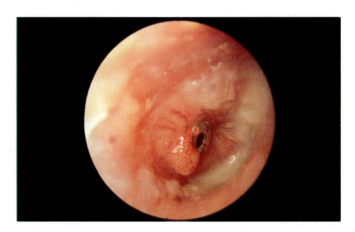

Figure 1.270
Tube granuloma

In approximately 1% of cases, the keratin collar that accumulates around a ventilation tube inserted in the tympanic membrane will incite a foreign body granulomatous reaction. This results in the local production of an exuberant mass of granulation tissue. The vascular lesion arising from the surface of the tympanic membrane and covering the inferior portion of the stainless steel ventilation tube is a tube granuloma. (The right ear is shown.)

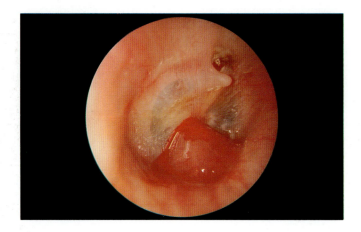

Figure 1.271

Tube granuloma

The larger polypoid granuloma present in this right tympanic membrane completely engulfed the stainless steel Reuter bobbin ventilation tube that had previously been inserted into the tympanic membrane.

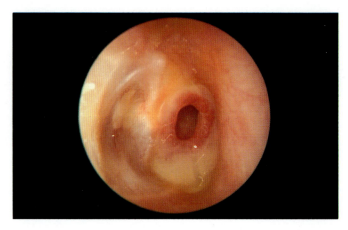

Figure 1.272

Chronic suppurative otitis media

Chronic suppurative otitis media is characterized by a painless persistent otorrhoea and a perforation in the tympanic membrane. Note the granulation tissue surrounding the margins of this anterior central perforation and the yellowish discharge within the canal. The organism cultured was *Staph. aureus*. (The right ear is shown.)

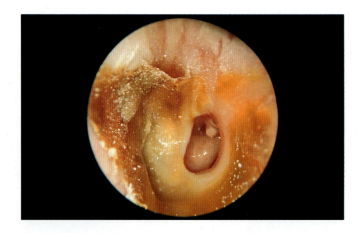

Figure 1.273

Chronic suppurative otitis media

In this patient's left ear there is a large perforation overlying the stapes. The entire membrane and deep canal are covered with a yellowish-green cast of inspissated mucus.

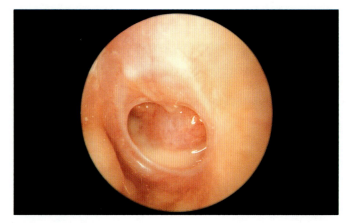

Figure 1.274

Chronic suppurative otitis media

This patient (left ear) with a large central perforation has developed an acute viral upper respiratory infection. The mucosa lining the middle ear has become infected and as a result has produced a creamy white, thick mucoid fluid.

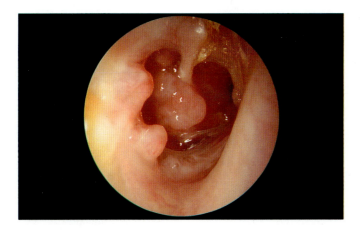

Figure 1.275

Chronic suppurative otitis media

In this patient (right ear), as a result of multiple episodes of acute otitis media, the mucosa lining the promontory has become thickened, hypertrophic and polypoid in nature. Note the large central perforation.

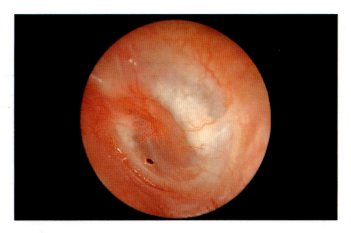

Figure 1.276

Pinpoint central perforation

This patient (left ear) has a small pinpoint perforation, which developed following an episode of acute otitis media.

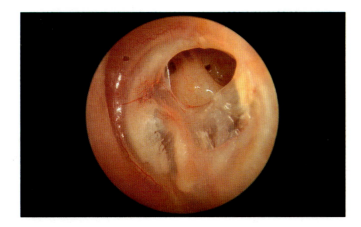

Figure 1.277

Medium central perforation

This patient (right ear) shows a medium-sized central perforation through which the round window niche can be seen in the posterior inferior quadrant.

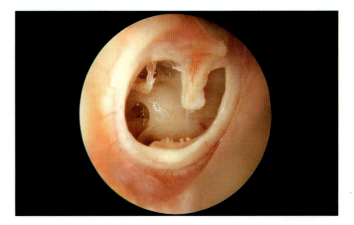

Figure 1.278

Subtotal perforation of the tympanic membrane

In this patient (right ear) almost the entire pars tensa has become perforated following an acute episode of otitis media. The medial wall of the middle ear can be clearly seen through the perforation. Note the fibrous band that attaches the remnant of the long process of the incus to the head of the stapes.

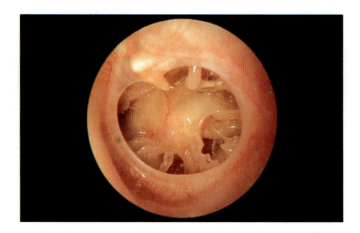

Figure 1.279

Total perforation of the tympanic membrane

In this patient (left ear) there is a total perforation of the tympanic membrane. Note how most of the handle of the malleus is missing.

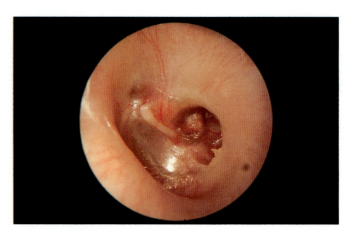

Figure 1.280

Cholesterol granuloma

This yellow-brown mass over the head of the stapes (left ear) is a small cholesterol foreign body granuloma.

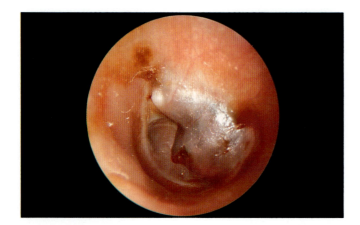

Figure 1.281

Cholesterol granuloma

This yellow-brown mass within the left middle ear, which is pushing the tympanic membrane laterally, is a cholesterol foreign body granuloma.

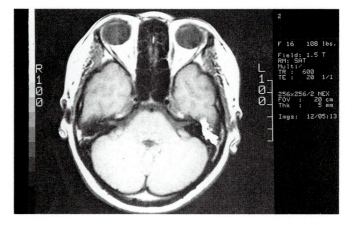

Figure 1.282

Cholesterol granuloma: MRI scan

The cholesterol crystals within a cholesterol granuloma are illuminated on an MRI scan and as a result a cholesterol granuloma is easily diagnosed with MRI.

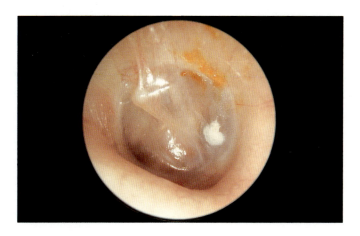

Figure 1.283
Tympanosclerosis

Tympanosclerotic plaques consist of collections of thickened hyalinized collagen located in the fibrous middle layer of the tympanic membrane. Tympanosclerotic plaques result from previous middle ear infections. The small discrete white spot in the 3 o'clock position of the tympanic membrane (left ear) is a tympanosclerotic plaque.

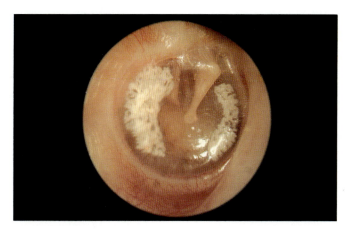

Figure 1.284
Tympanosclerosis

Note the chalky-white, crescent-shaped plaques on either side of the malleus in this right tympanic membrane.

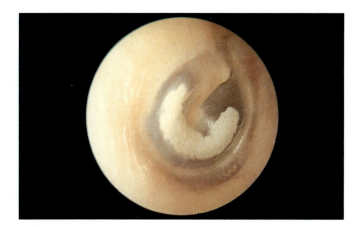

Figure 1.285
Crescent-shaped plaque of tympanosclerosis

In this patient (right ear) the tympanic membrane contains one large horseshoe-shaped tympanosclerotic plaque curving around the lower portion of the malleus.

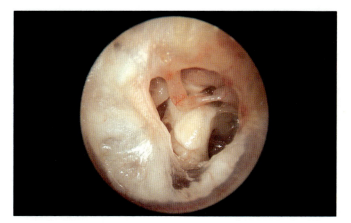

Figure 1.286
Tympanosclerosis of the middle ear

Tympanosclerotic plaques may develop in the mucosal lining of the middle ear. In this patient (left ear) a large tympanosclerotic plaque can be seen arising from the medial wall of the middle ear (the promontory). Middle ear tympanosclerosis may completely entrap the ossicles, causing a severe conductive hearing loss.

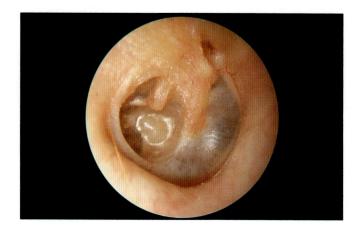

Figure 1.287

Retracted tympanic membrane

In this patient (right ear), because of chronic negative pressure within the middle ear, the posterior superior quadrant of the tympanic membrane has become retracted medially. Note how it is draped over the long process of the incus and also over the promontory.

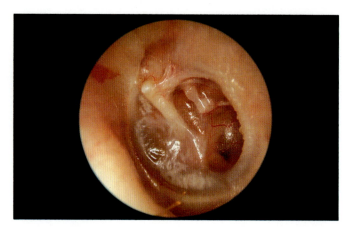

Figure 1.288

Myringostapediopexy

In this patient (left ear), as the result of chronic negative pressure, the tympanic membrane has become retracted over its posterior half. Note how the tympanic membrane is lying over the lateral surface of the incus and the head of the stapes.

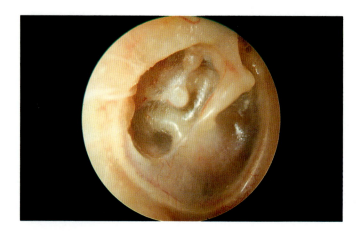

Figure 1.289

Myringostapediopexy

In this patient (right ear), with a similar pathology in the opposite ear, the lenticular process of the incus has eroded and the head of the stapes can be seen directly in contact with the tympanic membrane. This situation is known as a myringostapediopexy.

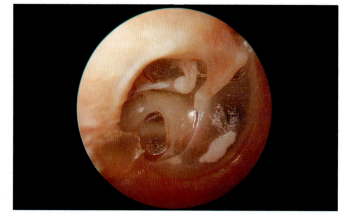

Figure 1.290

Self-cleansing retraction pocket

Chronic intratympanic negative pressure may cause the tympanic membrane to become retracted and thinned, forming a 'retraction pocket'. Retraction pockets occur most commonly in the posterior half of the tympanic membrane. As long as retraction pockets are self-cleansing they do not appear to be at risk for the development of a cholesteatoma. (The right ear is shown.)

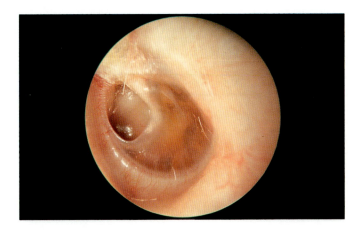

Figure 1.291
Retraction pocket

A deep retraction pocket may at first glance resemble a perforation. Note the apparent anterosuperior 'perforation' in this left tympanic membrane, which is in fact simply a deep self-cleansing retraction pocket, The orange discolouration of the tympanic membrane is the result of serous fluid within the middle ear.

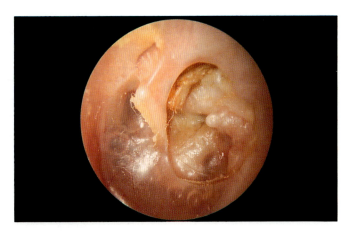

Figure 1.292
Non-self-cleansing retraction pocket

When the epithelium lining the retraction pocket loses its normal migratory abilities and consequently is no longer self-cleansing, keratin may accumulate within the retraction pocket. These patients are at risk for the development of a cholesteatoma in this area. (The left ear is shown.)

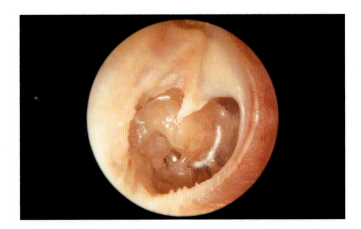

Figure 1.293
Middle ear atelectasis

Long-standing negative intratympanic pressure may cause almost complete resorption of the fibrous middle layer of the tympanic membrane. The result is an extensive retraction pocket, which may appear on first glance to be a large central perforation. (The right ear is shown.)

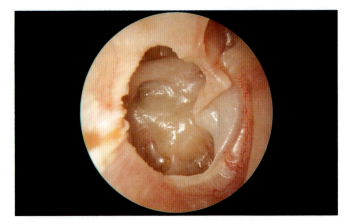

Figure 1.294
Adhesive otitis media

The last and most severe stage in the effect of chronic negative pressure on the middle ear is a condition known as adhesive otitis media. In adhesive otitis media, the medial surface of the tympanic membrane has become attached by adhesions to the medial wall of the middle ear. This is generally an irreversible condition. (The right ear is shown.)

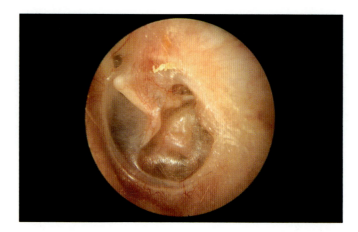

Figure 1.295

Pulsion hernia 1

The fibrous middle layer of that portion of a tympanic membrane involved in a retraction pocket usually becomes atrophic or completely resorbed. As a result this area of the tympanic membrane lacks strength. (The left ear is shown.)

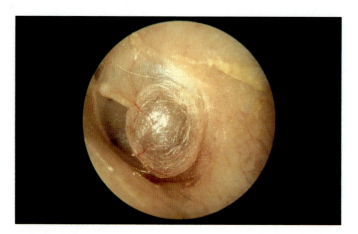

Figure 1.296

Pulsion hernia 2

If such a patient performs a Valsalva manoeuvre, this weakened area of the tympanic membrane may be displaced (herniate) laterally into the external canal. This is called a pulsion hernia. As the intratympanic pressure returns to normal, the tympanic membrane will return to its normal position. (The left ear is shown.)

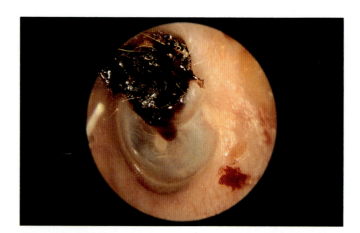

Figure 1.297

Attic cholesteatoma

Crusts overlying the attic frequently hide significant pathology and especially a cholesteatoma. (The left ear is shown.)

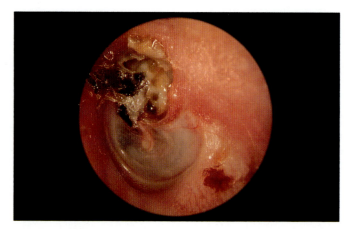

Figure 1.298

Attic cholesteatoma

This is the same patient as in Figure 1.297 following removal of the blood-stained serous crust. Note the collection of keratin debris arising from an attic cholesteatoma.

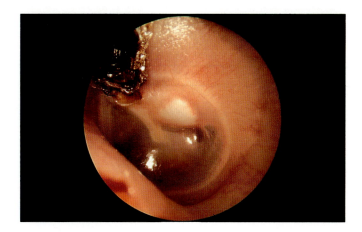

Figure 1.299
Middle ear cholesteatoma

In this patient (left ear) a cholesteatoma within the attic has extended down into the middle ear. Note the attic crust and the white mass of cholesteatoma behind the posterior quadrant of the tympanic membrane.

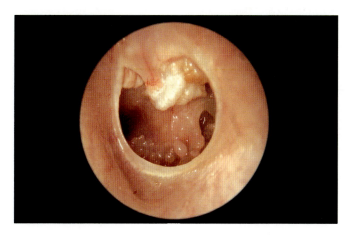

Figure 1.300
Middle ear cholesteatoma

In this patient (left ear) a cholesteatoma within the attic has extended down into the middle ear, and the accumulating keratin squames can be seen through a large central perforation.

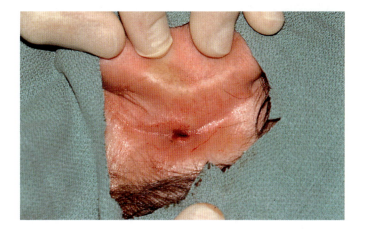

Figure 1.301
Mastoid fistula

This patient, who had an extensive cholesteatoma within the mastoid process, developed a fistula following an acute otitis media with mastoiditis.

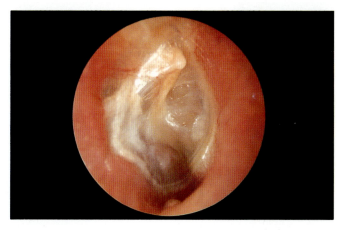

Figure 1.302
High jugular bulb

The blue dome-shaped mass arising from the floor of this right middle ear is an enlarged and unusually high but normal jugular bulb.

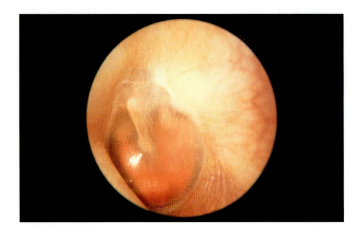

Figure 1.303

Aberrant internal carotid artery

The pink mass arising from the floor of this left middle ear and lying against the medial surface of the tympanic membrane is an aberrant internal carotid artery.

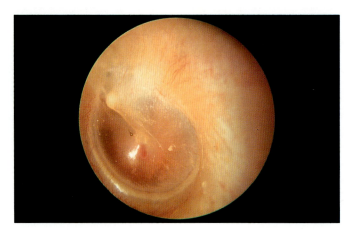

Figure 1.304

Glomus tympanicum

The small red mass lying against the medial surface of this left tympanic membrane just below the inferior tip of the malleus is a small glomus tympanicum.

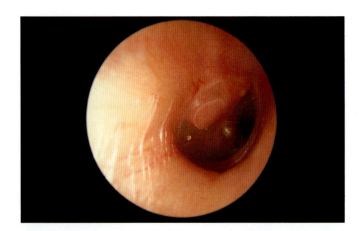

Figure 1.305

Glomus tympanicum

The red mass pressing against the posterosuperior quadrant of this right tympanic membrane is a medium-sized glomus tympanicum, which arose from the chorda tympani nerve.

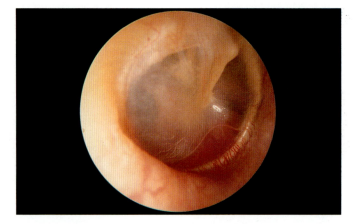

Figure 1.306

Glomus jugulare

The bright-red crescent-shaped mass pressing against the inferior portion of this right tympanic membrane is a glomus jugulare tumour.

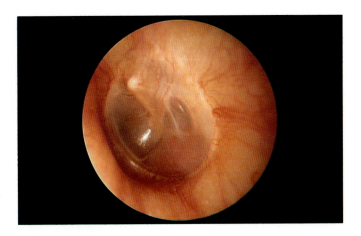

Figure 1.307

Glomus vagale

The larger pink mass pressing against the inferior quadrant of this left tympanic membrane arose from the vagus nerve. The portion of this glomus vagale that can be seen in the middle ear is just the 'tip of the iceberg'.

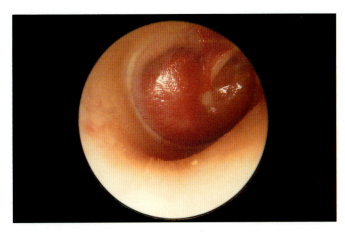

Figure 1.308

Glomus jugulare

The large red mass filling this right middle ear and pushing the tympanic membrane laterally is a huge glomus jugulare tumour, which filled this patient's middle ear.

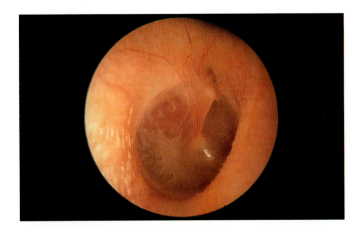

Figure 1.309

Facial nerve neuroma

The faint pink mass seen behind the posterosuperior quadrant of this patient's right tympanic membrane is a neuroma arising from the facial nerve.

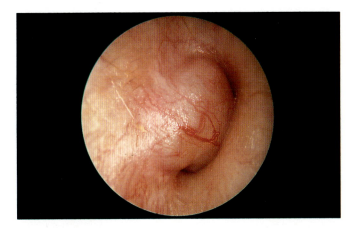

Figure 1.310

Facial nerve neuroma

Note how the benign tumour shown in Figure 1.309 has grown over 2 years.

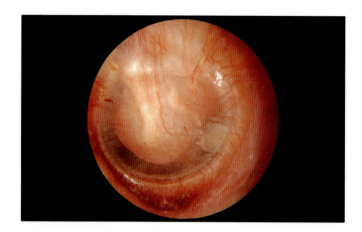

Figure 1.311

Facial nerve neuroma

The white discrete mass seen in this left middle ear is a facial nerve neuroma.

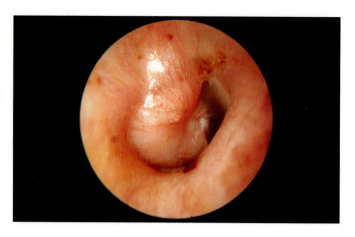

Figure 1.312

Primary adenoma of the middle ear

The creamy white mass filling the posterior four-fifths of this right middle ear was a primary adenoma arising from the middle ear mucosa.

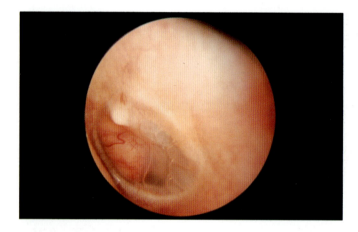

Figure 1.313

Acquired meningoencephalocele

The pinkish-yellow mass seen behind the anterior quadrant of this left middle ear was an acquired meningoencephalocele in a patient who had previously had a craniotomy for the removal of a meningioma.

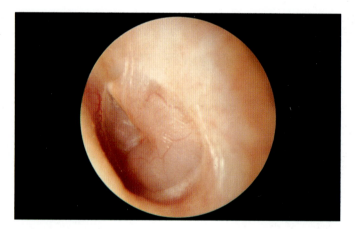

Figure 1.314

Acoustic neuroma

The pink-white mass filling this left middle ear is acoustic neuroma tissue that had extended into the middle ear via the stapes footplate.

2
The nose

Introduction

The symptoms of nasal disease are often mild and non-specific: they include nasal obstruction, nasal discharge and mid-facial pain. While the history and nature of these symptoms may suggest the area of the nose in which the problem lies, a complete nasal examination is always required to establish the diagnosis.

A rough clinical estimate of nasal airflow may be made by asking the patient to exhale through the nose onto a cool mirror and observing the extent of the misting thus produced upon the surface of the mirror.

A strong light source is required to illuminate the interior of the nasal cavity. A headlamp or headmirror allows the examiner the benefit of having both hands free!

The tip of the nose is everted and the nasal vestibule then carefully and completely inspected. All areas of the nasal vestibule must be completely examined in order to avoid missing a small malignant tumour or papilloma 'hidden' within the nasal vestibule. In children, eversion of the nasal tip may be all that is required to facilitate a thorough inspection of the anterior nasal cavity. In adults, dilatation of the nasal vestibule and separation of the nasal hairs with the insertion of a nasal speculum are usually required to allow inspection of the anterior nasal cavity. A systematic technique for the inspection of the nasal cavity (e.g. septum, nasal floor, inferior meatus, inferior turbinate, middle meatus, middle turbinate and roof of the nasal cavity) is helpful to identify all potentially visible pathology. To see the upper and lower portions of each nasal fossa the patient's head and the speculum must be angulated. A topical decongestant spray should then be applied to the nasal cavity to shrink down the inferior turbinate, thereby allowing a better inspection into the depths of the nasal cavity and the identification of deeper nasal pathology.

The office examination of the post-nasal space with a mirror and headlight is often difficult in adults and generally impossible in young children, even in the hands of experts. Fibreoptic nasal endoscopes, rigid rod endoscopes and radiology are all important methods of assessing the nasopharynx of a patient; a patient should, therefore, be referred to a specialist with access to these modalities when nasopharyngeal pathology is suspected.

An examination of the nose is never complete until the neck has been examined. Malignancy of the nose, paranasal sinuses and nasopharynx may have spread to the neck even when there are only minimal or even no nasal symptoms.

Facial scars from previous nasal and sinus surgery can often be missed and a careful inspection of the face and oral cavity is required. While it is reasonable to expect that most patients would remember details of previous nasal or sinus surgery, unfortunately this is not always the case!

Endoscopic examination of the upper airways has obtained a worldwide popularity since the early 1970s. The interior of the maxillary sinus was the initial focus of diagnostic interest. Endoscopic examination was soon extended to all the visible areas within the nasal cavity. Hopkins rigid rod nasal endoscopes enable the physician to examine the clefts and recesses of the nasal cavity in great detail, and the ability to pass these thin endoscopes into the middle meatus of the nose allows inspection of the region of the anterior ethmoid sinuses, which is the key area responsible for chronic paranasal sinus disease. Today, nasal endoscopic examination is an integral part of any routine otorhinolaryngological examination.

The role of Computed Tomography (CT) in the examination of the paranasal sinuses should be emphasized. Since an endoscopic examination can only show the 'surface' structures within the nasal cavity, a CT examination of the paranasal sinuses is now considered to be an essential component of the diagnostic evaluation of those patients who present with symptoms suggestive of paranasal sinus disease. CT provides the ideal technique for the examination of the delicate bony chambers of the ethmoidal labyrinth; and a CT scan can also demonstrate those anatomical variants which may compromise the ventilation and drainage of the paranasal sinuses and thus predispose a patient to recurrent episodes of sinusitis. A systematic endoscopic examination of the lateral nasal wall in conjunction with a CT examination of the nose and paranasal sinuses will allow a precise localization of the underlying disease processes and thus aid the clinician in planning appropriate therapy.

The recent increased interest in nasal endoscopy is a direct result of the dissemination of the technique of Functional Endoscopic Sinus Surgery. The concept of Functional Endoscopic Sinus Surgery was developed by Professor Walter Messerklinger in Graz, Austria, in the early 1970s, following extensive research into the anatomy and pathophysiology of the paranasal sinuses. Messerklinger's concepts have revolutionized, improved and radically altered the techniques used for the diagnosis and treatment of patients with paranasal sinus disease. His original research established that the health of the frontal and maxillary sinuses was subordinate to the anterior ethmoid and, in particular, to the prechambers (the frontal recess and the infundibulum) through which these sinuses receive ventilation and drain into the nasal cavity. He demonstrated that occlusion or narrowing of these prechambers was the prime cause

of recurrent sinus infection; and observed that, when infection developed in these larger paranasal sinuses, it was usually rhinogenic in origin (that is, it had spread from the nose through the anterior ethmoid to involve the frontal and maxillary sinuses secondarily).

Messerklinger noted in his patients that a limited endoscopic resection of the disease within the anterior ethmoid responsible for the obstruction of the ventilation and drainage pathways of these larger paranasal sinuses allowed re-establishment of ventilation and drainage through the natural pathways. Even mucosal pathology within the frontal and maxillary sinuses usually healed without direct surgical intervention into these larger sinuses. The key principle of Functional Endoscopic Sinus Surgery is thus that a minimal localized resection of the disease obstructing the ethmoidal prechambers allows restoration of normal mucociliary clearance and ventilation, which is followed by spontaneous resolution of the mucosal disease in the maxillary and frontal sinuses.

The endoscopic approach has also led to the realization that 'nasal polyposis' is not one disease entity. In contrast to the polyps in chronic rhinosinusitis, the diffuse nasal polyposis associated with sinobronchial syndrome, acetylsalicylic acid intolerance and hyperreactive airway disease is now seen as an immunological problem where surgery is only one part of the therapy. Less radical surgery, combined with topical corticosteroids, is today considered the state-of-the-art therapy to control this disease.

The majority of the photographs in this section were taken using the Karl Storz photographic system, the most important feature of which is Karl Storz Hopkins rigid rod nasal endoscopes. In order to obtain a high-quality photograph one needs a complete high-quality photographic system, which includes the endoscope, the camera, the light source, the light carrier, the film and the photographer. Details of the photographic system used in this section can be found in Heinz Stammberger, *Functional Endoscopic Sinus Surgery: The Messerklinger Technique* (BC Decker: Philadelphia 1991).

External nose

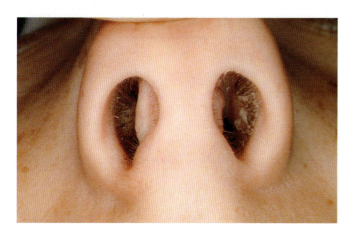

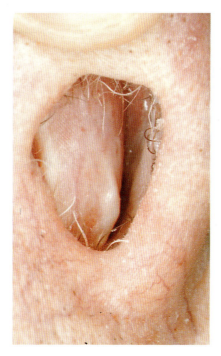

Figure 2.2

Severe caudal deviation of the nasal septum

The anterior end of the quadrilateral cartilage has deviated so extensively into this left nasal vestibule that a total nasal obstruction resulted.

Figure 2.1

Caudal deviation of the nasal septum

The anterior end of the nasal septum in this patient has become displaced from its normal position in the columella. Deviations of the anterior or caudal margin of the nasal septum are called 'caudal deviations'.

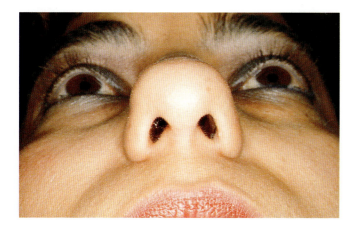

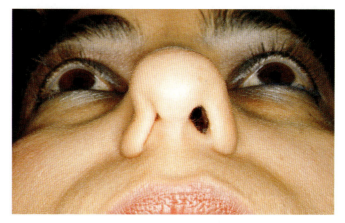

Figure 2.3

Alar collapse (during exhalation)

The alae nasi which make up the lateral walls of the nasal vestibule provide the rigid cartilaginous 'skeleton' that prevents the nasal vestibule from collapsing inwards during inspiration.

Figure 2.4

Alar collapse (during inspiration)

When the cartilaginous supporting framework within the ala nasi is weakened or deficient, the lateral wall of the nasal vestibule will be sucked inwards during nasal inspiration (alar collapse), as seen on this patient's right side.

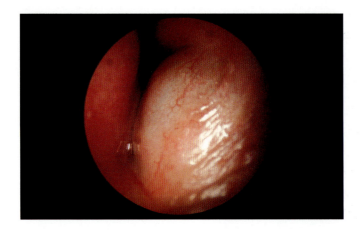

Figure 2.5

Nasoalveolar cyst (left nasal vestibule)

Nasoalveolar cysts form in the embryological line of fusion between the lateral nasal process and the maxillary process. Clinically, a nasoalveolar cyst presents as a smooth compressible swelling arising from the lateral portion of the floor of the nasal vestibule.

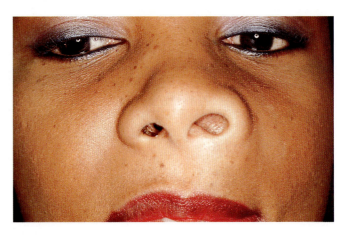

Figure 2.6

Nasoalveolar cyst

The large nasoalveolar cyst seen in this patient obstructs the nasal vestibule and displaces the left ala nasi and the nasolabial fold both laterally and anteriorly.

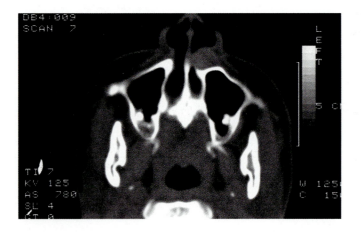

Figure 2.7

Nasoalveolar cyst

The relationship of the nasoalveolar cyst shown in Figures 2.5 and 2.6 to the ala nasi and the anterior wall of the maxilla can be seen in this coronal CT scan.

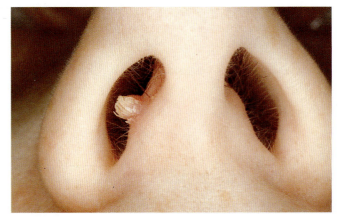

Figure 2.8

Benign squamous papilloma

Benign squamous papillomas are the most common benign tumours of the nasal vestibule. They not infrequently seed onto adjacent areas of the nasal septum, suggesting a viral aetiology.

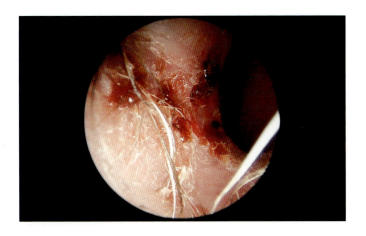

Figure 2.9
Nasal vestibulitis

Nasal vestibulitis is the term used to describe a chronic staphylococcal infection of the skin and hair follicles of the nasal vestibule. Nasal vestibulitis frequently develops as the result of local trauma to the skin of the nasal vestibule from repeated nasal picking. Yellowish crusts and scabs are usually seen starting at the base of the vibrissae and extending onto the adjacent vestibular skin and nasal mucous membranes.

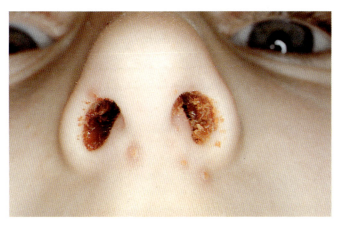

Figure 2.10
Impetigo

In impetigo contagiosa the causative organisms are usually either group A streptococci or *Staphylococcus aureus*. The thick yellowish crusts filling this right nasal vestibule and seeding onto the upper lip are characteristic of impetigo.

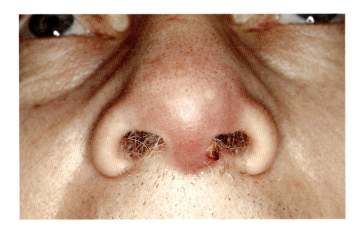

Figure 2.11
Cellulitis

The browny-red painful swelling affecting the skin over the tip of this patient's nose indicates the presence of cellulitis.

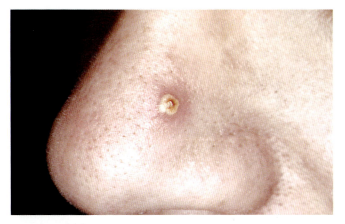

Figure 2.12
Furuncle

A furuncle is present in the skin of this patient's nose. All infections of the external nose must be treated aggressively to avoid the infection spreading to the cavernous sinus and producing a cavernous sinus thrombosis.

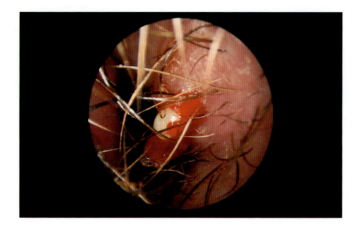

Figure 2.13

Furuncle of the nasal vestibule

A small but painful furuncle that developed at the base of a hair follicle has just been incised. Note the bead of pus draining from the tiny abscess cavity.

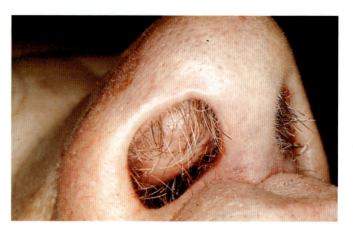

Figure 2.14

Abscess of the nasal vestibular skin

The large, tender and fluctuant swelling arising from the lateral wall of this right nasal vestibule is a nasal vestibular abscess.

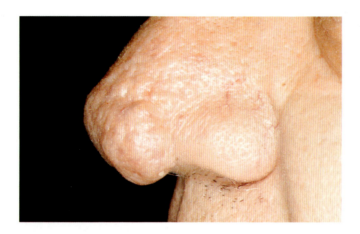

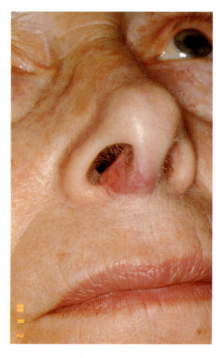

Figure 2.16

Sarcoidosis

The raised red infiltration of this patient's columella is the result of sarcoidosis.

Figure 2.15

Rhinophyma

Rhinophyma is the result of a massive hyperplasia of the sebaceous glands of the nasal skin, which is often associated with acne rosacea. The result is a thickening and coarsening of the skin covering the lower cartilaginous portion of the nose.

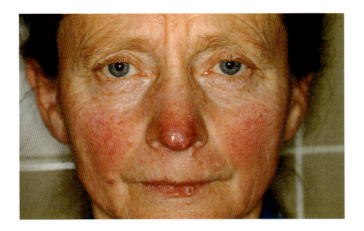

Figure 2.17

Sarcoidosis

The raised red infiltration of this nasal tip demonstrates the characteristic appearance of sarcoidosis.

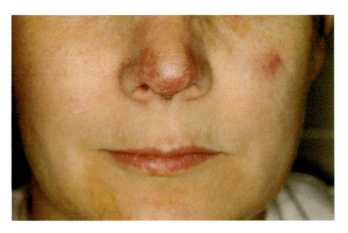

Figure 2.18

Sarcoidosis

In addition to generalized lymph node and mucosal involvement, this patient also has cutaneous sarcoidosis.

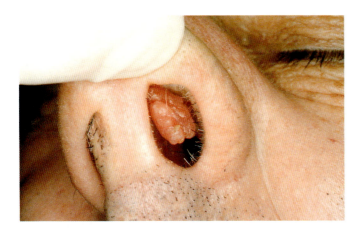

Figure 2.19

Inverting papilloma nasal vestibule

The exophytic lesion seen arising from the posterosuperior portion of this patient's left nasal vestibule is an inverting papilloma.

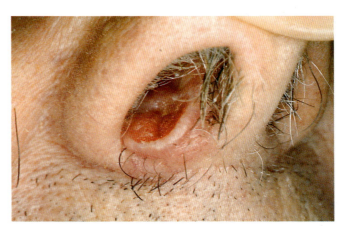

Figure 2.20

Squamous cell carcinoma of the nasal vestibule

The ulcerated 'sore' in the floor of the right nasal vestibule was initially treated as a case of nasal vestibulitis. A biopsy taken when the lesion failed to heal revealed the presence of an ulcerated squamous cell carcinoma.

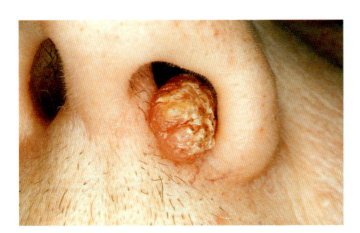

Figure 2.21

Carcinoma of the nasal vestibule

A biopsy is indicated for any persistent or non-healing cutaneous lesion. This relatively benign-appearing exophytic lesion arising from the floor of the left nasal vestibule was a well-differentiated squamous cell carcinoma.

The lateral nasal wall

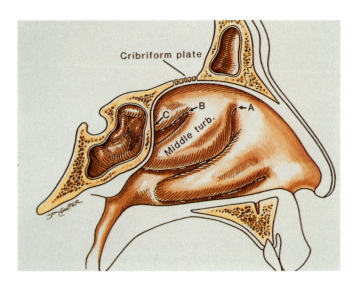

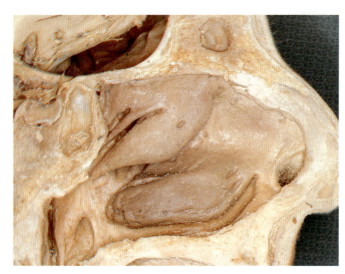

Figure 2.22

The lateral nasal wall

The nasal cavity's most important structures are situated on its lateral walls. Note the inferior turbinate, which occupies the inferior third of the lateral nasal wall. The middle turbinate and further superior subdivisions (the superior and the supreme turbinates) can be seen occupying the upper third of the lateral nasal wall. Note how the anterior end of the middle turbinate is located well behind and above the anterior end of the inferior turbinate. (Left) Diagram; (right) gross specimen.

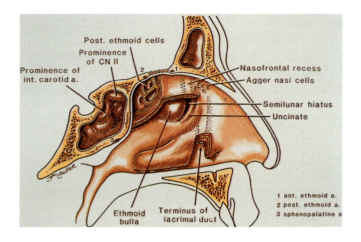

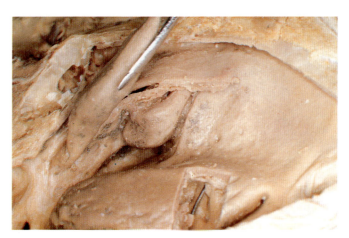

Figure 2.23

The lateral nasal wall

The key structures of the lateral nasal wall deep to the middle turbinate can be seen in these pictures. (Left) Diagram; (right) gross specimen.

Normal nasal cavity

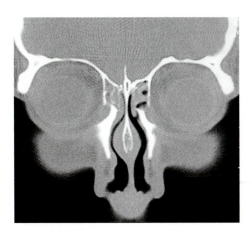

Figure 2.24

The nasal septal swell body

A discrete area of erectile tissue is present in the submucosa over the anterior cartilaginous nasal septum in some individuals. Vasodilatation of the septal swell body can be a cause of significant nasal obstruction. A septal swell body may initially be confused with a deviation of the nasal septum; however, the septal body can easily be identified by palpation, as the erectile tissue can readily be compressed, unlike the cartilage of a septal deviation.

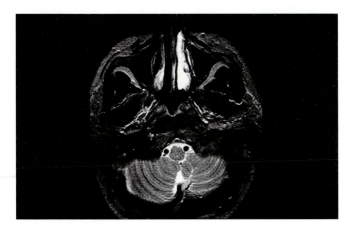

Figure 2.25

The normal nasal cycle

The state of vasodilatation (engorgement) and vasoconstriction of the erectile tissue of the inferior turbinate and of the nasal septal swell body normally alternates between the nasal cavities, i.e. as one side undergoes vasodilatation, the other becomes vasoconstricted. This is called the nasal cycle. In this T2-weighted magnetic resonance imaging (MRI) scan, note the bright areas, which represent vasodilatation of the right inferior turbinate and nasal septum.

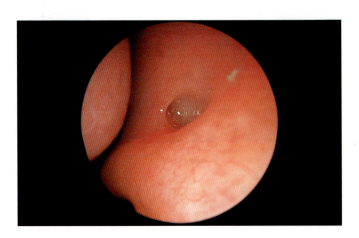

Figure 2.26

Jacobson's organ

A shallow circular pit or depression, which resembles a small ulcer or punched-out lesion, can sometimes be seen on the anterior cartilaginous nasal septum. This is Jacobson's organ, a vestigial olfactory organ that has no known function in humans. A Jacobson's organ should not be confused with a septal ulceration.

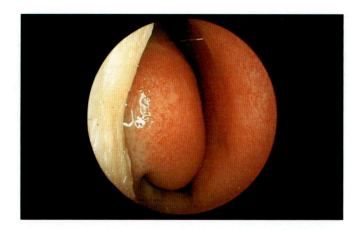

Figure 2.27
Normal inferior turbinate (right)

The inferior turbinate is the lowest and most anterior of the three scroll-shaped nasal turbinates (inferior, middle and superior). Its anterior border is the first intranasal structure encountered during a rhinoscopic examination. The submucosal layer of the inferior turbinate contains erectile tissue. The status of the nasal mucosa can be inferred from its colour. Normal nasal mucous membranes have a healthy pink colour and appear slightly moist.

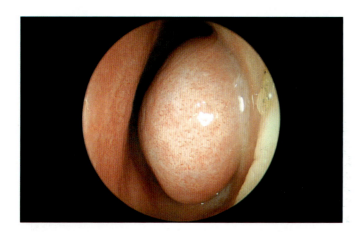

Figure 2.28
Swollen (vasodilated) inferior turbinate (left)

When the venous sinusoids within the inferior turbinate are dilated, the inferior turbinate may swell to such an extent that it comprises nasal respiration.

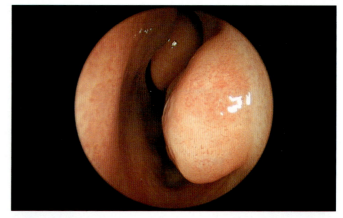

Figure 2.29
Vasoconstricted inferior turbinate (left)

A proper examination of the interior of the nose cannot generally be performed until the inferior turbinates have been vasoconstricted to allow access into the nasal cavity. Vasoconstriction can readily be achieved by the use of a topical decongestant nasal drop or spray such as 0.1% xylometazoline hydrochloride nasal solution USP. This is the same inferior turbinate seen in Figure 2.28 approximately 10 minutes later. Note that the front face of the middle turbinate can now be seen posterosuperiorly.

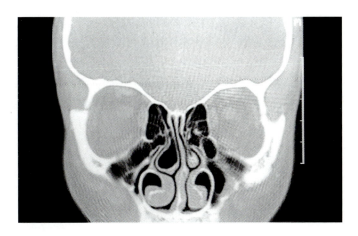

Figure 2.30

Normal vasodilatation of the inferior turbinates

The erectile tissue within the nasal cavity, which is located primarily in the inferior turbinates, is usually in a state of partial vasodilatation. Note the size of the normal inferior turbinates on this coronal CT scan. The right turbinate is grossly enlarged owing to the presence of an abnormal air cell (a concha bullosa), which compromises the left middle meatus.

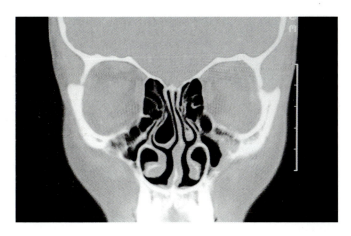

Figure 2.31

Vasoconstriction of the inferior turbinates

This is the same patient as shown in Figure 2.30 approximately 10 minutes later. Note the change in size in the inferior turbinates following the application of a topical vasoconstrictor. A large concha bullosa of the right middle turbinate and bilateral Haller's cells are also present.

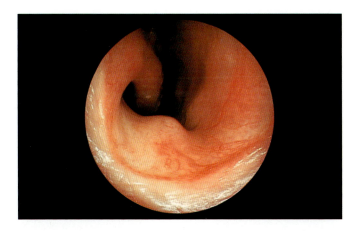

Figure 2.32

Erectile tissue on the floor of the nasal cavity (right)

Some patients have a discrete collection of erectile tissue located on the floor of the nasal cavity just behind the nasal vestibule. This area appears as a raised but compressible mound or swelling arising from the floor of the nose.

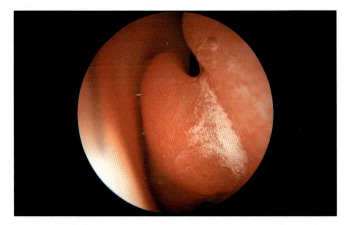

Figure 2.33

Bubbles from nasal spray

The application of a topical decongestant spray has caused the collection of frothy bubbles seen filling the left middle meatus.

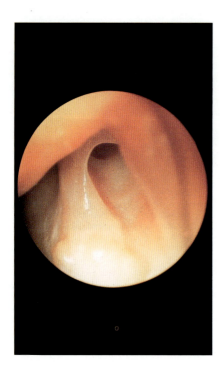

Figure 2.34
Nasolacrimal duct

The opening of the nasolacrimal duct and Hasner's valve can be clearly seen in this left inferior meatus.

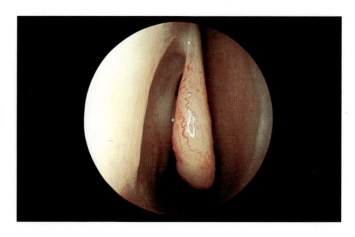

Figure 2.35
Normal right middle turbinate

The area lateral to the middle turbinate is called the middle meatus. Note the insertion of the middle turbinate (the neck of the middle turbinate) into the lateral nasal wall. A normal middle turbinate curves away from the lateral nasal wall. The raised portion of the lateral nasal wall which curves medially to join the neck of the middle turbinate is the lacrimal ridge.

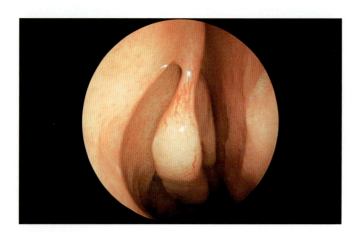

Figure 2.36
Normal right uncinate process

The curved structure that arises from the lacrimal ridge and extends posteromedially like a visor over the anterior aspect of the ethmoidal bulla is the uncinate process. The ethmoidal bulla can be seen just medial to the medial edge of the uncinate process.

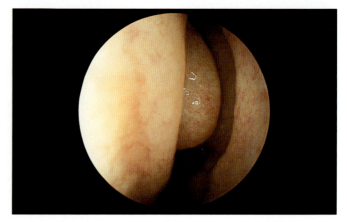

Figure 2.37
The ethmoidal bulla (right)

The anterior ethmoidal bulla arises from the lamina papyracea just behind the uncinate process. The space between the posterior free margin of the uncinate process and the anterior surface of the ethmoidal bulla is the hiatus semilunaris. In this patient the round structure seen behind the free margin of the uncinate process is a large ethmoidal bulla.

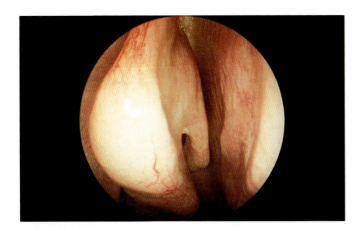

Figure 2.38

The superior turbinate and superior meatus (right)

Endoscopically, the superior turbinate appears to rise from the middle turbinate or to be a subdivision of it. From a developmental point of view, however, these are two very distinct structures connected to skull base and lamina papyracea each by their own ground lamella.

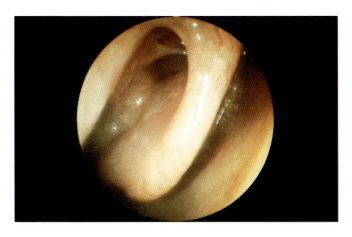

Figure 2.39

The superior meatus and sphenoethmoidal recess

A view into the superior meatus underneath a well-developed right superior turbinate. The ostia of ethmoidal clefts and cell openings can be seen in the superior meatus. The inferior border of the right superior turbinate can be seen running from 1 to 7 o'clock. The superior meatus lies lateral to the superior turbinate.

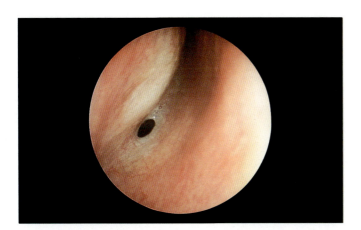

Figure 2.40

The sphenoid sinus ostium

The sphenoid sinus ostium is located in the posterosuperior portion of the nasal cavity just lateral to the insertion of the posterosuperior portion of the nasal septum into the anterior wall of the sphenoid. The right sphenoid sinus ostium can be seen between the nasal septum and the superior turbinate.

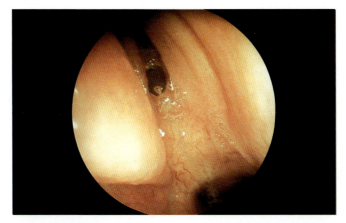

Figure 2.41

Sphenoethmoidal recess

A right sphenoethmoidal recess. Note the superior and supreme turbinates and the sphenoid sinus ostium. There is some thickened, non-purulent secretion coming from the posterior ethmoid and sphenoid sinuses.

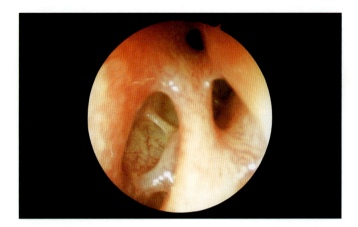

Figure 2.42

Normal frontal recess

A view into a normal left frontal recess with a 30° telescope. To the right, the lateral face of the middle turbinate is visible. The uncinate process is seen fading superiorly. Between 4 and 12 o'clock a small bony spur from the bulla reaches the skull base and fuses with the middle turbinate medially. The 'opening' at 12 o'clock opens into the frontal sinus, and the one at 2 o'clock into the lateral recess (recessus suprabullaris).

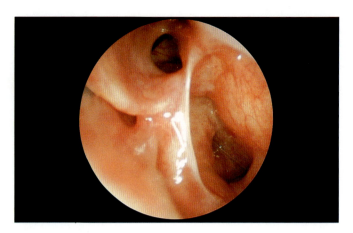

Figure 2.43

Normal postoperative frontal recess

A close-up view into the frontal recess area following endoscopic sinus surgery. The unobstructed passage into the frontal sinus can be clearly seen.

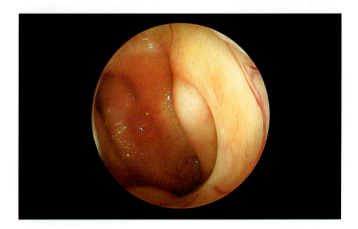

Figure 2.44

Eustachian tube (right)

The torus tubarius (Eustachian tube orifice) is formed by the medial end of the Eustachian tube, which projects into the lateral wall of the nasopharynx and consequently can only be seen by means of conventional posterior rhinoscopy (mirror examination of the nasopharynx) or, as in this case, by means of a nasal endoscope.

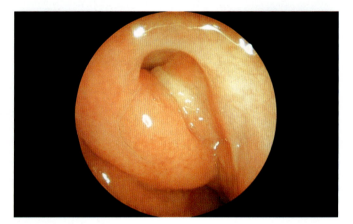

Figure 2.45

Eustachian tube orifice

The opening and closing of the torus tubarius can be observed as the patient swallows or performs a Valsalva manoeuvre.

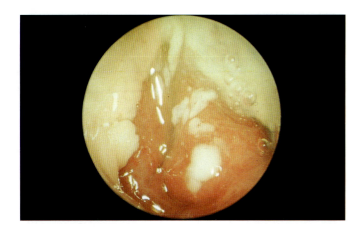

Figure 2.46

Eustachian tube ostium

A left Eustachian tube ostium seen during purulent rhinosinusitis. Note how the mucopurulent secretions are transported not only medially and laterally to the Eustachian tube, but also directly over the tubal ostium. The resultant inflammation and swelling of the torus may cause malventilation of the middle ear and a secondary otitis media.

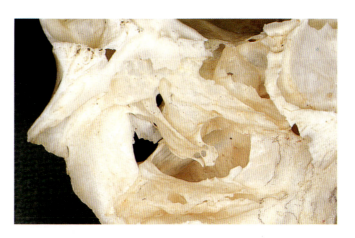

Figure 2.47

Nasal fontanelles

There are usually defects in the bony lateral wall of the nose located between the uncinate process and the inferior turbinate that in life are covered with a dense connective tissue that is a continuation of the periosteum. These defects in the bony skeleton of the medial wall of the maxillary sinus are the anterior and the posterior nasal fontanelles.

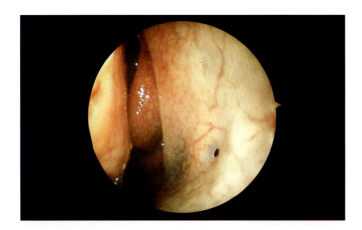

Figure 2.48

Accessory maxillary sinus ostium

Accessory maxillary sinus ostia located in the anterior or posterior nasal fontanelles are not infrequently seen in the middle meatus. A small accessory ostium is present in the anterior nasal fontanelle on the left side. The uncinate process is bent medially.

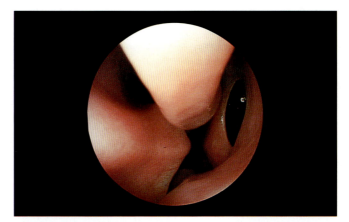

Figure 2.49

Accessory maxillary sinus ostium

A large accessory ostium is present through the posterior fontanelle of this left side. Note the prominent nasal septal spur protruding into the middle meatus and abutting against the inferior surface of the left middle turbinate.

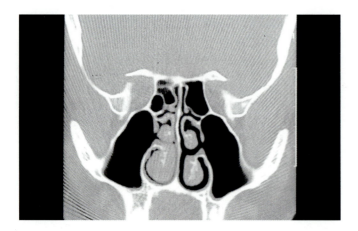

Figure 2.50
Accessory maxillary sinus ostium

The direct connection between the left maxillary sinus and the left middle meatus, seen on this coronal CT scan, is an accessory maxillary sinus ostium in the posterior fontanelle.

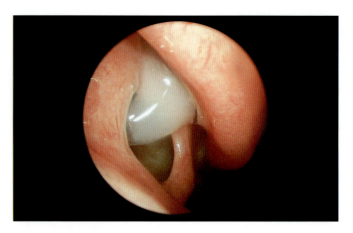

Figure 2.51
Accessory maxillary sinus ostium

Mucus may circulate back into a maxillary sinus via an accessory ostium as seen here. Note the thick white stream of mucus flowing down from the hiatus semilunaris and re-entering this right maxillary sinus through a large accessory maxillary sinus ostium located in the anterior nasal fontanelle.

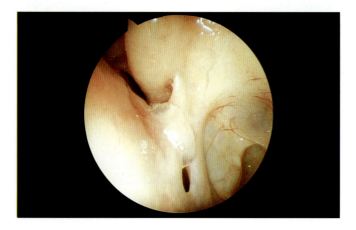

Figure 2.52
Accessory maxillary sinus ostium

Maxillary sinoscopy via the left canina fossa. There is an accessory ostium in the posterior fontanelle. Thick mucus can be seen being transported into the maxillary sinus through the accessory ostium from the nasal cavity. Transport continues within the maxillary sinus towards the natural ostium and the infundibulum (10–11 o'clock). The outward bound mucus is then transported back into the sinus via the accessory ostium and thereby recirculates.

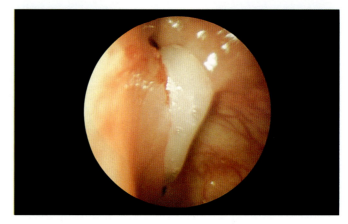

Figure 2.53
Accessory maxillary sinus ostium

Maxillary sinoscopy. Mucopus enters this maxillary sinus through an accessory ostium in the posterior fontanelle and leaves again via the natural ostium to recirculate. Note the slight oedematous inflammatory changes of the mucosa in the vicinity of the ostium. If the natural ostium or the infundibulum become blocked, this mechanism may lead to 'maxillary' sinusitis. The pathogens reaching the sinuses from the nasal cavity thereby indicate the rhinogenic nature of this disease.

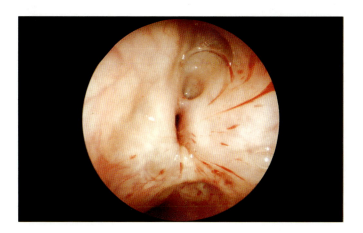

Figure 2.54

Maxillary sinus ostium

The natural ostium of the maxillary sinus is hidden behind the posterior and inferior portion of the uncinate process and cannot be seen during a routine diagnostic endoscopic examination. The medial surface of the maxillary ostium can be seen by maxillary sinoscopy. The star-like secretion routes are outlined by traces of blood staining the mucus on its way towards the ostium.

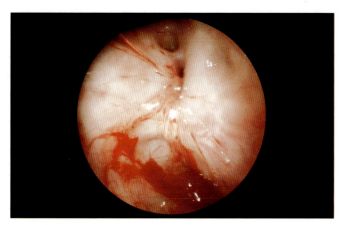

Figure 2.55

Maxillary sinus ostium

Note the mucociliary transport routes from the floor towards the natural ostium of this right maxillary sinus.

Nasal foreign bodies

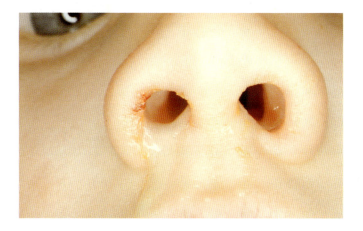

Figure 2.56

Foreign body

The presence of a persistent, unilateral, foul-smelling nasal discharge in a child often indicates the presence of a foreign body.

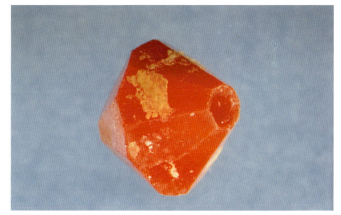

Figure 2.57

Foreign body

An inert foreign body such as this red plastic bead may remain inside the nasal cavity for a prolonged period of time without causing any symptoms.

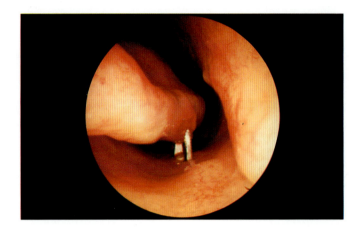

Figure 2.58

Foreign body nasal cavity

The metal 'roots' of a dental implant have perforated the hard palate and pierced into the inferior right turbinate. The patient complained of offensive smell and crusting.

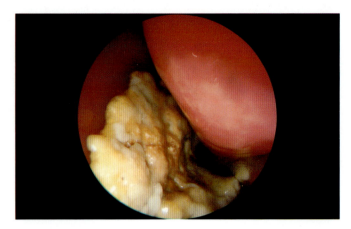

Figure 2.59

Rhinolith (left)

If an inert foreign body remains within the nasal cavity for many years it may become surrounded by a calcified coating. Such a 'nasal stone' is termed a rhinolith. Rhinoliths have a whitish-grey colour, and are hard and gritty to palpation.

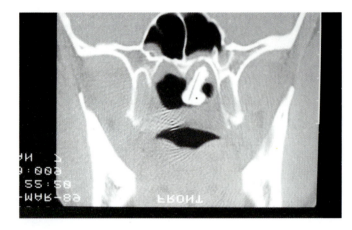

Figure 2.60

Rhinolith

Rhinoliths are radio-opaque and can be clearly seen on a CT scan. The radiolucent slit seen inside this large rhinolith identifies the location of the foreign body, which in this case was a plastic tiddlywink.

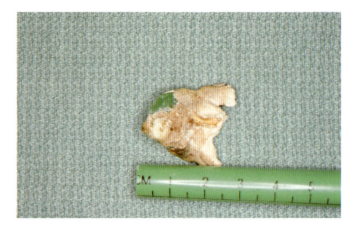

Figure 2.61

Rhinolith

Rhinoliths may 'grow' to a very large size. This was the rhinolith removed from the patient shown in Figures 2.59 and 2.60. Note the plastic tiddlywink, which was the nidus around which the rhinolith formed.

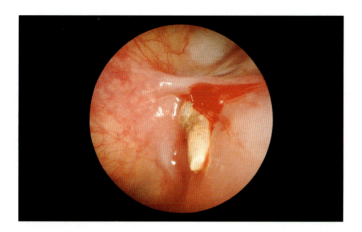

Figure 2.62

Foreign body in the maxillary sinus

Maxillary sinoscopy. A foreign body (aberrant dental filling material) has become impacted in the natural ostium of the maxillary sinus on the left.

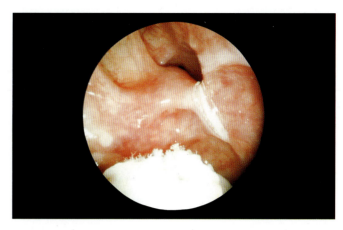

Figure 2.63

Maxillary sinus fungus ball

A fungus ball (non-invasive *Aspergillus fumigatus*) was encountered on the floor of this sinus at maxillary sinoscopy. Clearly visible are fungal spores mixed in the mucopus, which is being transported out of the sinus by the wide and patent natural maxillary sinus ostium.

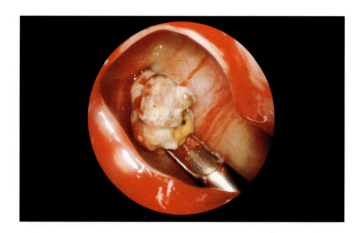

Figure 2.64

Maxillary sinus fungus ball

During endoscopic removal, a good view is achieved into this left maxillary sinus via the middle meatus. The trocar, which was inserted through the canina fossa, is used to help 'shovel' the fungal masses towards the enlarged natural ostium. All of the fungal masses were removed by this approach.

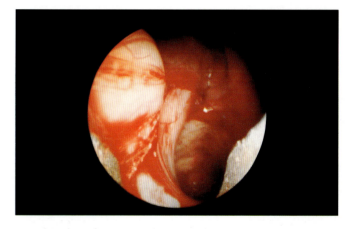

Figure 2.65

Maxillary sinus cyst

Maxillary sinoscopy on the left. There is a cyst over the lacrimal eminentia in the medial wall of the maxillary sinus. Mucus is transported over this small cyst without any difficulty toward the natural ostium.

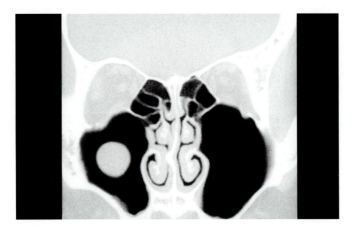

Figure 2.66

Maxillary sinus cyst

The round 'moon-like' structure seen in the centre of this right maxillary sinus was a simple cyst, which was filled with a clear golden-yellow watery fluid.

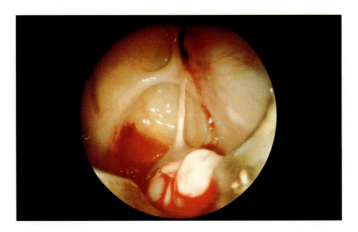

Figure 2.67

Maxillary sinoscopy

Maxillary sinoscopy (right side). A cystic polyp has been punctured with the insertion of the trocar. The stalk of the polyp can be seen hanging from the natural maxillary sinus ostium and the adjacent ethmoidal infundibulum, indicating its origin from this area.

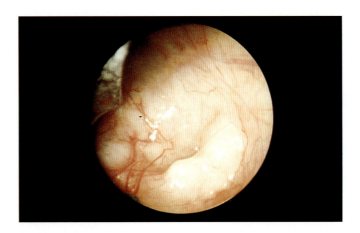

Figure 2.68

Dental roots

Left maxillary sinus view laterally and inferiorly onto the alveolar recess. The bulging of dental roots can be seen covered by thin mucosa.

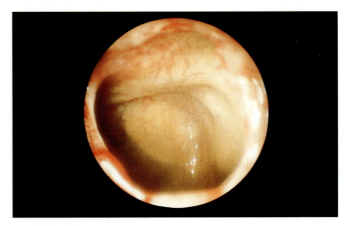

Figure 2.69

Course of infraorbital nerve in the maxillary sinus

A view into a left maxillary sinus through a large ostium in the middle meatus following previous ethmoid surgery. The course of the infraorbital nerve over the roof of the maxillary sinus can be seen. The mucosal lining of the sinus is normal.

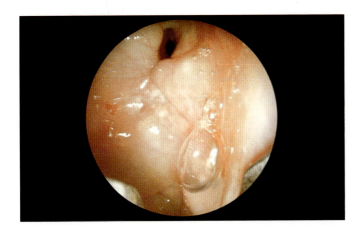

Figure 2.70

Kartagener's syndrome

Maxillary sinoscopy on the right. Despite a wide and unobstructed ostium, thick glassy mucus cannot leave the ostium apparently because of ciliary insufficiency. This patient had Kartagener's syndrome.

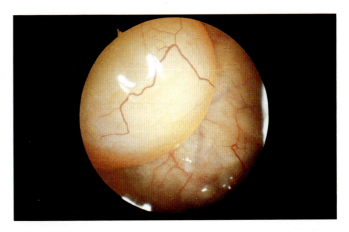

Figure 2.71

Maxillary sinus cyst

Maxillary sinoscopy. A large cyst can be seen arising from the roof of the maxillary sinus. The cyst was sitting on a dehiscent infraorbital nerve and caused midfacial pain.

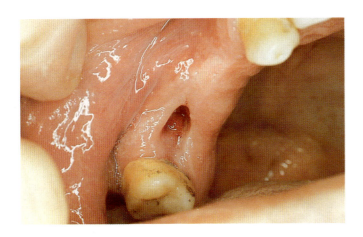

Figure 2.72

Oroantral fistula

This oroantral fistula seen from below was the cause of chronic suppurative maxillary sinusitis.

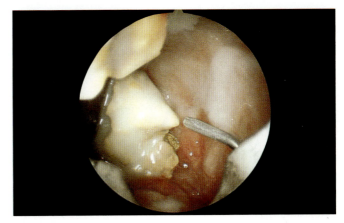

Figure 2.73

Oroantral fistula

Maxillary sinoscopy on the left. Following tooth extraction an oroantral fistula had developed that did not close spontaneously. The patient only visited the doctor weeks later, when an *Aspergillus* mycosis of the sinus had developed. The trocar sheath is visible at 7 and 5 o'clock; a probe is inserted through the fistula transorally. Note the pus-covered fungal concretions.

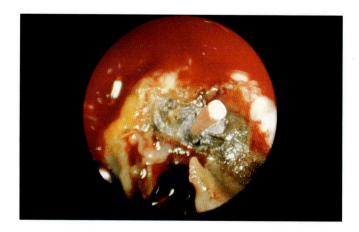

Figure 2.74

Maxillary *Aspergillus* mycosis

Maxillary *Aspergillus* mycosis following the extrusion of Gutta-percha dental root filling material into the sinus. The Gutta-percha stent placed into one root canal has pierced into the maxillary sinus and acted as a point of crystallization for the mycotic masses.

Rhinitis

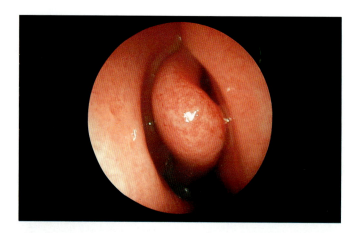

Figure 2.75

Acute viral rhinitis (URI)

During the prodromal phase of an acute upper respiratory infection (URI or coryza) the mucous membranes lining the nasal cavity are reddened, the nose is often abnormally patent, and the mucus is frequently scant and stringy in appearance. At this stage the patient usually complains of an itching or burning inside the nose. Shortly after, the mucosa becomes engorged and there is an outpouring of clear watery mucus.

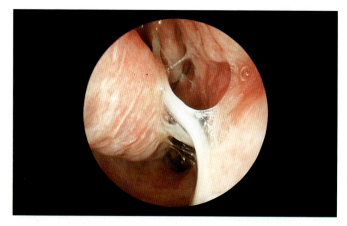

Figure 2.76

Acute viral rhinitis (URI)

If a bacterial superinfection develops, the mucus increases in amount and becomes coloured. As the acute phase resolves, the mucosa gradually returns to normal, although for a time there is still an overproduction of mucus, which at this stage is often abnormally viscid.

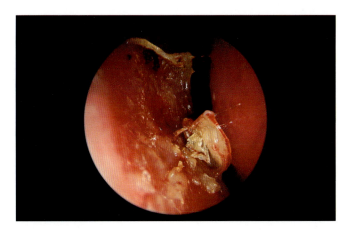

Figure 2.77

Chronic bacterial rhinitis

The mucosa of the nasal cavity may become chronically infected and colonized by bacteria. Note the yellow dry patches of exudate. A swab taken for culture and sensitivity is often of value.

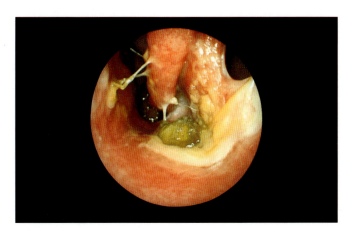

Figure 2.78

Chronic bacterial rhinitis

The thick yellow crust covering the floor of this left nasal cavity overlies an area of local bacterial rhinitis caused by *Pseudomonas aeruginosa*. Note the inferior meatal antrostomy.

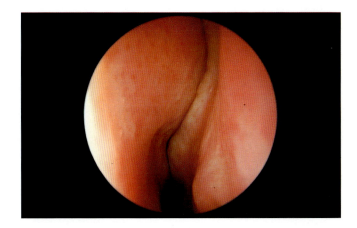

Figure 2.79

Rhinitis medicamentosa

The chronic use of topical nasal decongestants produces a state of chronic rhinitis, which is known as rhinitis medicamentosa. Topical vasoconstrictors cause such severe constriction of the blood vessels of the nasal mucosa that ischaemic mucosal damage develops. Consequently, when the vasoconstrictor's effect wears off, the nasal mucosa 'rebounds' becoming reddened and oedematous. The patient then experiences increased nasal obstruction and reapplies the decongestant thereby establishing a vicious cycle. On examination, the nasal mucous membranes are usually fiery-red and swollen. The history of topical decongestant abuse is usually freely given.

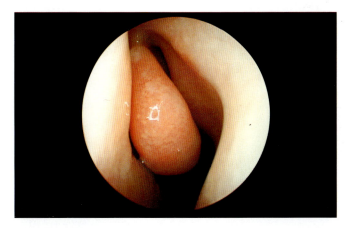

Figure 2.80

Vasomotor rhinitis

Vasomotor rhinitis is a common cause of chronic nasal congestion and rhinorrhoea, which is currently believed to be caused by an imbalance in the autonomic nerve supply to the nasal mucous membranes. Vasomotor rhinitis is characterized by chronic nasal congestion with engorgement of the inferior turbinates and by a troublesome profuse, clear and watery rhinorrhoea.

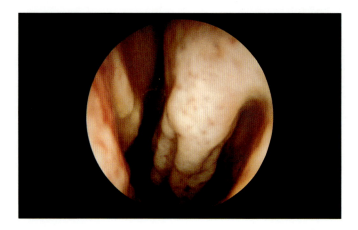

Figure 2.81

Post-laryngectomy atrophy

Following a laryngectomy, there is no longer any flow of air through the nasal cavity, and the mucosa atrophies and develops a pale purple discolouration. Note the characteristic shrunken appearance of the inferior turbinate in this patient's left nasal cavity.

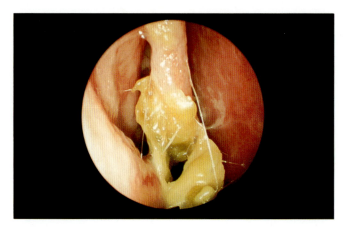

Figure 2.82

Atrophic rhinitis (ozena)

Atrophic rhinitis is an idiopathic, chronic degenerative disorder that affects both the nasal mucous membranes and the turbinates. The turbinates atrophy and the nasal cavities become abnormally patent. Atrophic rhinitis is characterized by the accumulation of large greenish-yellow crusts, as seen in this right nasal cavity, and severe fetor. Fortunately most of these patients are anosmic.

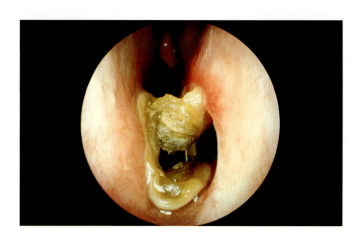

Figure 2.83

Atrophic rhinitis (ozena)

This patient has iatrogenic atrophic rhinitis, which developed following excessive electrocautery to the left interior turbinate.

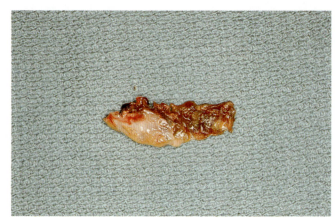

Figure 2.84

Atrophic rhinitis (ozena)

This large yellowish-green crust was removed from the nasal cavity of the previous patient. These foul-smelling crusts result from the associated acquired atrophy of the cilia, which prevents the mucous blanket from being carried normally into the nasopharynx. The stagnant infected mucus gradually dries into the crust.

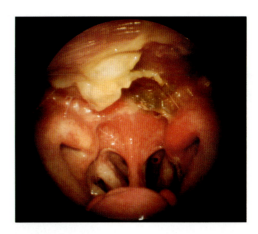

Figure 2.85

Atrophic rhinitis (ozena)

An endoscopic view of the nasopharynx of a female patient aged 44 years who presented with complaints of a stuffy nose and post-nasal drip. These symptoms were caused by an atrophic rhinopharyngitis.

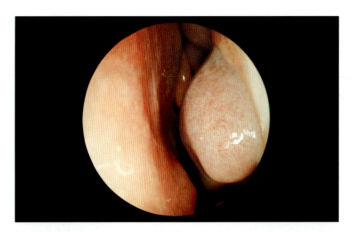

Figure 2.86

Allergic rhinitis

Because one of the main functions of the nose is the trapping and removal of particulate matter, it is not surprising that many individuals develop allergies to a variety of inspired substances. The allergic response within the nose results in a triad of symptoms: paroxysmal sneezing, nasal obstruction and a watery rhinorrhoea. This swollen bluish left inferior turbinate is pathognomonic for allergic rhinitis.

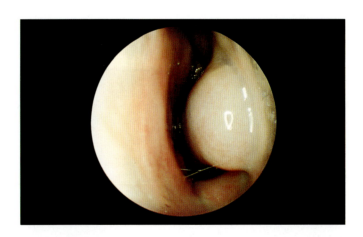

Figure 2.87

Allergic discolouration of the nasal mucous membranes

The nasal mucous membranes in patients with allergic rhinitis often have a pale blue, purple or even whitish colouration as seen in this swollen left inferior turbinate. Note the clear thin watery discharge.

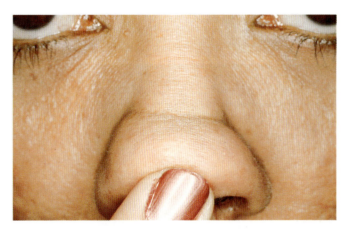

Figure 2.88

The allergic crease

The tendency of allergic individuals to rub their itchy nose repeatedly during childhood may produce a permanent horizontal skin crease above the bip of the nose. This has been called the 'allergic crease'.

Granulomatous diseases

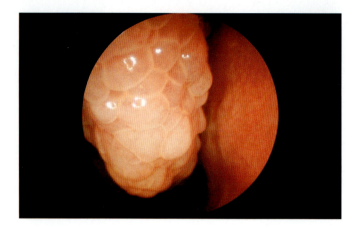

Figure 2.89

Tuberculosis of the inferior turbinate

The right inferior turbinate in a patient with open pulmonary tuberculosis.

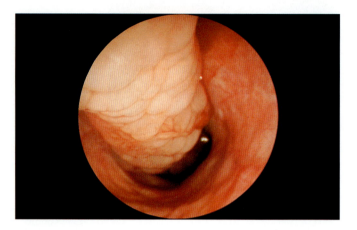

Figure 2.90

Sarcoidosis

Inferior turbinate in a case of sarcoidosis.

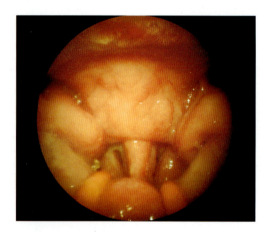

Figure 2.91

Sarcoidosis

Sarcoidosis in the roof of the nasopharynx in a 28-year-old woman.

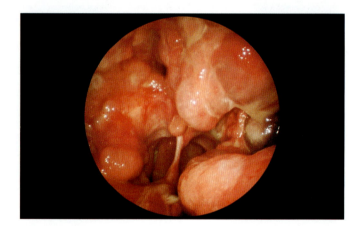

Figure 2.92

Wegener's granuloma

In this patient with extensive Wegener's granuloma, the nasal septum has been destroyed except for a small rim of the vomer.

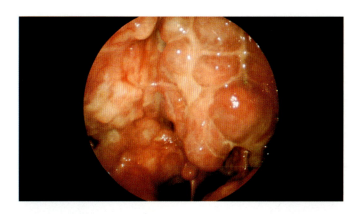

Figure 2.93
Wegener's disease

The late stage of Wegener's disease. Only posterior remnants of the nasal septum are visible. No other anatomical landmarks can be identified in the nasal cavity.

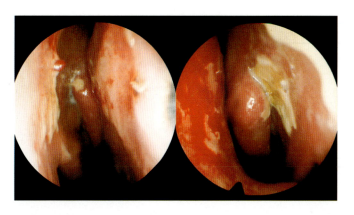

Figure 2.94
Pseudomembranous pemphigoid

This 78-year-old man with pseudomembranous pemphigoid presented with recurrent epistaxis.

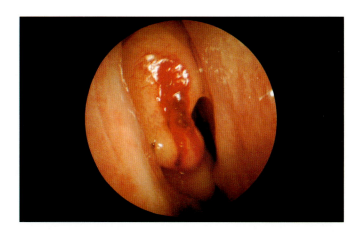

Figure 2.95
Endometriosis

This 51-year-old woman has a small patch of ectopic endometriosis in the head of the right inferior turbinate. Her menses were invariably preceded by a minor nose bleed by 1 day.

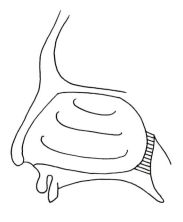

Figure 2.96
Choanal atresia

Choanal atresia is caused by a bony or membranous congenital occlusion of the posterior nasal opening: the choana. Bilateral choanal atresia is a severe and potentially life-threatening emergency in the newborn, as the newborn infant is an obligate nasal breather and cannot breath with the mouth closed.

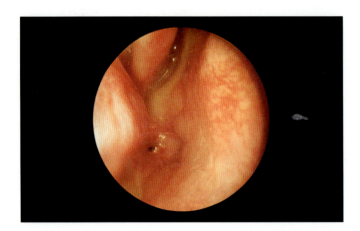

Figure 2.97

Choanal atresia

Choanal atresia in a neonate. The atresia plate on the right side has just been perforated (a 2.7 mm 0° telescope was used).

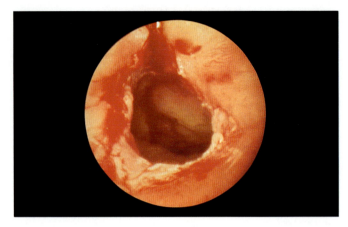

Figure 2.98

Choanal atresia

The situation after the opening in the atresia plate has been enlarged.

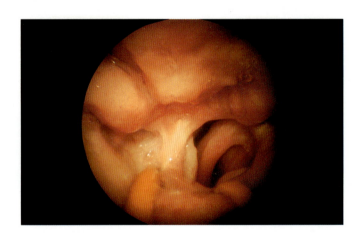

Figure 2.99

Unilateral choanal atresia

This patient has a unilateral choanal atresia.

Nasopharynx

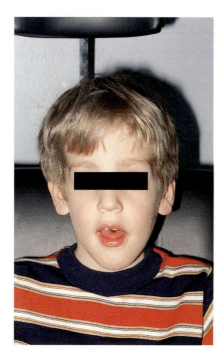

Figure 2.100
Adenoid facies

Hypertrophy of the nasopharyngeal pad of lymphoid tissue (the adenoids) is the most common cause of nasal obstruction in children. The most common presenting symptoms are chronic mouth breathing and snoring. The most dangerous symptom is sleep apnoea. Persistent mouth breathing due to nasal obstruction in childhood may result in the 'long face syndrome' (previously called 'adenoid facies').

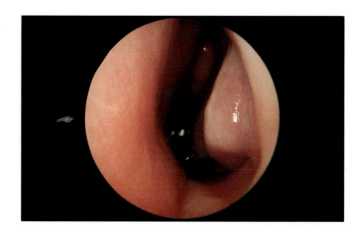

Figure 2.101
Anterior nasal mucosal changes secondary to nasopharyngeal obstruction from enlarged adenoids

When the air flow through the nasal cavity ceases as a result of enlarged adenoids, a characteristic secondary change in the mucosa of the anterior nasal cavity may be observed. This change consists of a state of vasoconstricton and purple discolouration of the mucosa of the anterior portion of the inferior turbinates. These changes result in a wider than normal anterior air space and pale-purple small inferior turbinates. Such changes should not be misinterpreted as an allergic rhinitis.

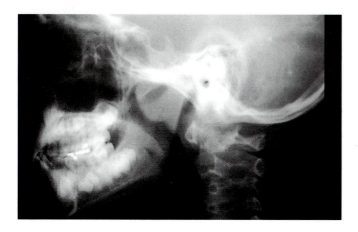

Figure 2.102
Adenoid hypertrophy (lateral radiograph)

Enlarged adenoids are not easily identified on physical examination. A lateral radiograph of the nasopharynx provides a simple and cost-effective method for assessing the size of the adenoids and the amount of post-nasal air space remaining.

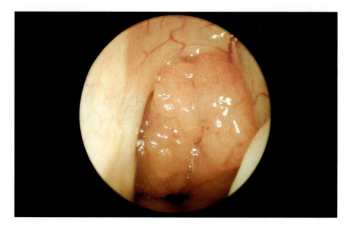

Figure 2.103
Adenoid hypertrophy (endoscopic view)

Enlarged adenoids extending anteriorly into and obstructing the left posterior choana are clearly seen on this endoscopic photograph of a 32-year-old man. While the adenoid tonsil usually undergoes spontaneous involution around puberty, the hypertrophy may persist into adult life. Adenoid hypertrophy in adults may be associated with HIV positivity.

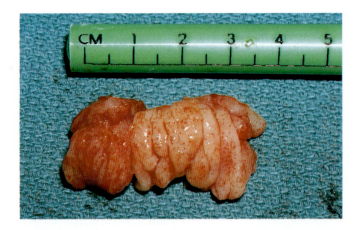

Figure 2.104

Adenoids (surgical specimen)

When obstruction of the nasopharynx causes total nasal obstruction, snoring, recurrent otitis media, secondary dental problems or sleep apnoea, then adenoidectomy is indicated. This huge adenoid tonsil was removed from the nasopharynx of a 6-year-old child.

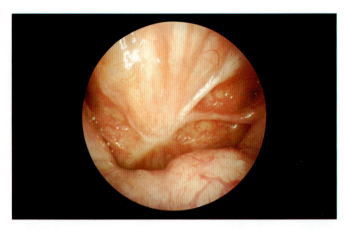

Figure 2.105

Post-adenoidectomy scarring of the nasopharynx

These fibrous bands and scars are the result of a previous adenoidectomy.

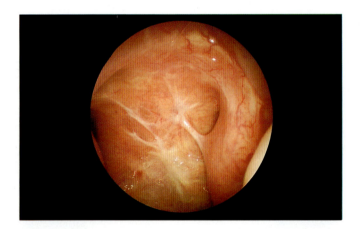

Figure 2.106

Post-adenoidectomy scarring of the nasopharynx causing autophonia

The fibrous band of scar tissue that has tethered this left Eustachian tube cushion to the posterior nasopharynx kept the torus in an 'open' position, producing a patulous Eustachian tube and autophonia. Endoscopic division of the band cured the autophonia.

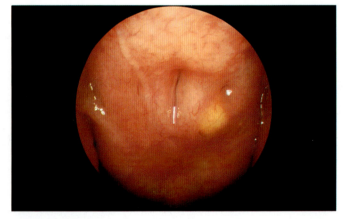

Figure 2.107

Tornwaldt's bursa

A small midline pit or opening may be seen in the posterior nasopharyngeal wall. This represents the opening of a Tornwaldt's bursa.

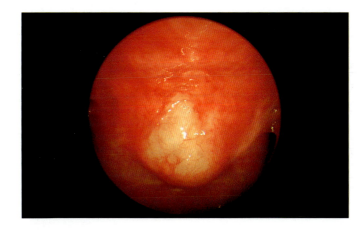

Figure 2.108

Tornwaldt's cyst

If the opening of a Tornwaldt's bursa becomes occluded, a midline cyst may develop; this is a Tornwaldt's cyst.

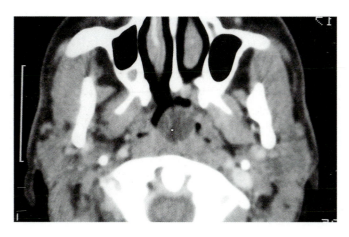

Figure 2.109

Tornwaldt's cyst

This axial CT scan demonstrates the presence of a midline cyst in the nasopharynx.

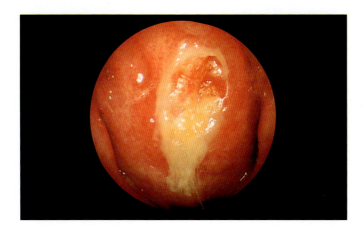

Figure 2.110

Chronic nasopharyngitis

Chronic mucosal infection of the nasopharynx is uncommon. The yellowish crust and central area of infection in the nasopharynx of this patient suggests the presence of an area of 'chronic adenoiditis', which in some cases is due to a focus of infection in a Tornwaldt's bursa.

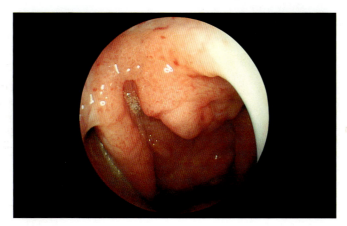

Figure 2.111

Carcinoma of the nasopharynx

This 48-year-old man presented with a history of blood-tinged nasal mucus. The area of 'adenoid tissue' in the vault of the left nasopharynx was proven to be a carcinoma of the nasopharynx by biopsy.

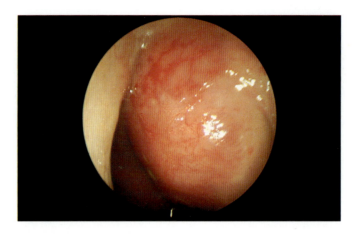

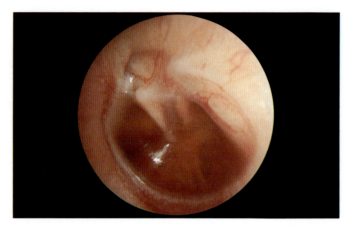

Figure 2.112

Carcinoma of the nasopharynx

This 40-year-old Chinese man presented with a persistent serous effusion in the left ear (right). The torus tubarius is grossly swollen by submucosal carcinoma.

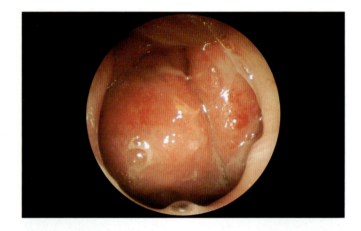

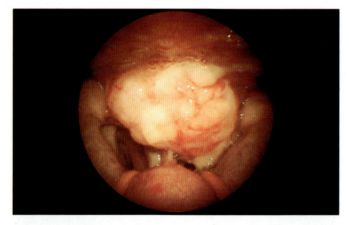

Figure 2.113

Carcinoma of the nasopharynx

Transnasal view onto the choana on the left side, displaying a large nasopharyngeal carcinoma.

Figure 2.114

Carcinoma of the nasopharynx

This large squamous cell carcinoma of the nasopharynx caused a unilateral conductive hearing loss in this 64-year-old man.

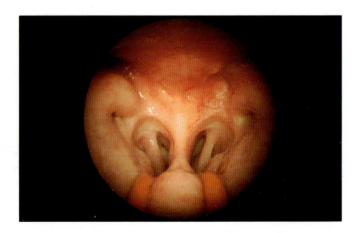

Figure 2.115

Carcinoma of the nasopharynx

This 55-year-old man presented with grossly enlarged cervical lymph nodes. The cervical lymphadenopathy was caused by the very small primary squamous cell carcinoma seen in the nasopharynx.

Nasal septum

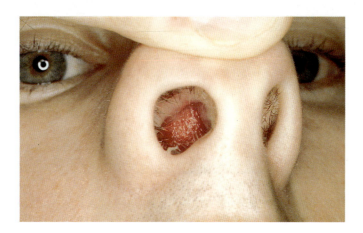

Figure 2.116
Nasal septal haematoma

Subperichondrial bleeding following trauma to the nose may produce a collection of blood between the perichondrium and the underlying cartilage of the nasal septum. The nose is characteristically blocked and tender to palpation, especially when the nasal tip is elevated. Prompt surgical drainage is required, because if the haematoma persists or becomes infected, the cartilage will become necrotic and the support provided by the anterior septal cartilage of the nose will be lost.

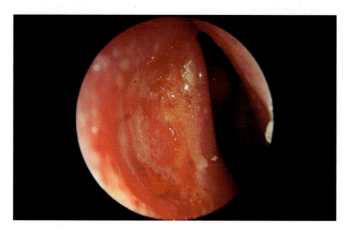

Figure 2.117
Nasal septal ulceration

The mucosa of the nasal septum may become ulcerated, most commonly from repeated local trauma (usually finger picking). The result is a localized ulceration of the mucosal surface which may ultimately spread to involve the underlying perichondrium resulting in a perforation through the nasal septum.

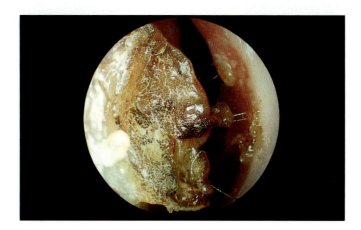

Figure 2.118
Nasal septal ulceration and crusting

Exudate from the ulcerated mucosa may accumulate over the site of the ulceration to form yellow-green crust as seen on this left nasal septum.

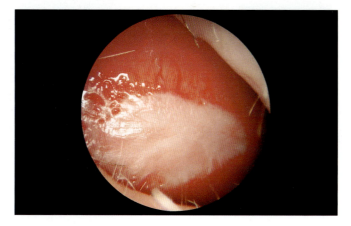

Figure 2.119
Hyperkeratosis of the nasal septum

Chronic local trauma to the anterior nasal septum from picking has caused the mucosa to undergo squamous metaplasia producing a thickened white hyperkeratotic area.

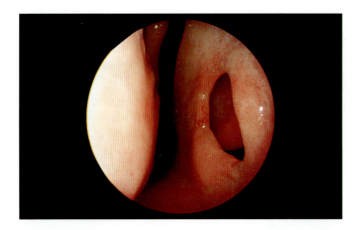

Figure 2.120

Nasal septal perforation

Perforations of the nasal septum may occur from a variety of causes. The most common cause is previous septal surgery. Other causes include nose picking, repeated cauterization of the nasal septum for epistaxis, exposure to industrial chemicals such as chromium, repeated cocaine abuse, nasal granulomas, and as a result of chronic infections such as syphilis or tuberculosis. Smaller septal perforations are usually asymptomatic, although they are more likely to produce a whistling noise during nasal respiration.

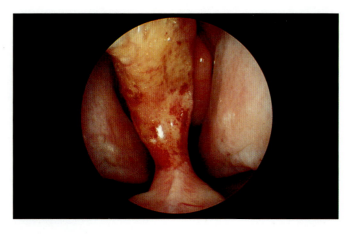

Figure 2.121

Large nasal septal perforation

Large septal perforations often produce a sensation of nasal stuffiness which is probably due to air flow disturbance. The drying effect of the inspired air on the posterior margin of the perforation frequently causes crust formation, and epistaxis as the crusts separate. The mucosa of the margins of the perforation frequently undergo squamous metaplasia and thus appear clinically to be hyperkeratotic.

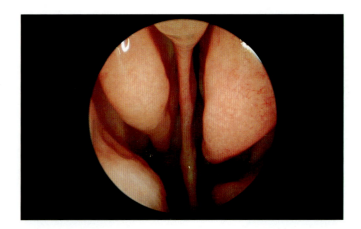

Figure 2.122

Subtotal nasal septal perforation

This patient has a huge nasal septal perforation involving most of the nasal septum. Both sides of the nose can be seen on either side of the posterior remnant of the nasal septum. The spontaneous development of a nasal septal perforation should always raise the possibility of one of the two potentially fatal non-healing granulomas of unknown origin that may occur in the nasal cavity: Wegener's granulomatosis and Stuart's malignant non-healing granuloma.

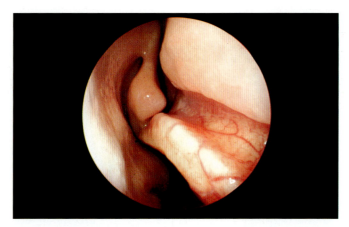

Figure 2.123

Deviated nasal septum

While the 'ideal' nasal septum is located in the midline of the nasal cavity, most normal nasal septa deviate to a slight extent from the midline. Such minimal deviations do not interfere with airflow through the nose and should not be considered abnormal. Nasal septal deviations that are severe enough to affect nasal airflow are relatively common and usually involve the anterior half of the nasal septum.

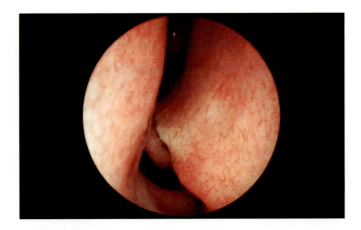

Figure 2.124

Severely deviated nasal septum

This patient's quadrilateral cartilage has deviated into the right nasal fossa to such an extent that nasal respiration has become severely limited. Any additional mucosal swelling (e.g. from allergic rhinitis or from an upper respiratory infection) will totally block the left nasal cavity.

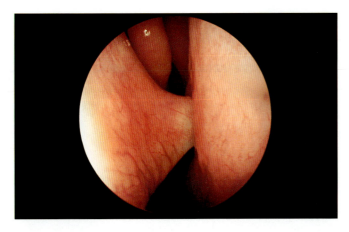

Figure 2.125

Nasal septal spur

In this patient, probably as the result of a local growth disorder, the vomer has developed a spur, which presses into the left inferior turbinate and which was responsible for recurrent unilateral headaches.

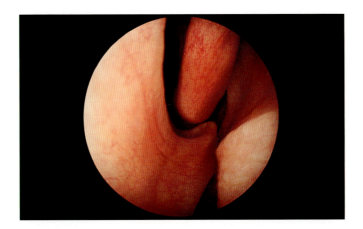

Figure 2.126

Nasal septal spur

Note the large vomerine spur that projects into the left middle meatus and impinges against the lower portion of the uncinate process.

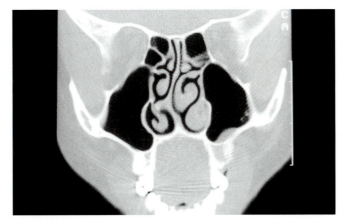

Figure 2.127

Nasal septal spur

This CT scan shows a large septal spur abutting against the right inferior turbinate.

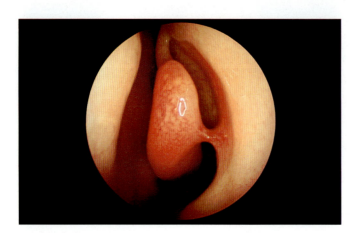

Figure 2.128

Synechiae

Synechiae are red or pale-pink fibrous adhesions that usually run across the nasal cavity between the nasal septum and the inferior turbinate. Synechiae develop following an injury that creates opposing raw surfaces on the lateral nasal wall and the nasal septum. The tiny synechia running between this left middle turbinate and the lacrimal ridge is of no clinical significance.

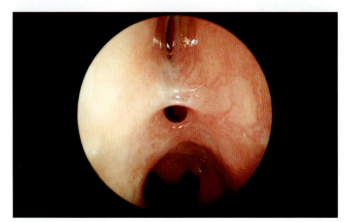

Figure 2.129

Postoperative synechiae

While most synechiae are small and asymptomatic, on some occasions synechiae may be large enough to interfere with nasal respiration. Note the extensive synechiae between the septum and the right lateral nasal wall that developed after endonasal surgery.

Lateral nasal wall

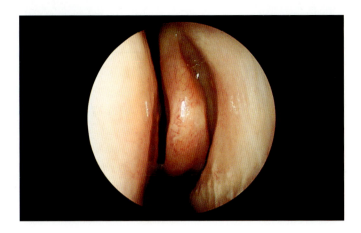

Figure 2.130
Elongated middle turbinate

The inferior border of a normal middle turbinate stops well above the insertion of the inferior turbinate into the lateral nasal wall. The inferior border of an elongated middle turbinate extends up to or overlaps the insertion of the inferior turbinate.

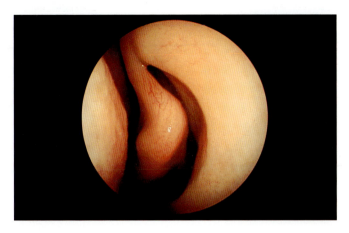

Figure 2.131
Paradoxically curved middle turbinate

A normal middle turbinate curves away from the lateral nasal wall, i.e. the concavity of the middle turbinate is directed laterally. This results in a wide middle meatus. The concavity of a paradoxically bent middle turbinate is directed medially, with the convexity of the middle turbinate curving into the lateral nasal wall, thereby narrowing the middle meatus.

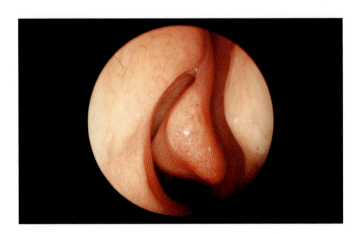

Figure 2.132
Paradoxically bent concha bullosa

Note how the convexity of this widened right middle turbinate curves paradoxically into the lateral nasal wall. A CT scan revealed that this was a paradoxically bent concha bullosa.

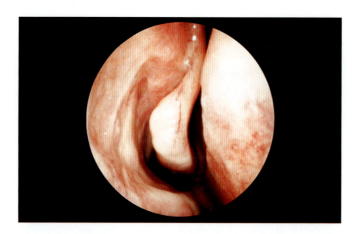
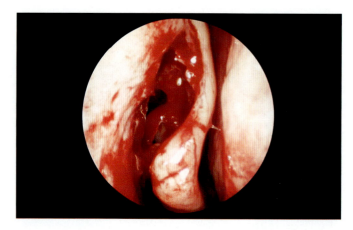

Figure 2.133
Paradoxically curved middle turbinate

If a paradoxically curved middle turbinate is associated with anterior ethmoidal pathology (left), then the ethmoid usually can be approached endoscopically by resecting the uncinate process without harming the middle turbinate, as seen in the photograph on the right.

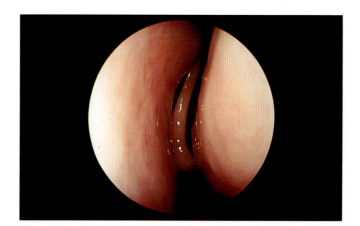
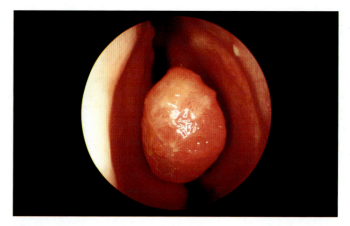

Figure 2.134
Lateralized middle turbinate

The middle turbinate may lateralize or collapse laterally. In this case, an atrophic right middle turbinate appears to have been 'pushed' laterally by a deviated nasal septum. The middle turbinate has lateralized to such an extent that the entrance to the middle meatus is closed off.

Figure 2.135
Anterior extending middle turbinate

The anterior face of the middle turbinate usually extends about 1 cm or less anterior to the point at which the turbinate inserts into the lateral nasal wall. In this patient, the head of the left middle turbinate extends anteriorly almost into the nasal vestibule.

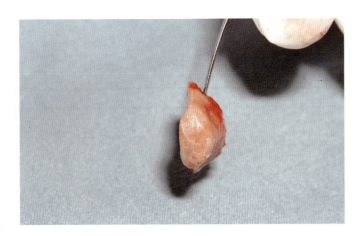

Figure 2.136
Anterior extending middle turbinate

The anterior end of the left middle turbinate shown in Figure 2.135 was resected because it was causing significant obstruction to nasal respiration. The anterior face of the turbinate is seen on the left. The probe points to the level at which the turbinate inserted into the lateral nasal wall.

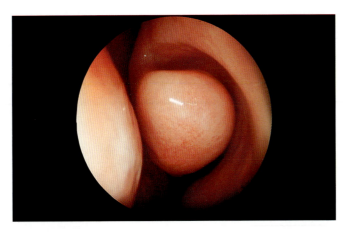

Figure 2.137
Concha bullosa

The body of this left middle turbinate is abnormally enlarged and widened. The reason for the enlargement was revealed by a CT scan, which showed that the bone of the middle turbinate contained a large air cell.

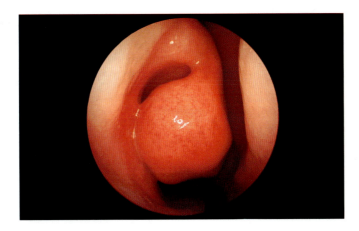

Figure 2.138
Concha bullosa

The air cell within this right middle turbinate is so large that the turbinate has expanded to such an extent that the lateral side of the turbinate has come into contact with the lateral nasal wall.

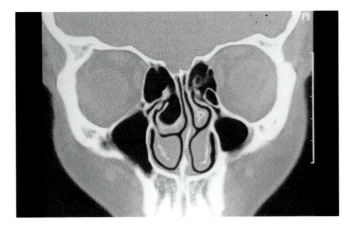

Figure 2.139
Concha bullosa

The large air cell within the right middle turbinate of the patient shown in Figure 2.138 is clearly seen on the CT scan.

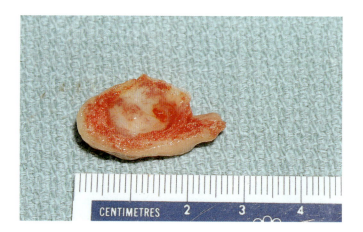

Figure 2.140

Concha bullosa

The lateral half of the concha bullosa shown in Figures 2.138 and 2.139 was resected endoscopically. Note its size.

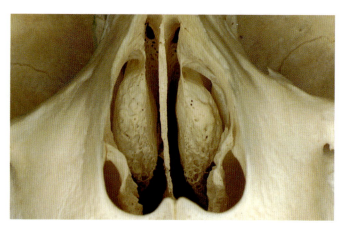

Figure 2.141

Concha bullosa

This specimen has bilateral large concha bullosa. Note the balloon-like shape of both middle turbinates.

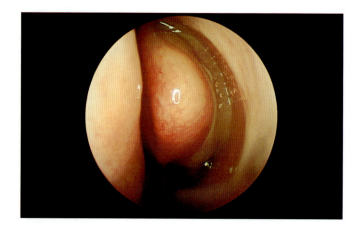

Figure 2.142

Concha bullosa

The air cell in this left middle turbinate has expanded to such an extent that the lateral surface of the middle turbinate is now in direct contact with the lateral nasal wall. The middle meatus is obliterated by oedematous polypoid mucosa that developed at the site of contact.

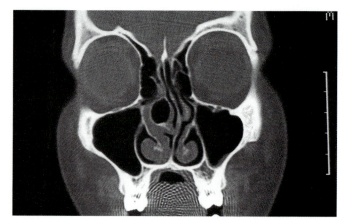

Figure 2.143

Concha bullosa

Note in this CT scan how the large concha bullosa bulges into the lateral nasal wall. It is from these contact areas that the localized mucosal oedema that precedes nasal polyp formation frequently begins.

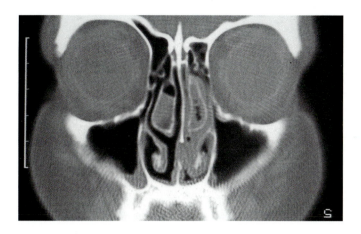

Figure 2.144
Concha bullosa

The air cells within a middle turbinate can be affected by any of the diseases that appear in the other paranasal sinuses. Note the bilateral mucoceles in these aerated middle turbinates.

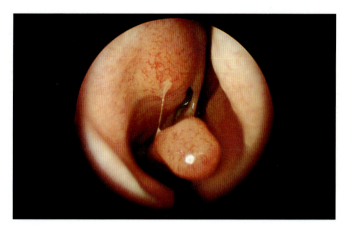

Figure 2.145
Agger nasi

A pneumatized agger nasi mound appears as a distinct bulge anterior to the insertion of the middle turbinate into the lateral nasal wall. The agger nasi mound is so enlarged in this patient that it completely obscures the insertion of the turbinate. Note the unusual club-shaped middle turbinate.

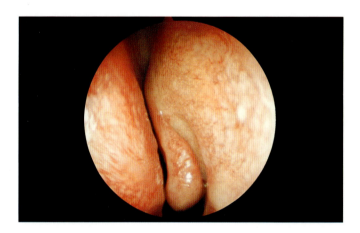

Figure 2.146
Agger nasi

An enlarged or diseased agger nasi may compromise the frontal recess and cause frontal sinus disease. This enlarged left agger nasi cell was responsible for recurrent episodes of frontal sinusitis.

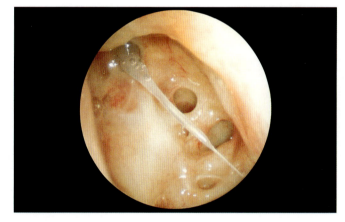

Figure 2.147
Postoperative agger remnant

A view into a left middle meatus 8 weeks after endoscopic surgery. Note the viscous, non-purulent mucus in the frontal recess. On revision remnants of an agger nasi cell were found still obstructing the frontal sinus ostium.

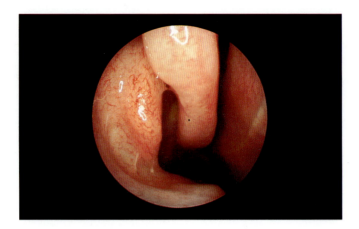

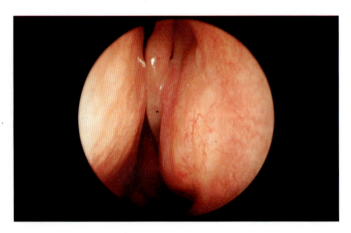

Figure 2.148

Medially bent uncinate process

In this patient the right uncinate process is medially bent (rotated) to such an extent that it is lying at right angles to the long axis of the nasal cavity. The medial end of the uncinate process is in actual contact with the lateral surface of the right middle turbinate.

Figure 2.149

Enlarged and medially bent uncinate process

In this patient with a left maxillary sinus mucocele, the left uncinate process is grossly enlarged and rotated medially so that it lies at right angles to the long axis of the nasal cavity. The uncinate process is so large that it obscures the anterior surface of the ethmoidal bulla.

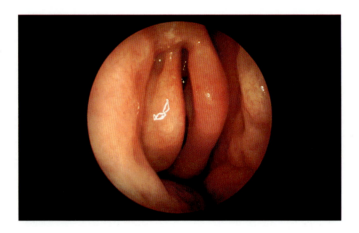

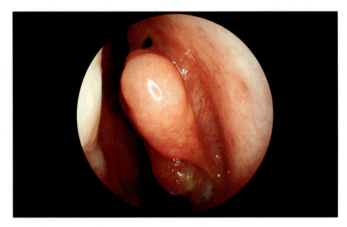

Figure 2.150

Anteriorly bent uncinate process

In some patients the uncinate process is rotated almost 180°, so that its posterior border faces anteriorly. When the uncinate process is also enlarged, as in this patient, the middle turbinate appears to be 'doubled'. The lateral 'extra middle turbinate' is actually the anteriorly rotated and enlarged uncinate process, which protrudes out of the middle nasal meatus.

Figure 2.151

Anteriorly bent uncinate process

This left uncinate process is both anteriorly bent and grossly enlarged. At first glance the uncinate process could easily be mistaken for the middle turbinate, the inferior border of which can just be seen behind and below the inferior margin of the uncinate process.

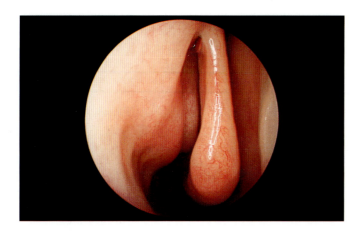

Figure 2.152

Enlarged ethmoidal bulla

The ethmoidal bulla may be grossly enlarged. In this patient the uncinate process is both medially bent and enlarged. The enlarged ethmoidal bulla can be seen behind the medial end of the uncinate process.

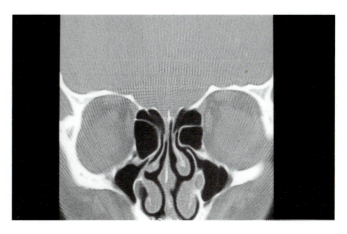

Figure 2.153

Enlarged ethmoidal bulla

Grossly enlarged ethmoidal bullae are seen narrowing the ethmoidal infundibulum bilaterally on this coronal CT scan.

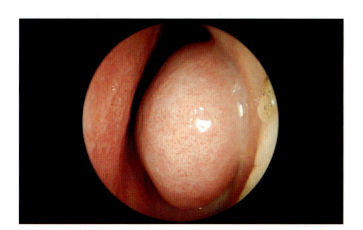

Figure 2.154

Enlarged inferior turbinate

'Enlargement' of the inferior turbinate is a common cause of nasal obstruction. In most cases, the apparent enlargement is primarily due to vasodilatation. Dilatation of the mucosa of the inferior turbinate may be the result of an acute or chronic rhinitis, or a reflex response to a focus of chronic infection or inflammation within the anterior ethmoid.

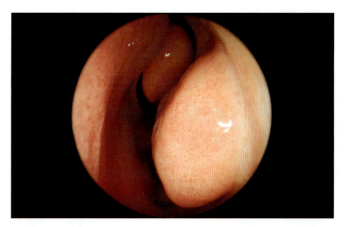

Figure 2.155

Enlarged inferior turbinate

In rare cases the underlying bone of the inferior turbinate is truly enlarged, as seen after vasoconstriction.

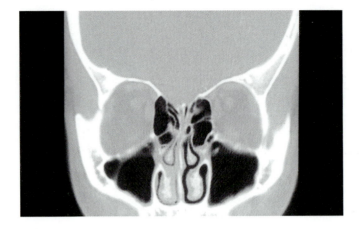

Figure 2.156
Enlarged inferior turbinates

Both bony inferior turbinates are grossly enlarged on this coronal CT scan.

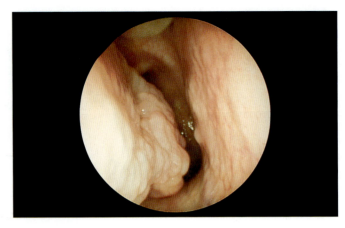

Figure 2.157
Enlarged posterior end of the inferior turbinate

The hypertrophied posterior end of an inferior turbinate may obstruct the choana to such an extent that severe nasal obstruction results. Note the 'mulberry' hypertrophy of the posterior end of this right inferior turbinate.

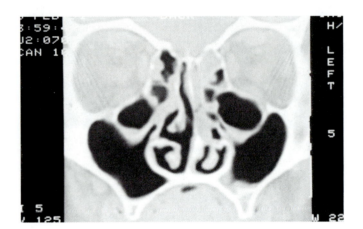

Figure 2.158
Haller's cells

Note the unusually large bilateral Haller's cells, which narrow the ethmoidal infundibulum and the maxillary sinus ostium on both sides.

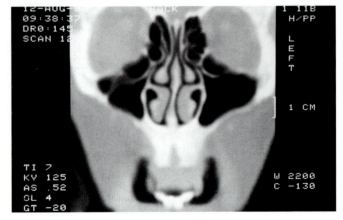

Figure 2.159
Haller's cells

Haller's cells can be seen bilaterally arising from the floor of the orbit and narrowing the infundibulum.

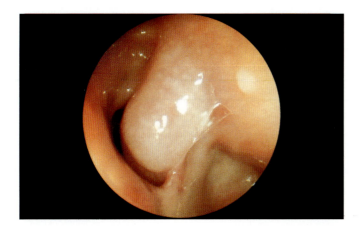

Figure 2.160
Haller's cells

A Haller's cell can be seen at maxillary sinoscopy narrowing the left maxillary sinus ostium and the infundibulum. This situation may predispose to recurring maxillary sinusitis.

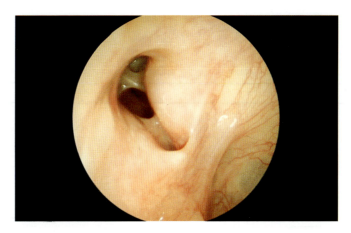

Figure 2.161
Haller's cells

The same patient seen by maxillary sinoscopy 3 months after endoscopic sinus surgery and removal of the Haller's cell. One can now see through the infundibulum into the anterior ethmoid.

Epistaxis

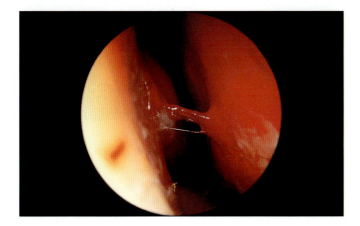

Figure 2.162
Epistaxis

Nosebleeds are extremely common and usually minor. Most nosebleeds originate from the anterior nasal septum in the region of Little's area.

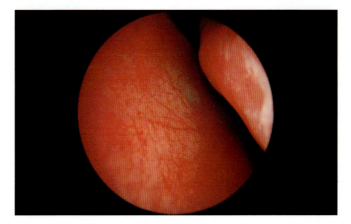

Figure 2.163
Epistaxis

A highly vascular region, Kiesselbach's plexus of vessels arises in Little's area of the nasal septum, from the termination of the major feeding systems: the anterior and posterior ethmoidal arteries, the septal branch of the superior labial artery and the sphenopalatine artery.

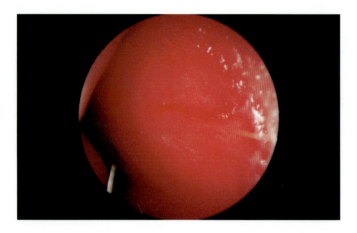

Figure 2.164

Kiesselbach's plexus

Sometimes the vessels in Kiesselbach's plexus may become quite large and, by virtue of their superficial location, susceptible to damage from the most minimal trauma. The result is spontaneous recurrent episodes of epistaxis.

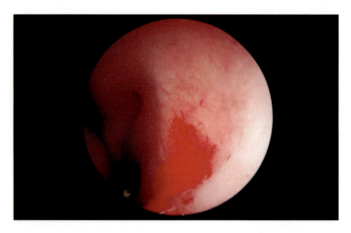

Figure 2.165

Epistaxis

The origin of the bleeding is not always obvious. In this case the removal of any clots or crusts by gentle rubbing of Little's area with a cotton-tipped applicator may reveal the source of the bleeding.

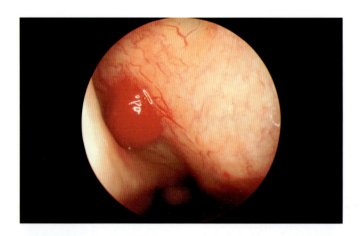

Figure 2.166

Epistaxis

Nasal endoscopes have proven invaluable for identification of the site of bleeding and for the application of site-specific cauterization. This small cherry-red haemangioma located on the anterior medial surface of this left ethmoidal bulla was the source of recurrent severe epistaxis. Once the haemangioma was identified, it was readily destroyed by suction electrocautery.

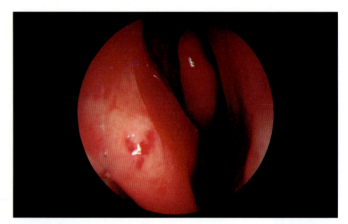

Figure 2.167

Rendu–Osler–Weber disease

Recurrent and troublesome epistaxis is a feature of congenital haemorrhagic telangiectasia (Rendu–Osler–Weber disease). Note the multiple telangiectatic spots on the anterior surface of this left inferior turbinate.

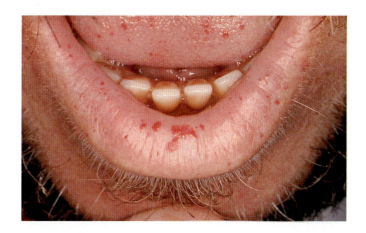 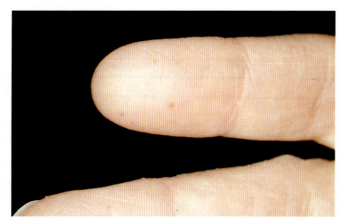

Figure 2.168

Rendu–Osler–Weber disease

Telltale telangiectatic spots may also be found on the surface of the lips, tongue and fingertips.

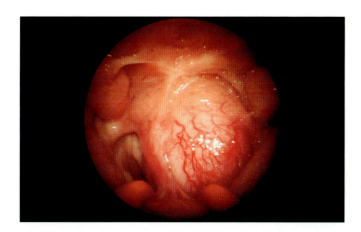

Figure 2.169

Juvenile angiofibroma

Recurrent episodes of epistaxis in adolescent males should alert the examiner to the possibility of a juvenile angiofibroma. The left choana of this 13-year-old boy is completely blocked by an angiofibroma. Note how the nasal septum has been displaced to the right.

Sinusitis

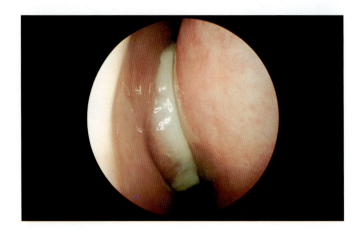

Figure 2.170
Acute maxillary sinusitis

Recurrent episodes of acute maxillary and frontal sinusitis are usually associated with significant anatomical abnormalities of the lateral nasal wall and ostiomeatal complex. Note the creamy-white purulent discharge in the left middle meatus of this patient with acute bilateral maxillary sinusitis.

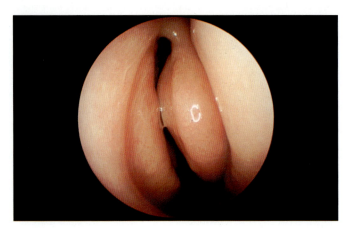

Figure 2.171
Acute maxillary sinusitis

The administration of a suitable broad-spectrum antibiotic is still the treatment of choice for acute, uncomplicated bacterial sinusitis. This is the same patient as shown in Figure 2.170, 5 weeks later. The predisposing anatomical abnormalities can now be clearly identified: a medially bent uncinate process and a concha bullosa.

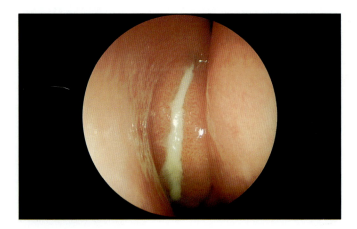

Figure 2.172
Acute maxillary sinusitis

When medical therapy is unable to cure a sinus infection, then a functional endoscopic sinus surgical approach using the Messerklinger technique may be required. Despite 8 weeks of a suitable broad-spectrum antibiotic, chosen on the basis of culture and sensitivity studies, this patient still has a chronic right maxillary sinus mucopyocele. Note the oedematous medially bent uncinate process. He was successfully treated by means of an endoscopic procedure.

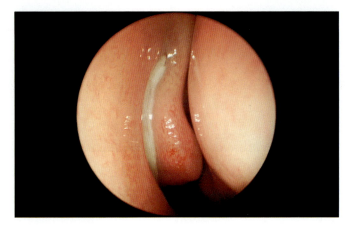

Figure 2.173
Acute maxillary sinusitis

This patient's chronic right maxillary and frontal sinus infections were associated with a paradoxically bent aerated right middle turbinate.

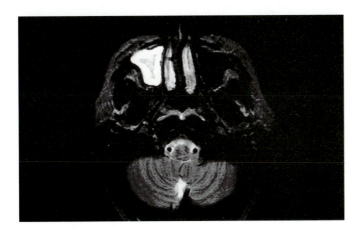

Figure 2.174
Acute maxillary sinusitis

The pathology with the maxillary sinus during an acute sinusitis is well demonstrated on this T2-weighted MRI scan. Note the massive oedema of the mucosal lining (the brightest area) and the collection of purulent material within the sinus (less brightly illuminated).

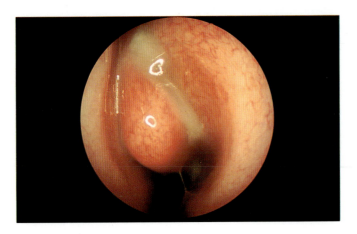

Figure 2.175
AIDS-associated chronic sinusitis

The acquired immune deficiency syndrome (AIDS) is associated with an increased incidence of unusual and potentially serious opportunistic infections. This patient with AIDS suffered from chronic pansinusitis. Note the widened oedematous middle turbinate and the purulent mucus in the left middle meatus.

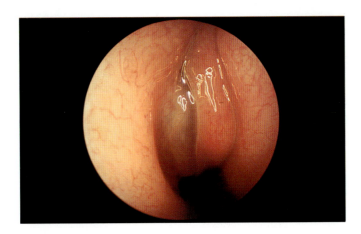

Figure 2.176
AIDS-associated chronic sinusitis

On the opposite side, oedematous mucosa can be seen herniating anteriorly from the hiatus semilunaris.

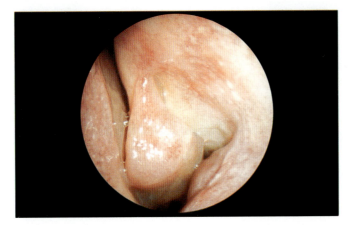

Figure 2.177
Anterior ethmoid disease

On endoscopic examination a hypertrophic inferior turbinate is bypassed and the diseased middle meatus becomes visible. Note the medially deflected and bulging uncinate process and its inflamed mucosa.

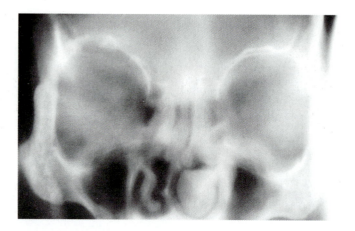

Figure 2.178
Anterior ethmoid disease 2

Conventional tomography indicated bilateral anterior ethmoidal disease. The inferior turbinate on the left appears to be 'enlarged'.

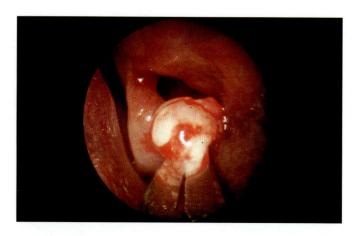

Figure 2.179
Anterior ethmoid disease 3

The uncinate process was resected, and a large mass of polypoid mucosa is being removed from the anterior ethmoid.

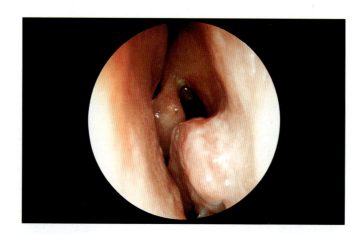

Figure 2.180
Anterior ethmoid disease 4 (postoperative appearance)

Eight days after the endoscopic procedure, the inferior turbinate has shrunk back to its normal size without having been touched. The enlargement of the left inferior turbinate seen in Figure 2.178 was the result of a reflex vasodilatation, probably stimulated by the chronic inflammation within the anterior ethmoid. Once the ethmoid infection was cured, the inferior turbinate returned to its normal size.

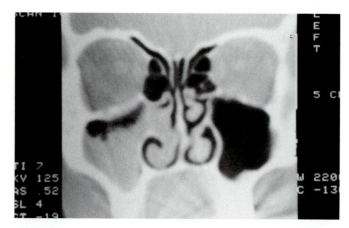

Figure 2.181
Recurrent maxillary sinusitis

This patient's recurring episodes of maxillary sinusitis were due to infundibular obstruction.

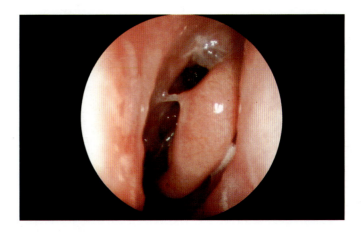

Figure 2.182

Recurrent maxillary sinusitis

The appearance of the middle meatus of the patient whose CT scan is shown in Figure 2.181, 1 week following functional endoscopic sinus surgery.

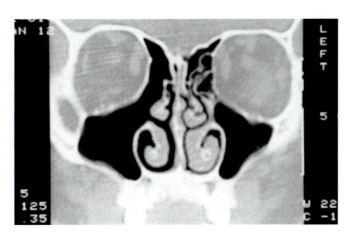

Figure 2.183

Recurrent maxillary sinusitis

The control CT scan of the patient shown in Figures 2.181 and 2.182, 1 year after surgery, showing normal healing.

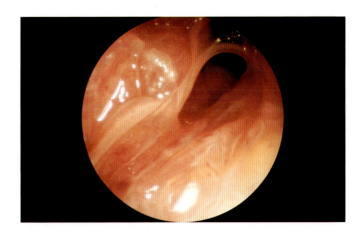

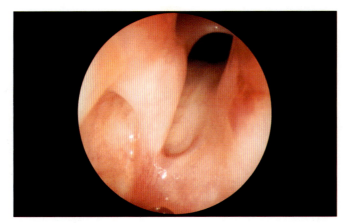

Figure 2.184

Frontal recess: postoperative appearance

(Left) The view into a left frontal recess 3 weeks after endoscopic surgery for massive polyposis. There is still some diffuse oedema and thickish secretions. A little crusting can be seen at the entrance of the frontal sinus. On close-up view, some mucopus was encountered. Note the lymph vessels in the tissue. This was an allergic fungal sinusitis, which healed (right) only after being treated with oral itraconazole and corticosteroids combined with antihistamines.

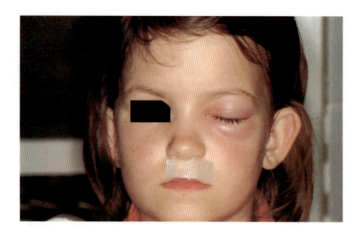

Figure 2.185
Orbital cellulitis 1

This young girl shows the characteristic appearance of developing orbital complications due to acute sinusitis.

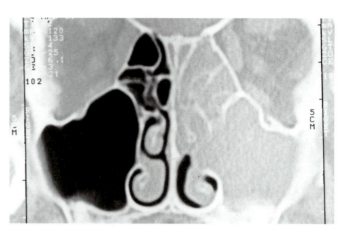

Figure 2.186
Orbital cellulitis 2

The CT scan of the patient shown in Figure 2.185 reveals orbital infiltration.

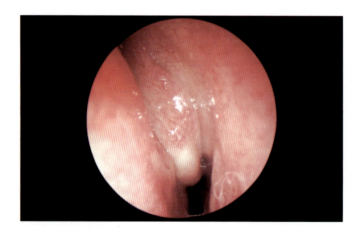

Figure 2.187
Orbital cellulitis 3

Endoscopically, the uncinate process was found pressing against the middle turbinate, and there was no free pus visible.

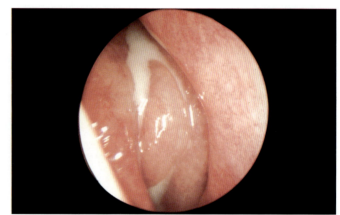

Figure 2.188
Orbital cellulitis 4

After cotton swabs soaked with a decongestant solution (adrenaline 1:1000) were placed high up into the middle meatus under endoscopic control, pus started to flow. Continuous intravenous antibiotic therapy was administered, and complete resolution occurred.

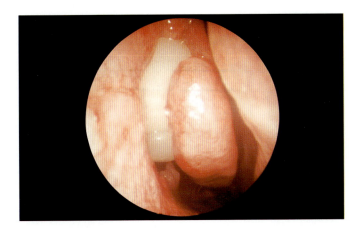

Figure 2.189
Early orbital cellulitis

When the right uncinate process of this patient with early orbital complications of acute sinusitis was resected, masses of pus under pressure drained.

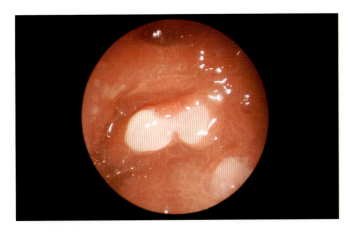

Figure 2.190
Maxillary sinusitis of dental origin

Note the two small intramucosal abscesses in the floor of the sinus causing this denteriginous infection of the left maxillary sinus.

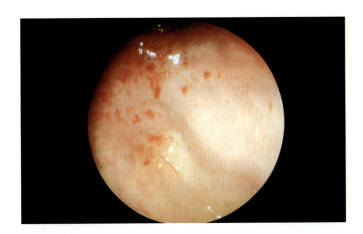

Figure 2.191
Barotraumatic maxillary sinusitis

Note the intramucosal and submucosal petechial bleeding in a diver following barotrauma as seen by maxillary sinoscopy.

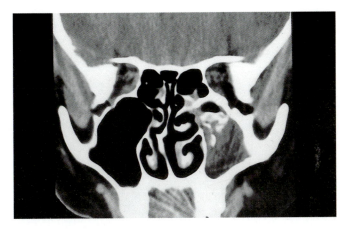

Figure 2.192
Fungal sinusitis

The presence of an area of increased radio-opacity on CT within the paranasal sinuses indicated the presence of a fungal sinusitis (usually due to *Aspergillus* species).

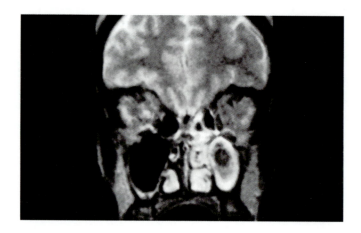

Figure 2.193

Fungal sinusitis

MRI can be used to confirm the presence of a fungal ball within a sinus cavity. The bright areas on this MRI scan of a left maxillary sinus represent inflamed and vascular mucosa. The central dark signal void area represents the actual fungal ball.

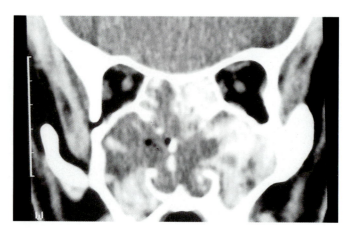

Figure 2.194

Allergic fungal sinusitis

While the aetiology of nasal polyps has yet to be fully understood, the role of allergy is undisputed. This patient with the ASA triad has had four endonasal polypectomies in the past 14 months. After each polypectomy, the polyps recurred within 6 weeks. The reason for this rapid recurrence is suggested on this coronal CT scan. The streaky areas of increased radio-opacity within the maxillary sinuses and posterior ethmoid sinuses represent fungal elements.

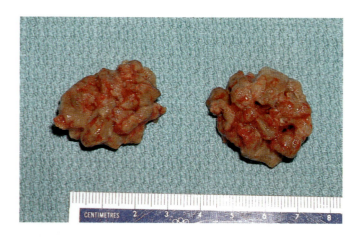

Figure 2.195

Allergic fungal sinusitis

This photograph shows the contents of the maxillary sinuses seen in Figure 2.194. These khaki-coloured rubbery masses contained numerous entrapped elements of the fungus *Aspergillus*. This material is characteristic of patients with allergic fungal sinusitis. The allergic reaction to the entrapped fungal elements was responsible for the rapid recurrence of the nasal polyps. Not surprisingly, these nasal polyps were highly steroid sensitive.

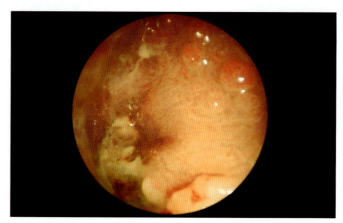

Figure 2.196

Osteomyelitis of the maxilla with secondary sinusitis

This female patient, aged 76 years, has severe maxillary sinusitis on the left side with granulations, accompanying an underlying osteomyelitis.

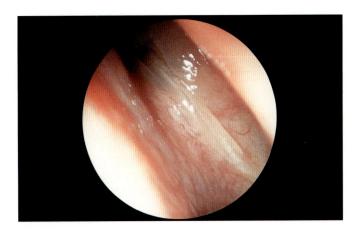

Figure 2.197

Sphenoid sinusitis

The mucopus draining from this right sphenoid sinus ostium indicates the presence of chronic sphenoid sinusitis.

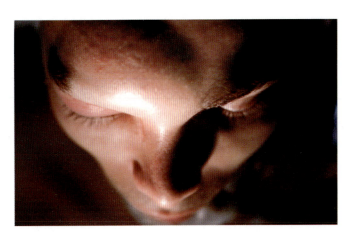

Figure 2.198

Frontal bone osteomyelitis

The 'Pott's puffy tumour' affecting this 21-year-old man's right frontal bone was the result of acute ethmoidal and frontal sinusitis with osteitis.

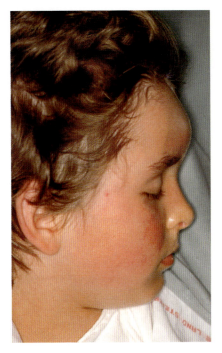

Figure 2.199

Frontal bone osteomyelitis

Note the swollen forehead in this 9-year-old girl with frontoethmoidal sinusitis that has extended into the frontal bone causing osteomyelitis.

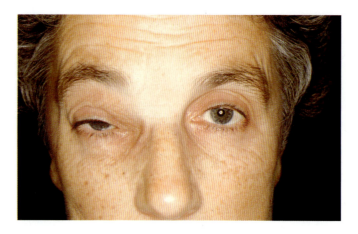

Figure 2.200

Frontal sinus mucocele with extension into the orbit

The lateral and inferior displacement of this patient's globe was caused by a frontal sinus mucocele that had extended inferiorly into the anterior orbit and superiorly through the anterior skull base.

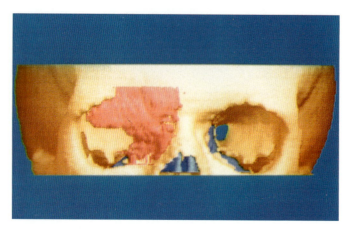

Figure 2.201

Frontal sinus mucocele with extension into the orbit

A three-dimensional reconstruction of the mucocele shown in Figure 2.200. The mucocele was decompressed by means of an endoscopic approach 5 years ago. To date, there has been no recurrence.

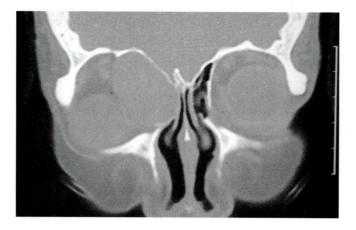

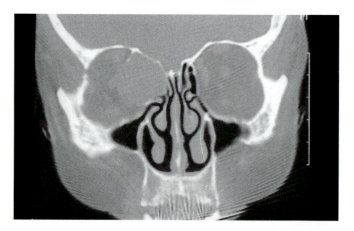

Figure 2.202

Anterior ethmoidal mucocele with extensive intraorbital extension

Note the large mucocele of the anterior ethmoid which has extended extensively into the right orbit and caused severe displacement of the globe.

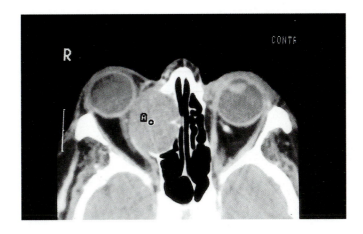

Figure 2.203

Anterior ethmoidal mucocele with extensive intraorbital extension

Note the severe displacement of both the right globe and the optic nerve in this coronal CT scan of the patient shown in Figure 2.202.

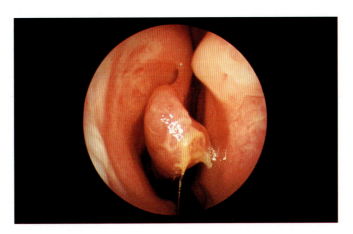

Figure 2.204

Anterior ethmoidal mucocele with extensive intraorbital extension

The endoscopic photograph of the patient shown in Figures 2.202 and 2.203. While there is a large agger mound and a paradoxically bent right middle turbinate, the middle meatus appears otherwise to be unremarkable.

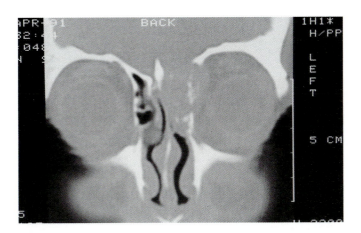

Figure 2.205

Frontoethmoidal mucocele

There is a mucocele of the left anterior ethmoid and frontal sinus, which has caused osteolysis of the anterior skull base.

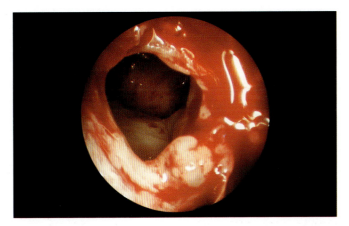

Figure 2.206

Frontoethmoidal mucocele

The endoscopic appearance of the patient shown in Figure 2.205 after endonasal surgery. There was a mycotic mucocele (non-invasive *Aspergillus fumigatus*), which was treated endoscopically. The endoscope is looking into the left frontal sinus with the anterior contour of the frontal lobe visible. There was no leak of cerebrospinal fluid (CSF).

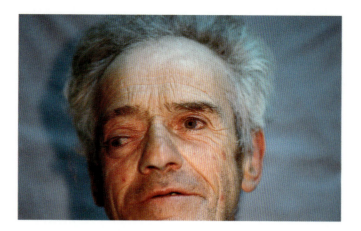

Figure 2.207

Frontoethmoidal mucocele

This patient has a frontoethmoidal mucocele with massive displacement of the right eyeball.

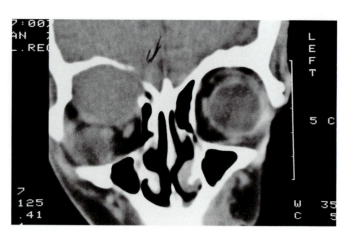

Figure 2.208

Frontoethmoidal mucocele

The CT scan of the patient shown in Figure 2.207. The eyeball has been pushed towards the inferior lateral corner of the orbit. Note the osteolysis of the skull base.

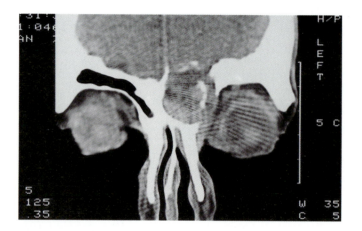

Figure 2.209

Frontoethmoidal mucocele

A frontoethmoidal mucocele on the left side contains a secondary fungal growth (non-invasive *Aspergillus fumigatus*), as evidenced by the areas of increased radio-opacity within the mucocele.

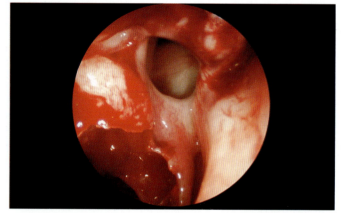

Figure 2.210

Frontoethmoidal mucocele

The appearance of the sinus shown in Figure 2.209 during endoscopic removal. The frontal sinus has been opened below and the fungal masses have been aspirated and irrigated. Note the bulging of the dura over the frontal lobe at the anterior table of the frontal sinus, where the bone was eroded. There was no CSF leak.

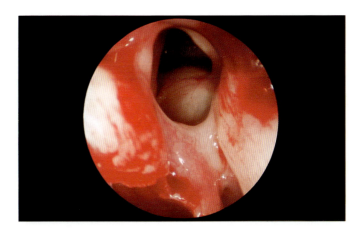

Figure 2.211

Frontoethmoidal mucocele

Approaching with a 30° endoscope allows an even better view into the frontal sinus and provides a higher magnification without switching lenses.

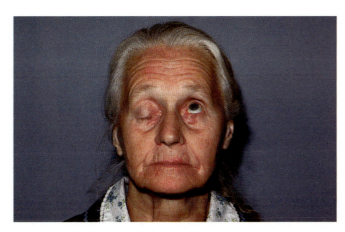

Figure 2.212

Posterior ethmoid and sphenoid mucocele

This 77-year-old patient developed complete ophthalmoplegia and blindness from a mucocele of the posterior ethmoid and sphenoid sinuses.

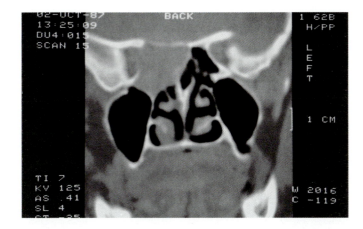

Figure 2.213

Posterior ethmoid and sphenoid sinus mucocele

The CT scan of the patient shown in Figure 2.212. Note the destruction of the lamina papyracea and the optic tubercle and the thinning of the bone at the sphenoidal/posterior ethmoidal roof. After endoscopic drainage, the ophthalmoplegia resolved; unfortunately, however, the vision did not return.

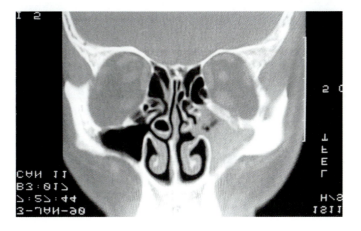

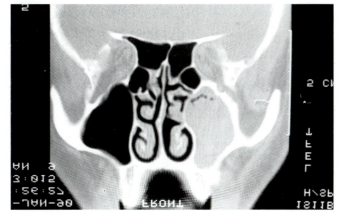

Figure 2.214

Maxillary sinus mucocele

(Left) Obstruction of the infundibulum has produced a left maxillary sinus mucocele in this patient. Note the entrapped air bubbles within the thick collection of mucus in the scan on the right.

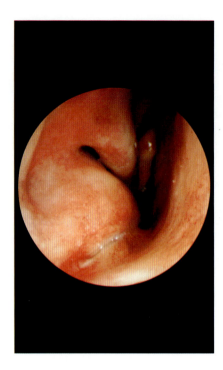

Figure 2.215

Maxillary sinus mucocele

The medial wall of the right maxillary sinus is bulging massively into the right inferior meatus. The patient had undergone a Caldwell–Luc procedure almost 30 years previously.

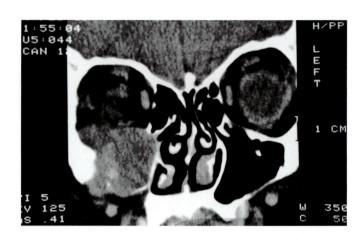

Figure 2.216

Maxillary sinus mucocele

The CT scan of the patient shown in Figure 2.215. There is a large septated mucocele of the maxillary sinus causing the endoscopic appearance seen in Figure 2.215.

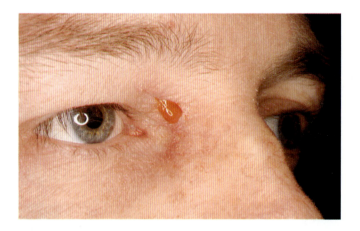

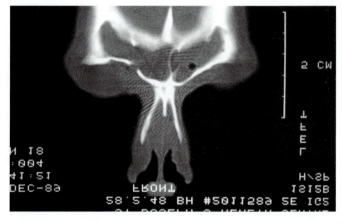

Figure 2.217

Frontal sinus fistula

(Left) A fistula tract has developed through the floor of the right frontal sinus at the site of a previous frontal sinus trephine performed for the treatment of a frontal sinus mucocele. As the obstruction of the frontal recess was not treated, the mucocele promptly recurred, become infected and drained through the site of the previous trephination. The CT scan (right) shows the defect in the bony floor of the left frontal sinus.

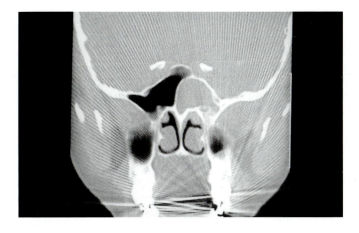

Figure 2.218

Sphenoid sinus mucocele

The mucocele filling this left frontal sinus presented as chronic posterior occipital headaches.

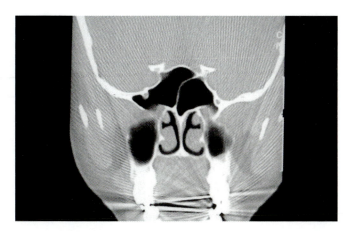

Figure 2.219

Spontaneous resolution of a sphenoid sinus mucocele

A repeat CT scan 3 months later shows that the mucocele has resolved spontaneously. The occipital heads were still present and obviously were not due to the sphenoid sinus mucocele.

Nasal polyps

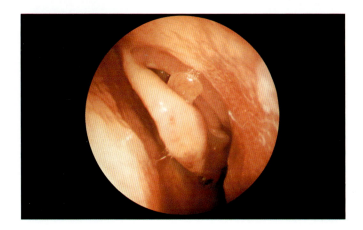

Figure 2.220

Small nasal polyp

A small nasal polyp is arising from the area of contact between the left middle turbinate and the uncinate process.

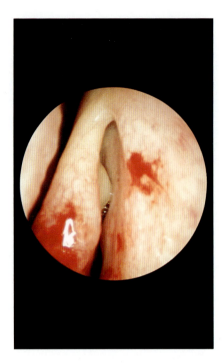
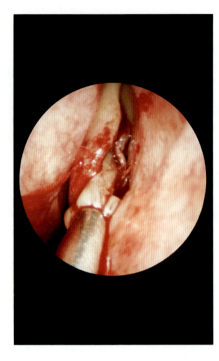

Figure 2.221

A sentinel or 'iceberg' nasal polyp

(Left) The tiny polyp seen 'peeking' out of this left middle meatus is so small that it seems of no clinical significance. However, after resection of the uncinate process the entire anterior ethmoid was found filled with polypoid and oedematous mucosa (right).

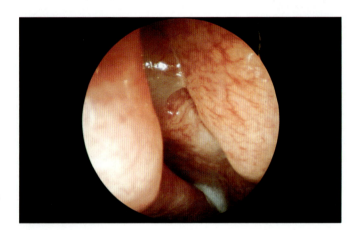

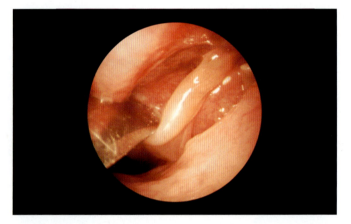

Figure 2.222

Nasal polyps: early polyp formation

The localized area of mucosal oedema protruding out of the hiatus semilunaris on this left side is turning into a polyp. This patient presented with a history of headaches and a sensation of nasal obstruction. The foamy secretion in the posterior nasal cavity is the result of spraying the nose with a topical anaesthetic and decongestant.

Figure 2.223

Nasal polyps

In this left middle meatus a broad-based oedema has developed over the ethmoidal bulla between the middle turbinate and the uncinate process. This is another example of the earliest stage of polyp formation.

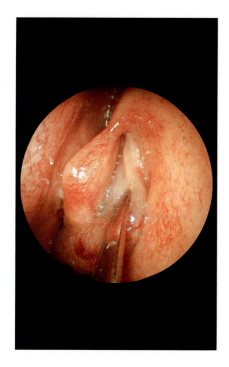 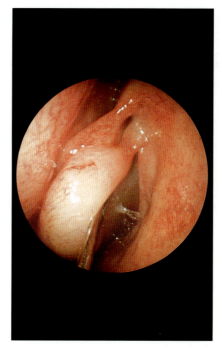

Figure 2.224
Nasal polyps

A large polyp is seen blocking the entire anterior middle nasal meatus. When pushed medially, its origin from the contact area between the uncinate process and middle turbinate superiorly, with a broad root from the anterior face of the ethmoidal bulla, is apparent. The patient's symptoms were recurring maxillary sinus empyemas.

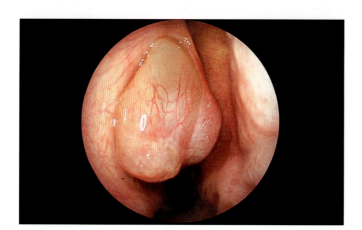 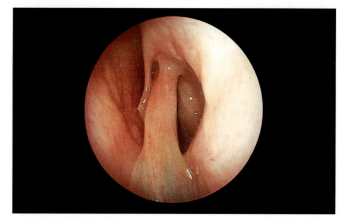

Figure 2.225
Nasal polyp

The large polyp extending anteriorly out of the right middle meatus has pushed the middle turbinate medially. The polyp has thinned the middle turbinate, apparently as a result of constant pressure against the septum. This polyp originated with a broad base from the free margin of a medially deflected uncinate process. No other pathology was encountered in the entire ethmoid during surgery.

Figure 2.226
Nasal polyp

This large, oedematous, solitary nasal polyp arose by a small stalk from the superior portion of the uncinate process at its insertion into the middle turbinate.

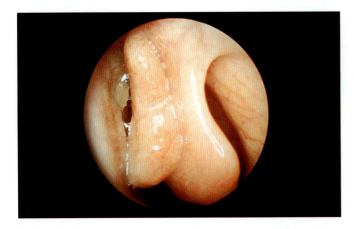

Figure 2.227

Nasal polyp

These polyps arising from the olfactory sulcus bilaterally (the left side is shown) were responsible for anosmia.

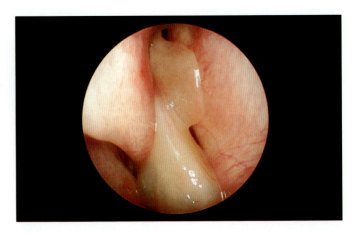

Figure 2.228

Nasal polyp

These two discrete oedematous nasal polyps arise from the left sphenoethmoid recess.

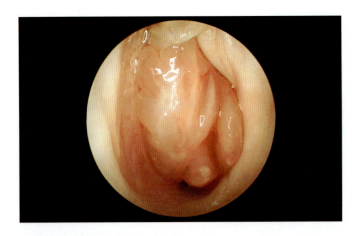

Figure 2.229

Steroid-sensitive nasal polyposis

The left nasal cavity of this patient with massive nasal polyposis is completely filled with oedematous nasal polyps.

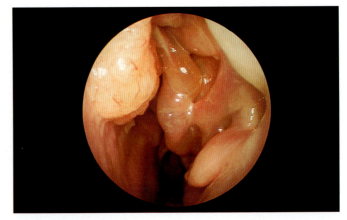

Figure 2.230

Steroid-sensitive nasal polyposis

Following a short course of high-dose prednisone, the nasal polyps have almost disappeared.

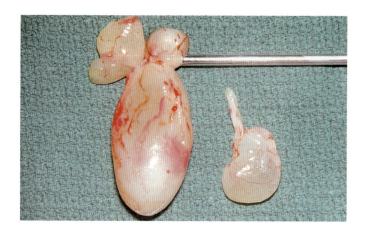

Figure 2.231

Nasal polyps

Nasal polyps can be removed endoscopically. Unfortunately, no matter what technique is used for their removal, some nasal polyps have a tendency to recur. The long-term use of a topical nasal spray seems to slow their reformation.

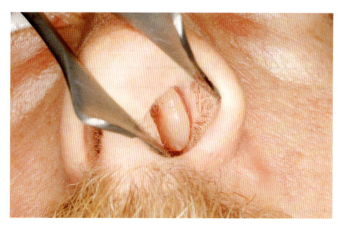

Figure 2.232

Severe diffuse polyposis

This patient with cystic fibrosis had so many nasal polyps that they extended into the nasal vestibule.

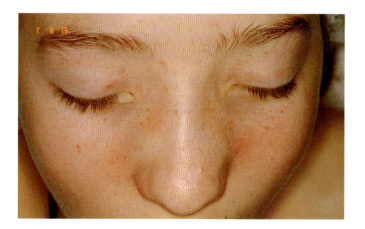

Figure 2.233

The ASA triad and hypertelorism

The facial appearance of a 16-year-old girl with the ASA (acetylsalicylic acid) triad (asthma, nasal polyps and ASA sensitivity) and hypertelorism due to massive polyposis.

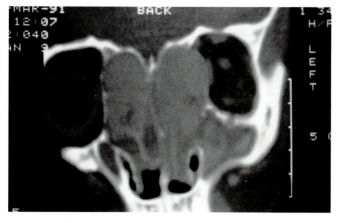

Figure 2.234

The ASA triad and hypertelorism

The coronal CT scan of the patient shown in Figure 2.233, showing the lateral displacement of the orbits.

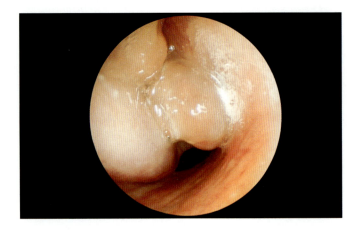

Figure 2.235

Nasal polyps and the ASA triad

The typical appearance of the diffuse polypoid rhinosinopathy encountered in sinobronchial syndrome with aspirin intolerance (the triad of nasal polyps, asthma and ASA sensitivity).

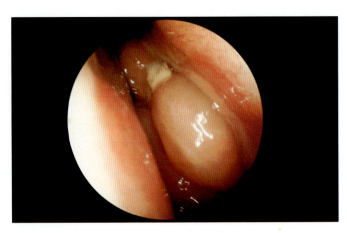

Figure 2.236

Diffuse polypoid rhinosinopathy

Diffuse polypoid rhinosinopathy in a patient with ASA intolerance. There are massive, sometimes glue-like, thick secretions between the polyps.

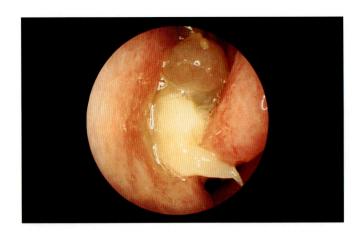

Figure 2.237

Aggressive diffuse nasal polyposis

Patients with the ASA triad often have the most aggressive nasal polyps. Note the abnormally thick yellowish mucus that is often associated with this condition. The mucus may be so thick and rubbery in consistency that it may initially be confused with a nasal polyp.

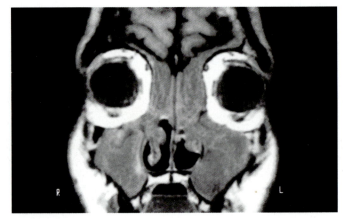

Figure 2.238

Aggressive diffuse nasal polyposis

Diffuse nasal polyposis represents a diffuse mucosal disease (as opposed to an area of diseased mucosa) and as such it affects the mucosa lining the entire nasal cavity and adjacent paranasal sinuses. The diffuse nature of this disease can be seen on this T1-weighted MRI scan.

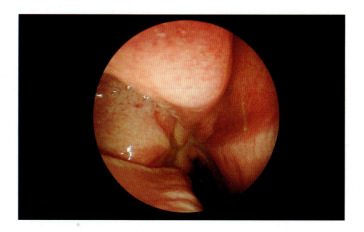

Figure 2.239

Hypoplastic maxillary sinus

The presence of a deeply retracted or lateralized posterior fontanelle suggests the presence of a hypoplastic maxillary sinus. Note the deeply retracted posterior fontanelle in this right middle meatus.

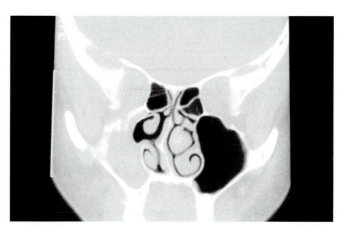

Figure 2.240

Hypoplastic maxillary sinus

This is a coronal CT scan of the patient shown in Figure 2.239. Note the type II hypoplasia of the right maxillary sinus.

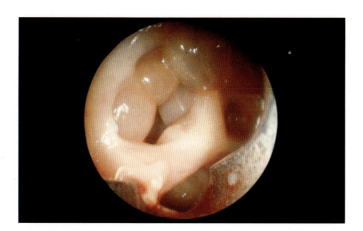

Figure 2.241

Nasal polyps: postoperative appearance

The endoscopic appearance in the vicinity of the maxillary sinus ostium 6 months after surgery in the patient shown in Figure 2.240. There is a cobblestone appearance of the mucosa, which required topical corticosteroids to be controlled. Attempts to resect nasal polyps alone without any corticosteroid therapy resulted in early regrowth of the polypoid oedema.

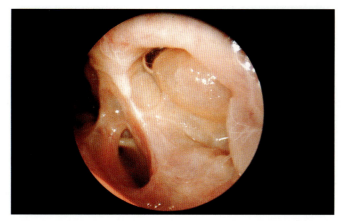

Figure 2.242

Nasal polyps: postoperative appearance

One solitary granulation type of polyp is present in this maxillary sinus ostium following endonasal surgery. Note that the mucosa of the surrounding area and of the other ethmoid compartments appears microscopically normal. Here, simple resection of the polyp without any further therapy resulted in complete healing.

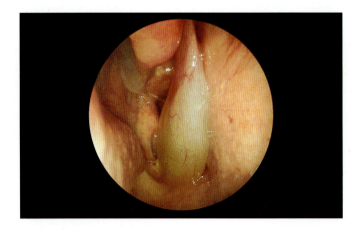

Figure 2.243

Choanal polyp

A choanal polyp is seen originating from the medial surface of the left middle turbinate.

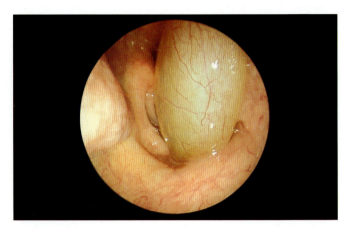

Figure 2.244

Choanal polyp

The inferior portion of the polyp shown in Figure 2.243 extended posteroinferiorly into the left nasal choana.

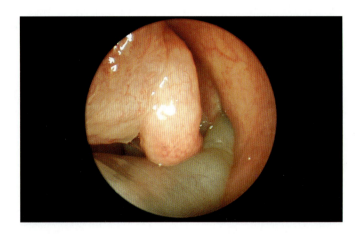

Figure 2.245

Choanal polyp

This patient had four or five discrete large nasal polyps in each nasal cavity. On the right side one of these large nasal polyps can be seen extending posteriorly along the floor of the nose and blocking the choana.

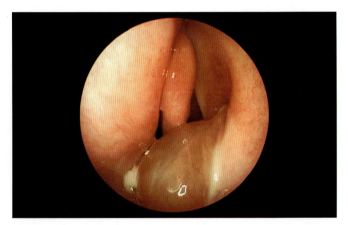

Figure 2.246

Antrochoanal polyp

This antrochoanal polyp originated from within the left maxillary sinus. Note the stalk of the polyp as it enters the nasal cavity via an accessory maxillary sinus ostium located in the anterior nasal fontanelle.

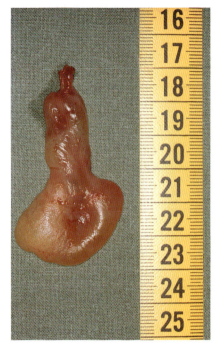

Figure 2.247
Antrochoanal polyp

The solid intranasal portion of an antrochoanal polyp after endoscopic removal.

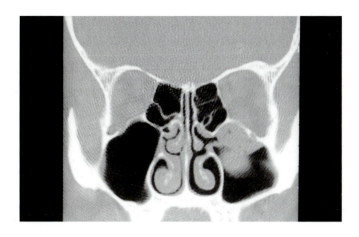

Figure 2.248
Antrochoanal polyp

The CT scan of an antrochoanal polyp. Note the cystic portion of the antrochoanal polyp within the left maxillary sinus.

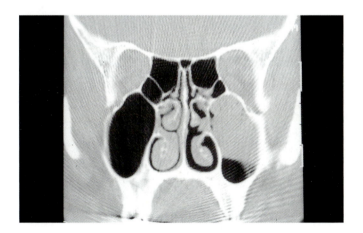

Figure 2.249
Antrochoanal polyp

A slightly more posterior coronal CT scan of the patient shown in Figure 2.248. The cystic intrasinus portion is again seen. Note the stalk of the polyp leaving the maxillary sinus via an accessory maxillary sinus ostium and entering the left middle meatus.

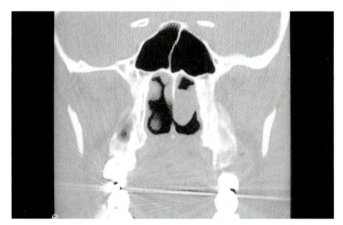

Figure 2.250
Antrochoanal polyp

A slightly more posterior coronal CT scan of the patient shown in Figures 2.248 and 2.249. The solid intranasal portion of the antrochoanal polyp is seen extending into the left choana.

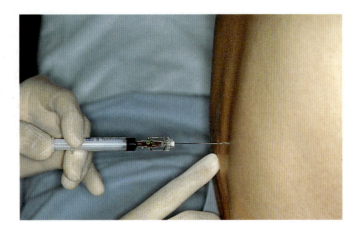

Figure 2.251

The fluorescein test for CSF rhinorrhoea

The injection of 0.5 ml of a 5% sodium fluorescein solution intrathecally.

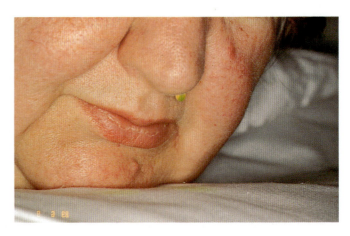

Figure 2.252

The fluorescein test for CSF rhinorrhoea

In this positive fluorescein test, fluorescein-stained CSF is seen dripping from the patient's left nostril after 45 minutes.

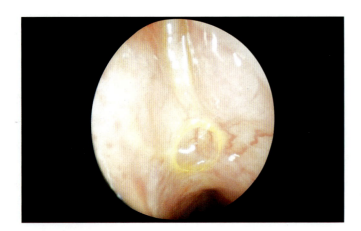

Figure 2.253

The fluorescein test for CSF rhinorrhoea

The fluorescein stain was traced back endoscopically to the sphenoethmoidal recess, indicating a defect in the posterior ethmoidal and/or sphenoidal sinuses.

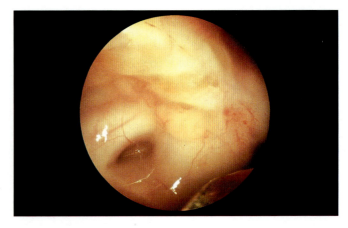

Figure 2.254

CSF fistula

The patient had suffered from recurrent episodes of purulent meningitis. Direct endoscopy of the sphenoid sinus on the right. The optic nerve is clearly visible from 8 o'clock towards the centre with the carotid artery underneath. From the roof of the sinus the mucosa bulges as if filled with water. These 'watercushions' proved to be CSF. There was a crack in the roof of the sphenoid not discovered before this investigation.

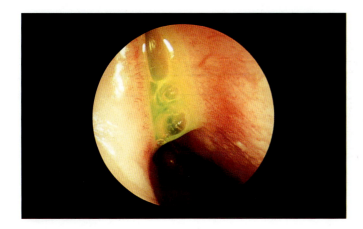

Figure 2.255
CSF rhinorrhoea

Fluorescein test, right nasal cavity. Yellowish-green fluorescein-stained CSF appears between the superior turbinate and the septum on the right side.

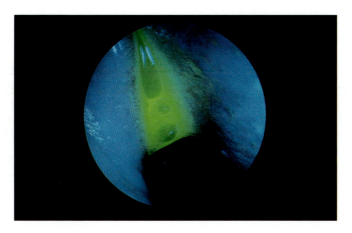

Figure 2.256
CSF rhinorrhoea

With blue light, fluorescence is induced and the CSF shines with a neon-like colour. The fluorescein was followed into the sphenoethmoidal recess close to the sphenoid sinus ostium.

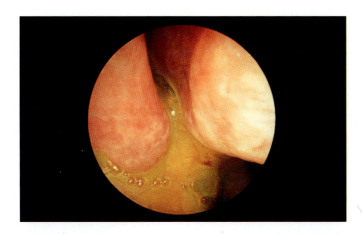

Figure 2.257
CSF rhinorrhoea

A massive CSF leak can be seen pouring from the right sphenoethmoidal recess into the choana and covering the Eustachian tube.

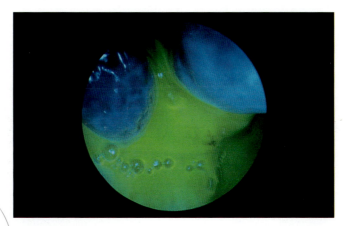

Figure 2.258
CSF rhinorrhoea

Same situation under blue light conditions.

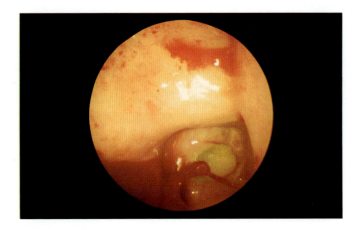

Figure 2.259
CSF rhinorrhoea

The intraoperative findings in the patient shown in Figure 2.258. A pea-sized meningoencephalocele can be seen protruding through the posterior wall of an extensively well-pneumatized right sphenoid sinus. Note the bulge of the sella above and over the carotid siphon to the (patient's) right. Medially, between 1 and 4 o'clock, the intersphenoidal septum can be seen.

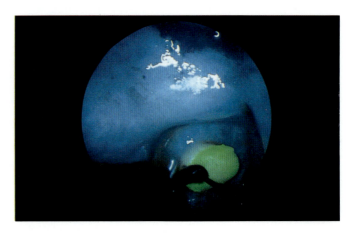

Figure 2.260
CSF rhinorrhoea

The same situation under blue light conditions. Note how clearly the fluorescent CSF shines through the meninges.

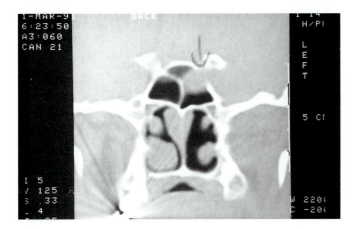

Figure 2.261
Sphenoid sinus cysts

The CT scan of a patient referred because of a suspected meningoencephalocele in the right sphenoidal sinus. The patient was referred with 'proven' CSF rhinorrhoea.

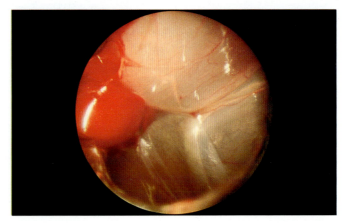

Figure 2.262
Sphenoid sinus cysts

The endoscopic view into the right sphenoid sinus of the patient shown in Figure 2.261. The fluorescein test was negative and no CSF was encountered. This was simply a case of 'secreting' sphenoid sinus cysts.

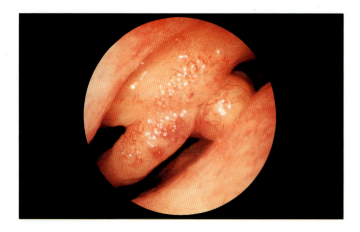

Figure 2.263
Meningoencephalocele

In the right side of the nose, a large polyp protrudes out of the middle meatus, and a smaller 'polyp' appears medially between the insertion of the middle turbinate and the septum.

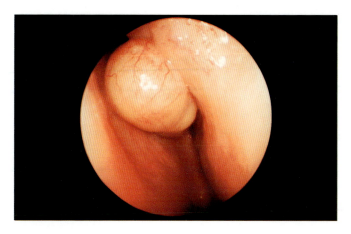

Figure 2.264
Meningoencephalocele

A close-up of the smaller polyp reveals some atypical vascular structures and the origin of the lesion from the junction of the cribriform plate and the nasal septum. This was a meningoencehalocele without CSF rhinorrhoea.

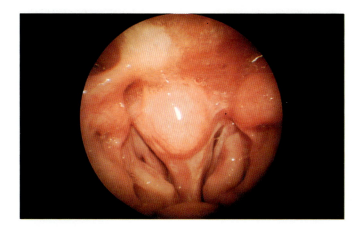

Figure 2.265
Meningocele

The smooth round mass arising from the posterosuperior aspect of the nasal septum in this 26-year-old woman is a meningocele. This photograph was taken with the patient in the upright position.

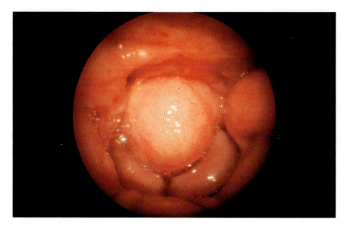

Figure 2.266
Meningocele

The same patient as shown in Figure 2.265, photographed in the supine position. Note how the higher intracranial pressure in the supine position causes the meningocele to swell.

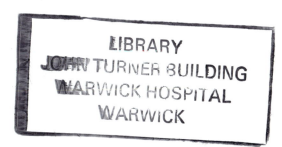

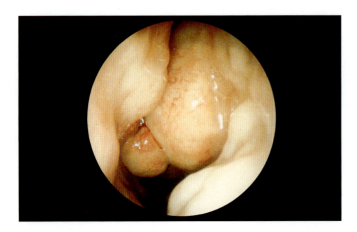

Figure 2.267

Intranasal meningioma

The unusual 'polypoid' lesion in the left middle meatus was an extradural meningioma, which originated from a thin stalk that was removed endoscopically. The lamella of the middle turbinate has been thinned out by the lesion and pressed tightly against the nasal septum.

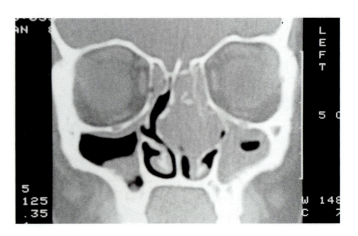

Figure 2.268

Intranasal meningioma

The preoperative CT scan of the patient shown in Figure 2.267.

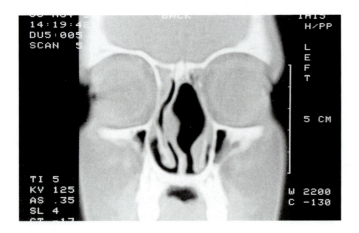

Figure 2.269

Intranasal meningioma

The postoperative CT scan of the patient shown in Figure 2.267.

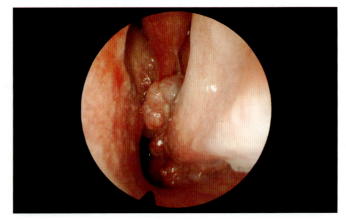

Figure 2.270

Intranasal spread of a meningioma

The tumour seen behind the left inferior turbinate is a meningioma that has spread into the nose from the infratemporal fossa, arising from the pterygoid region.

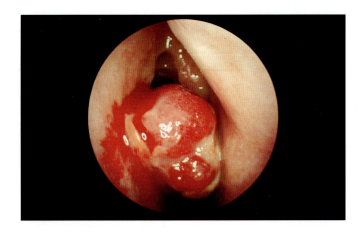

Figure 2.271

Pyogenic granuloma

The large red granulation tissue mass arising from this right anterior ethmoid is a pyogenic granuloma that developed 1 week after endoscopic sinus surgery.

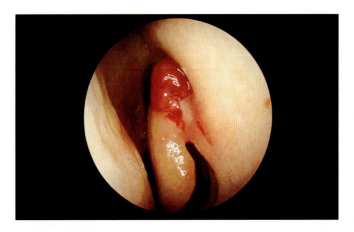

Figure 2.272

Capillary haemangioma

The cherry-red mass arising from the anterior surface of this left middle turbinate was a benign capillary haemangioma.

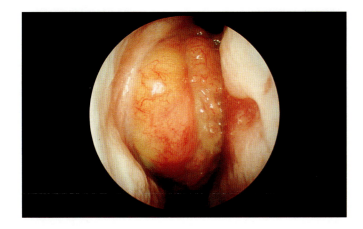

Figure 2.273

Inverting papilloma

This 37-year-old physician presented with a history of left-sided nasal polyps, which had been removed three times in the past year. On close inspection, the anterior surface of the middle turbinate had a knobbly appearance suggestive of an inverting papilloma.

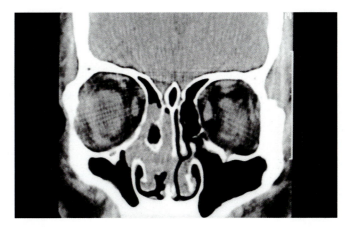

Figure 2.274

Inverting papilloma

The CT scan of the patient shown in Figure 2.273. There is a large discrete soft-tissue mass, which appears to be arising from an aerated left middle turbinate.

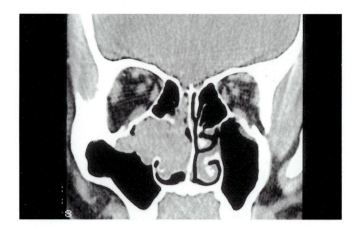

Figure 2.275

Inverting papilloma

A more posterior coronal CT scan of the patient shown in Figures 2.273 and 2.274. Note how the soft-tissue mass has extended into the posterior nasal cavity and is projecting into the widened ostium of the maxillary sinus.

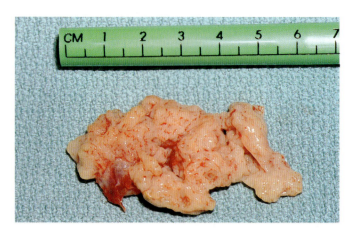

Figure 2.276

Inverting papilloma

The inverting papilloma from the patient in Figures 2.273–2.275 and its site of origin (the middle turbinate) were removed endoscopically. The excised specimen shows the characteristic knobbly appearance of an inverting papilloma.

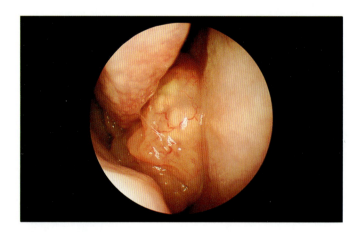

Figure 2.277

Inverting papilloma

This 45-year-old woman presented with a history of bilateral nasal obstruction. Endoscopic examination revealed an irregular polypoid mass arising from the left superior turbinate and extending anteriorly into the nasal cavity.

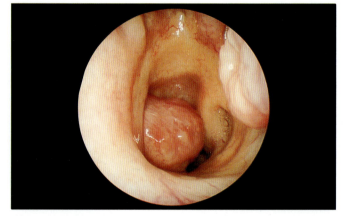

Figure 2.278

Inverting papilloma

The inverting papilloma show in Figure 2.277 also extended through the nasopharynx to enter the right posterior choana.

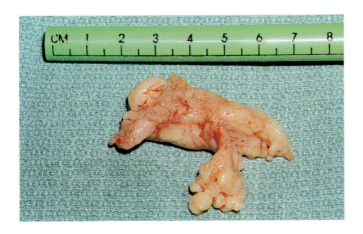

Figure 2.279
Inverting papilloma

The inverting papilloma shown in Figures 2.277 and 2.278 was resected endoscopically.

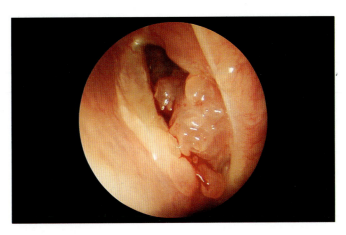

Figure 2.280
Inverting papilloma of the sphenoid sinus

The irregular 'polypoid' growth extending from the ostium of this left sphenoid sinus is an inverting papilloma.

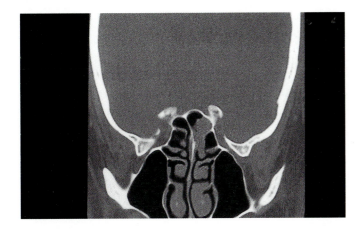

Figure 2.281
Inverting papilloma of the sphenoid sinus

This soft-tissue mass extending into the superior portion of the nasal cavity is an inverting papilloma arising from the mucosa of the left sphenoid sinus.

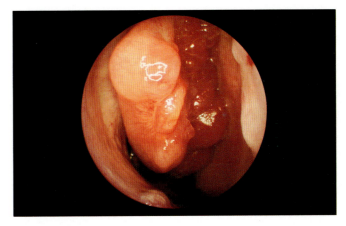

Figure 2.282
Olfactory aesthesioneuroblastoma

The salmon-coloured tumour seen arising from the roof of the nasal cavity and extending medial to this right middle turbinate is an olfactory aesthesioneuroblastoma.

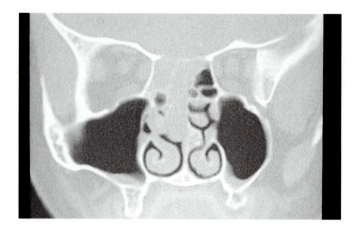

Figure 2.283

Olfactory aesthesioneuroblastoma

The origin of the olfactory aesthesioneuroblastoma from the cribriform plate is shown on this CT scan.

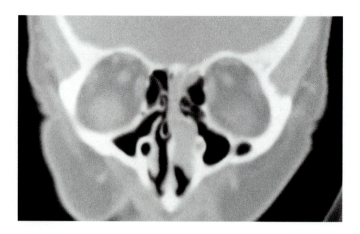

Figure 2.284

Neuroblastoma

This unusual origin of an alleged nasal polyp turned out to be a neuroblastoma, which due to its exclusively extracranial origin was endoscopically resected.

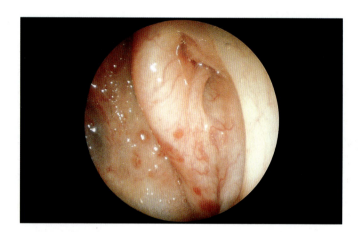

Figure 2.285

Kaposi's sarcoma

The petechial vascular lesions seen around this left tubal ostium turned out to be the early stages of Kaposi's sarcoma in an HIV-positive patient.

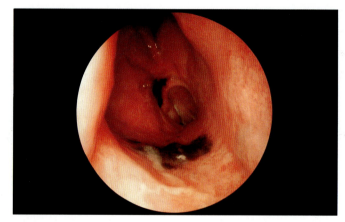

Figure 2.286

Metastatic malignant melanoma

Metastatic spread of a (primary) malignant melanoma of the nasal mucosa towards the choana.

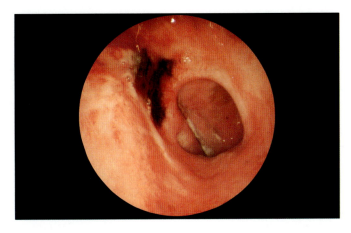

Figure 2.287

Metastatic malignant melanoma

Note the multiple micrometastases, which reach back even to the adenoid area.

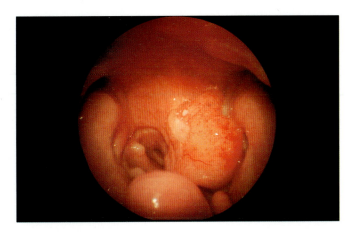

Figure 2.288

Adenoid cystic carcinoma

Unilateral left choanal obstruction caused by an adenoid cystic carcinoma in a 42-year-old woman.

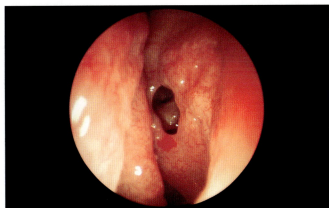

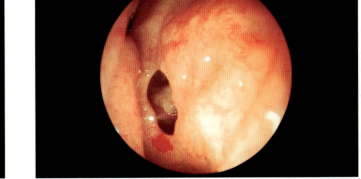

Figure 2.289

Metastatic squamous cell carcinoma

A submucous metastasis of a pulmonary squamous cell carcinoma in the left agger nasi region: open agger cell ostium.

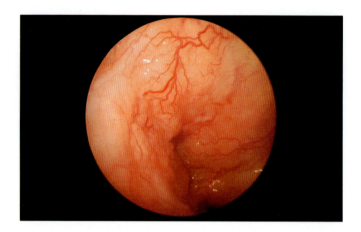

Figure 2.290

Submucosal spread of an adenoid cystic carcinoma

The submucosal spread of an adenoid cystic carcinoma from the left lateral wall of the nasopharynx into the left maxillary sinus.

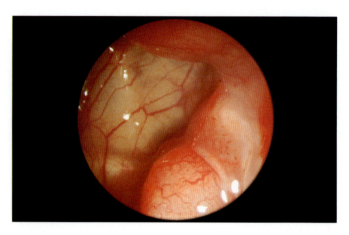

Figure 2.291

Invasive carcinoma

A transitional cell carcinoma has grown from the pterygopalatine fossa into the right maxillary sinus.

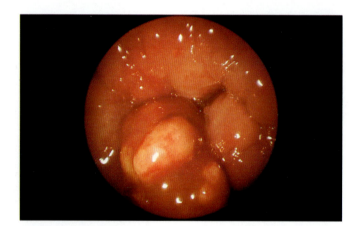

Figure 2.292

Non-Hodgkin's lymphoma

Manifestations in the left maxillary sinus of an anaplastic non-Hodgkin's lymphoma.

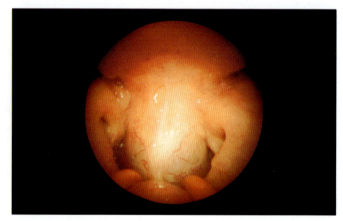

Figure 2.293

Chromophobe adenoma

A large recurrence of a chromophobe adenoma of the pituitary gland blocks both nasal passages.

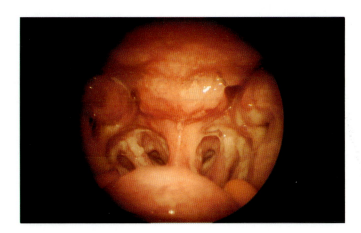

Figure 2.294

Oxyphil adenoma

An oxyphil adenoma in the roof of the nasopharynx. The patient consulted an otorhinolaryngologist because of complaints resulting from a large cyst in the vallecula.

Postoperative appearances

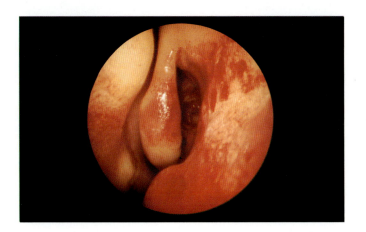

Figure 2.295

Postoperative appearance

The left middle meatus immediately after endoscopic ethmoid surgery.

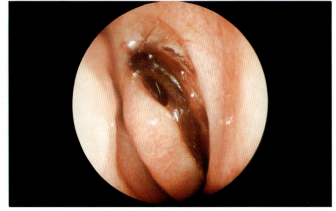

Figure 2.296

Postoperative appearance

The entrance of a left middle meatus 6 days following functional endoscopic sinus surgery (FESS); there is normal healing. The secretions and crust are usually removed 1 week postoperatively.

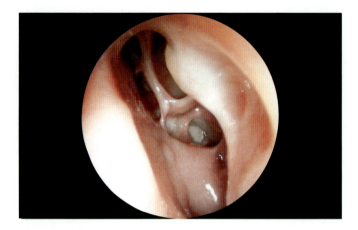

Figure 2.297
Normal postoperative appearance

A view into the left anterior ethmoid, the frontal recess and the frontal sinus 10 weeks after FESS for chronic recurring frontal sinusitis. Even without radical surgery being performed, there is perfect healing of all the areas previously diseased.

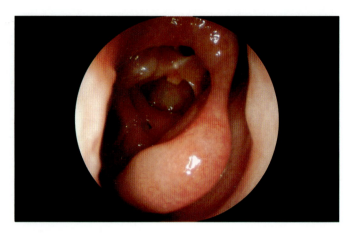

Figure 2.298
Postoperative appearance

A right side showing the status 1 year after FESS. The frontal and maxillary sinuses now have free drainage and ventilation.

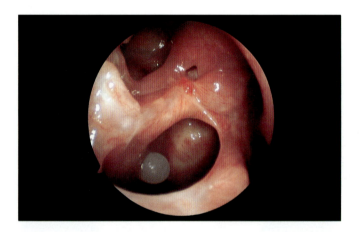

Figure 2.299
Postoperative appearance

A view into a right maxillary sinus through an enlarged natural maxillary sinus ostium, 1 year after endoscopic sinus surgery. A small ball of mucus is being transported out of the sinus. The mucosa is normal and the patient is free of symptoms.

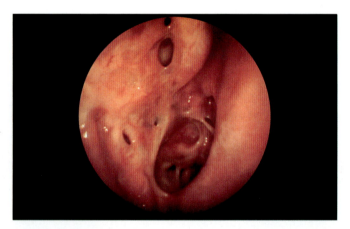

Figure 2.300
Postoperative appearance

A left nasal cavity viewed with a 30° lens, 10 weeks after the endoscopic resection of a neuroblastoma of the olfactory ridge and after gamma knife irradiation.

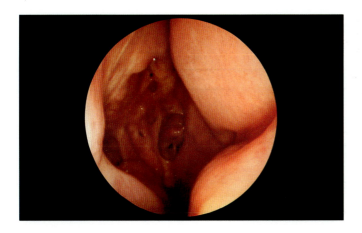

Figure 2.301

Postoperative appearance

The view towards the sphenoid sinus in the patient shown in Figure 2.300.

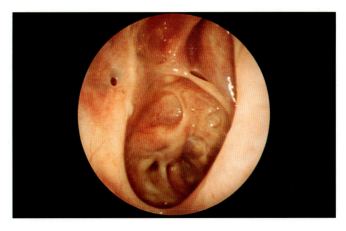

Figure 2.302

Postoperative appearance

A view up toward the frontal recess area in the patient shown in Figures 2.300 and 2.301. The middle and superior turbinates have been resected. The CSF leak resulting from resection of the olfactory plate was patched with lyophilized dura and fibrin glue during the endoscopic resection. There is good healing, no CSF leak and no recurrence of the neuroblastoma.

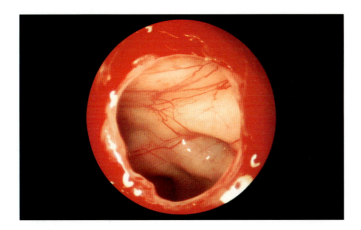

Figure 2.303

Postoperative sphenoid sinus anatomy

The situation after opening the anterior wall of the sphenoid sinus in a case of chronic pansinusitis. The optic nerve and the carotid artery are clearly visible. The mucosa lining the sinus appears to be normal.

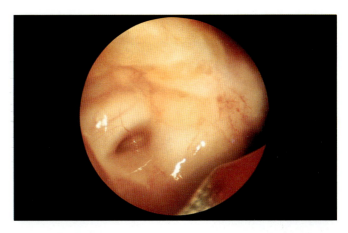

Figure 2.304

Sphenoid sinus

Direct sphenoid sinus endoscopy on a right sphenoid sinus. The optic nerve is visible from 9 o'clock towards the centre, the carotid artery bulges underneath. From 4 to 6 o'clock the lip of the trocar is visible.

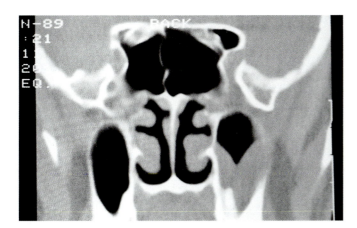

Figure 2.305

The optic nerve in the sphenoid sinus

This coronal CT scan demonstrates an optic nerve travelling 'free' through the left sphenoid sinus. Note the pneumatization lateral to the optic nerve extending into the anterior clinoid process.

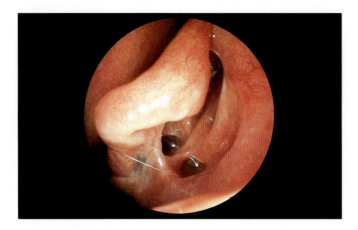

Figure 2.306

Postoperative scarring

A left middle meatus following endoscopic sinus surgery. Some scars have developed, but despite this the patient is free of symptoms. There is a free view into the maxillary sinus.

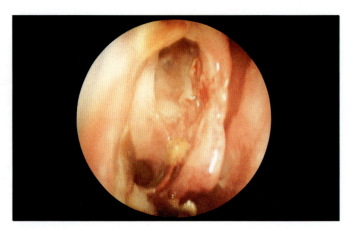

Figure 2.307

Postoperative osteitis

Massive persistent inflammation and granulation following endoscopic sinus surgery. There was an underlying osteitis, which was resolved after resection of the diseased bulla and intravenous antibiotic therapy combined with oral corticosteroids.

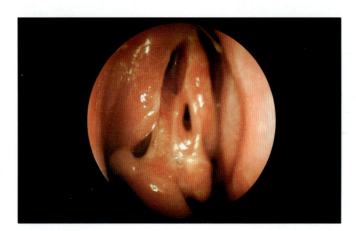

Figure 2.308

Postoperative scarring and distortion of the anatomical structures

This confusing situation was encountered in a patient 10 years after a transmaxillary approach to the ethmoids for chronic sinusitis. The ethmoidal structures and parts have been pushed medially and are scarred and partially fused with the septum. In cases like this, the CT scan and the surgeon's experience must be combined to avoid trouble.

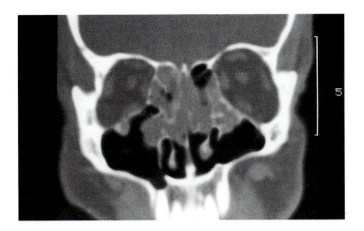

Figure 2.309

Inferior meatal antrostomy window with persistent anterior ethmoid disease

The CT scan of a patient who has undergone bilateral inferior meatal antrostomy (fenestration). The underlying pathology in the ethmoids, which was never treated, is clearly visible.

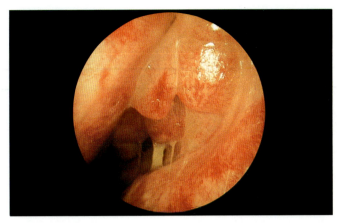

Figure 2.310

Inferior meatal antrostomy window with persistent anterior ethmoid disease

A view into the left middle meatus of the patient shown in Figure 2.309. The uncinate process is visible from 2 to 7 o'clock, and the middle turbinate from 8 to 12 o'clock. Massive polyps arising from the anterior ethmoid are seen in the middle meatus.

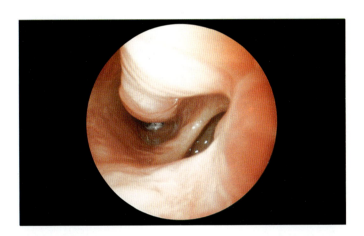

Figure 2.311

Inferior meatal antrostomy

On this left side, the inferior turbinate has been partially resected. Note the inferior meatal window opening into the maxillary sinus.

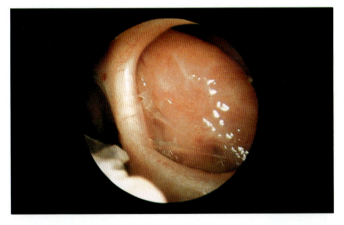

Figure 2.312

Inferior meatal antrostomy

On closer inspection with a 30° lens, massive granulation tissue can be seen in the maxillary sinus despite the wide fenestration.

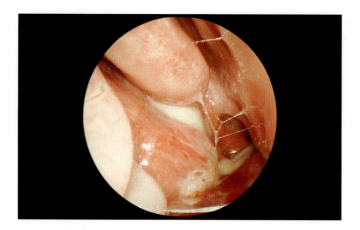

Figure 2.313

Chronic ethmoid sinusitis

The right middle meatus of a patient who continued to suffer from recurrent episodes of sinusitis despite a previous inferior meatal antrostomy and partial resection of the inferior turbinate. Photographed at the time of an acute episode. Polyps, granulation tissue and pus can be seen in the middle meatus. Note how the pus moves directly over the ostium of the Eustachian tube.

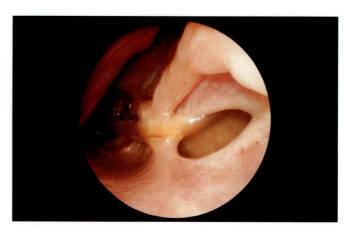

Figure 2.314

Inferior meatal antrostomy

The left side of the patient shown in Figure 2.313. The inferior turbinate has been partially resected and there is a patent inferior meatal window. The maxillary sinus contains a thick, highly viscous mucus, which the patient can only clear with forced inspiration. When looking into the maxillary sinus, the mucus was observed being transported towards the (blocked) natural ostium. There are two forces working on this plug of mucus: the cilia trying to transport it towards the natural ostium and the forces of inspiration trying to pull the mucus into the nasopharynx.

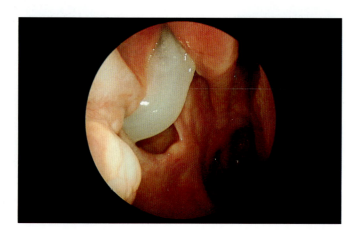

Figure 2.315

Inferior meatal antrostomy

A stream of white thick mucus can be seen recycling through this right maxillary sinus. The mucus leaves the sinus by its natural ostium, exits the hiatus semilunaris, and then slides inferiorly to re-enter the sinus by the inferior meatal window.

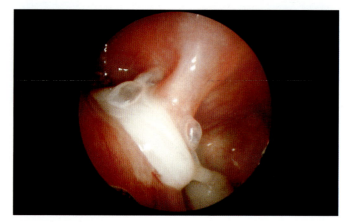

Figure 2.316

Inferior meatal antrostomy

Maxillary sinoscopy via the canine fossa in a patient who had previously undergone a left inferior meatal nasoantral window. Thick white mucopus is being transported up from the floor of the sinus towards its natural ostium (at 10 o'clock). The mucus is unable to leave the sinus via the blocked natural ostium, and after a while gravity causes it to slide back down to the floor of the sinus. Only minor amounts of the mucus leave the sinus through the previously created inferior meatal window, and then the process repeats itself once again.

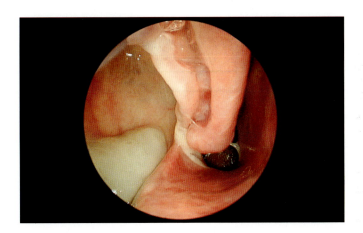

Figure 2.317
Inferior meatal antrostomy

Despite the presence of a wide inferior meatal window, persistent disease within this maxillary sinus caused the accumulation of large amounts of thick green mucus within the sinus cavity, much to the patient's distress.

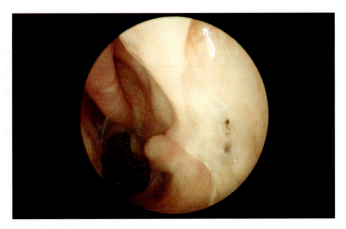

Figure 2.318
Inferior meatal antrostomy

Not all nasoantral windows remain patent, as seen in this patient in whom the inferior meatal antrostomy has stenosed down to two tiny pinholes.

3
The oral cavity

Introduction

The oral cavity, or mouth, is in many ways one of the more important 'organs' of the body. The oral cavity consists of the lips, teeth, gums, oral mucous membranes, palate, tongue and oral lymphoid system (Waldeyer's ring). The mouth plays essential roles in many key bodily functions, including nutrition (mastication and swallowing), respiration and communication. The mouth also provides the individual with a major source of pleasure and gratification.

Numerous different groups may be called upon to diagnose and treat diseases of the oral cavity, including general practitioners, nurse practitioners, dentists, oral surgeons, otorhinolaryngologists, rheumatologists, venereal disease specialists, dermatologists and dermatopathologists. It is important that these specialities all have an adequate knowledge of those diseases of the oral cavity that they are likely to encounter during the course of their practice.

The most important diagnostic tools for the examination of the mouth are the examiner's eyes, aided by a source of illumination (and perhaps also by magnification), a tongue depressor and, when indicated, the use of the technique of palpation by the examiner's glove-covered fingers. As with the examination of any area of the body, the key is the examiner's ability to inspect directly and systematically all areas of the oral cavity. The patient's dentures must be removed not only so that the areas under the dentures can be inspected but also so that the dentures themselves can be examined.

While most diseases of the oral cavity can be diagnosed by visual inspection, some disorders can be perplexing and their diagnosis may be elusive. Over the past decade, a new multidisciplinary approach has been developed to assist in the diagnosis and management of the problem patient: The Mouth Clinic. The Mouth Clinic provides a patient with access to a multidisciplinary team of specialists, all of whom are interested in disorders of the mouth. The specialities represented in a mouth clinic usually include dentistry, oral surgery, otolaryngology, dermatology and pathology.

Photographic technique

Photography of the oral cavity has its own special problems and thus requires suitable equipment. The oral cavity is 'deep and dark' and, as with any area, the photographer must be able to see and illuminate the structure that is to be photographed. A macrolens is required in order to bring the light source (the flash) as close to the subject as possible. A through-the-lens exposure system is most desirable because at least 50% of the light from the flash will not enter the mouth and the calculation of the correct exposure is both highly complicated and empirical. We prefer to use a 35 mm camera with a medical macrolens and a ring light to provide a source of soft white daylight-type illumination that can be brought quite close to the subject matter. The only disadvantage of a ring flash is a lack of surface modelling. For film, we prefer to use a compromise colour transparency film such as Ektachrome Professional 100 or Ektachrome Professional 200. The relatively high speed (100–200 ASA) allows the lens to be set at a relatively high F stop (F 16–F22) for greater depth of field. A through-the-lens exposure system provides great convenience, especially if the photographer has previously taken the time to establish the correct exposure compensation. It is important for the photographer to bracket both the exposure and the focusing.

Special plastic oral retractors are available to retract the lips laterally and thus open the oral cavity for the camera. One disadvantage of such retractors is that their use requires an extra pair of hands (although the extra hands may be the patient's). A laryngeal or dental mirror can be used to photograph the posterior surface of some structures. One must remember that the use of a mirror will cause a lateral reversal of structures.

One of the photographic systems that we have used with great success over the past decade consists of the following.

An Olympus model 2n 35 mm camera is a good example of the previous generation of 35 mm cameras, which measure exposure by reading the amount of light reflected directly off the emulsion or film surface. This 'off the film' or 'OTF' system provides an accurate and reproducible exposure. An Olympus Zuiko 50 mm F3.5 automacrolens is used. For close-up photographs, a 25 mm autoextension tube can be added. The Olympus OM 2n system allows the photographer to change the focusing screen. For macrophotography, a type 1-10 checker mat screen is used. This type of focusing screen, has vertical and horizontal engraved lines, which allow more accurate orientation and alignment of the structure photographed.

The illumination is provided by an Olympus T10 (model 1) ring flash, which is powered by a dedicated electronic flash 'T' power control (model 1). When the correct level of exposure has been reached, the 'OTF' sensor extinguishes the flash. The through-the-lens 'OTF' automatic flash system compensates automatically for changes in magnification and subject distance, thereby allowing a free choice of lens apertures. The 'T' power control has two signal lights, one located on the back of the control panel and the other visible through the camera view finder. These signal lights blink immediately after an exposure to indicate that a correct exposure has been obtained. The T10 ring flash has eight small tungsten illuminators, which (using a separate 6 V portable battery powered pack) provide illumination on the subject for the purpose of composition and focusing.

Lips

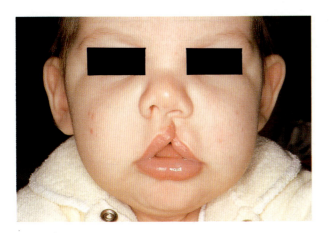

Figure 3.1
Cleft lip

A cleft lip is frequently associated with a cleft palate. Deformities of the nasal tip and of the anterior nasal septum are commonly found in association with a cleft lip. Note the flattening of the right lower lateral cartilage and the deviation of the nasal septum to the patient's left.

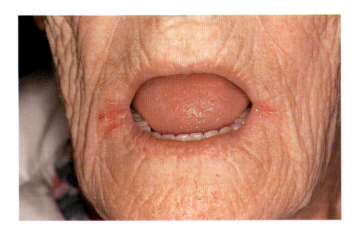

Figure 3.2
Angular cheilitis

The fissures at the corner of the mouth have developed as a result of overclosure of the mouth in a woman with ill-fitting dentures. Local maceration of the skin and a monilial infection at the corner of the mouth produced the angular cheilitis.

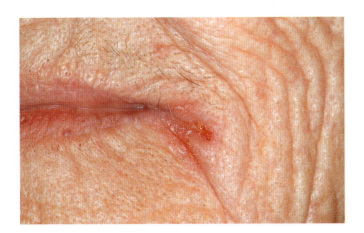

Figure 3.3
Angular cheilitis

A closer view of the patient seen in Figure 3.2.

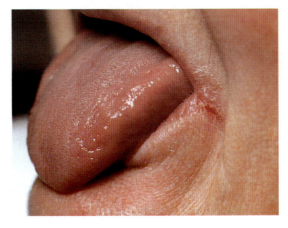

Figure 3.4
Angular cheilitis

The beefy red tongue of atrophic glossitis is seen in association with an angular cheilitis due to iron deficiency anaemia. In this example the 'beefy' appearance is located predominantly on the lateral border of the tongue.

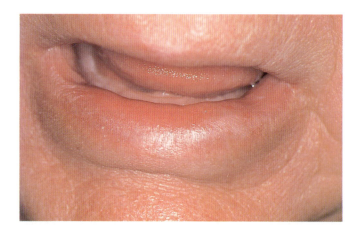

Figure 3.5
Actinic cheilitis

The lower lip has a thinned, white, atrophic epithelium with some pinhead-sized erosive areas. These changes are the result of excessive exposure to sunlight in a fair-skinned person.

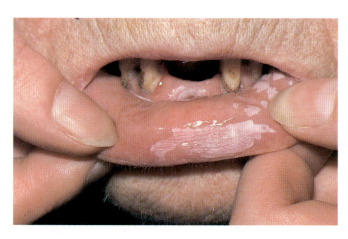

Figure 3.6
Hyperkeratosis of the lip (leukoplakia)

Leukoplakia is the general term used to describe a white patch of the oral cavity that cannot be wiped off and is not susceptible to any other clinical diagnosis. Biopsy is always required to reach a histological diagnosis. Leukoplakia on the vermilion surface of the lip typically arises from excessive exposure to sunlight or from the chronic thermal injury caused by the heat of a pipe stem.

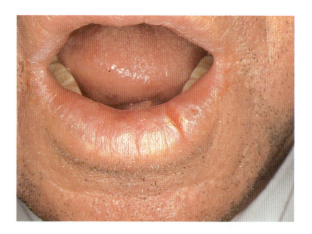

Figure 3.7
Lip fissure

This patient developed a split of the lower lip as a result of exposure to extreme weather. The lips are also dry and white as a result of exposure to the dry atmosphere.

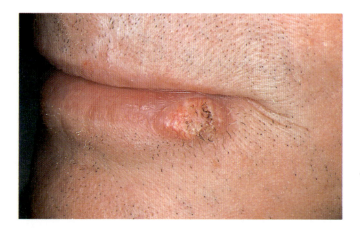

Figure 3.8
Squamous cell carcinoma of the lip

Squamous cell carcinoma of the lip is characterized by a painless, infiltrative and hard ulcer occurring most typically on the lower lip. A high index of suspicion should be maintained for those lip ulcers or nodules that persist for more than a month. This illustration shows a characteristic squamous cell carcinoma.

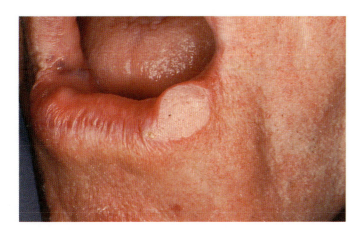

Figure 3.9

Squamous cell carcinoma of the lip

This example of squamous cell carcinoma of the lip shows a more discoid appearance than that shown in Figure 3.8.

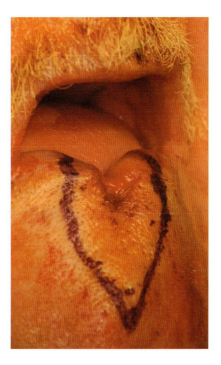

Figure 3.10

Squamous cell carcinoma of the lip

This illustration shows a very indurated ulcer of the lip. This was a squamous cell carcinoma. The yellow discolouration of the lip is due to the antiseptic skin preparation. The outline plan for the wedge excision is shown.

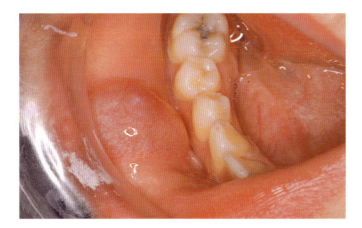

Figure 3.11
Mucocele of the lip

The firm, indentable and somewhat translucent swelling of this lower lip is a mucocele. Prominent blood vessels are commonly seen on the surface of a mucocele.

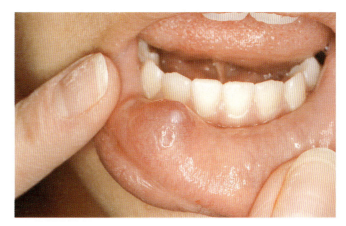

Figure 3.12
Mucocele of the lip

The dome of a large mucocele can be seen elevating the mucosa of the lingual surface of this lower lip.

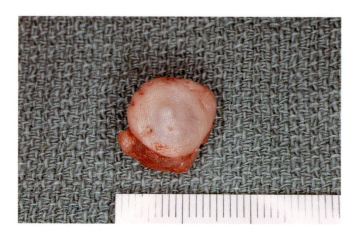

Figure 3.13
Mucocele of the lip

This is the excised mucocele shown in Figure 3.12. The entire mucocele has been removed intact.

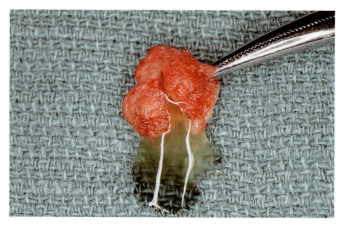

Figure 3.14
Mucocele of the lip

The posterior wall of the mucocele has been incised. Note the thick opalescent mucoid contents, which represent retained secretions of the minor salivary gland from which the mucocele arose.

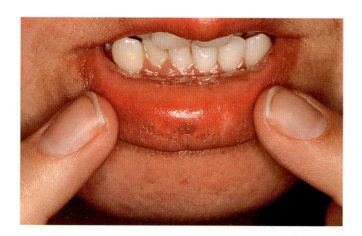

Figure 3.15
Melanonaevus

Pigmented lesions of the lip occur in hereditary haemorrhagic telangiectasia, Peutz-Jegher's syndrome, Addison's disease and in vascular malformations of the lip. In this illustration the pigmented lesion of the lower lip is a simple benign melanonaevus. Such a melanonaevus is not uncommon.

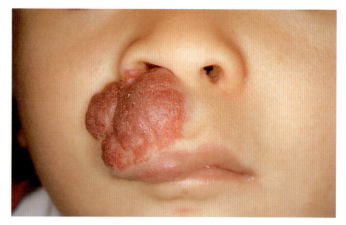

Figure 3.16
Haemangioma

A haemangioma is a congenital vascular abnormality. This child has a strawberry haemangioma of the upper lip. A strawberry haemangioma is raised above the surrounding tissue, blanches on pressure and is the most common type of haemangioma. Most strawberry haemangiomas are capillary in nature and tend to involute spontaneously by the fifth year of age.

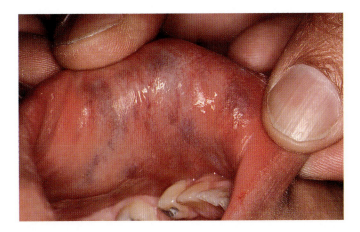

Figure 3.17

Vascular malformation of the lip and palate

Vascular malformations of the lip and palate are rare. In this adult patient the swelling and discolouration of the upper lip are due to a large congenital vascular malformation.

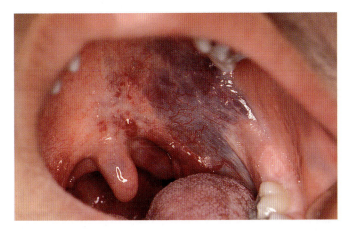

Figure 3.18

Vascular malformation of the lip and palate

This photograph shows the extension of the vascular malformation shown in Figure 3.17 as it extends into the hard and soft palate.

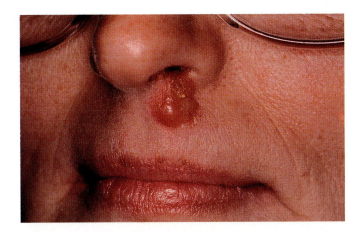

Figure 3.19

Herpes labialis (cold sore)

The cluster of clear vesicles on the lip of this woman is caused by the herpes simplex virus and is known as herpes labialis or cold sore.

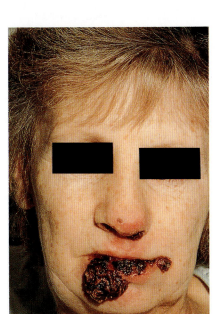

Figure 3.20

Herpes labialis (cold sore)

This is a severe example of herpes labialis that developed in an immuno-compromised patient who was being treated for a non-Hodgkin's lymphoma. Note the presence of vesicles around the nasal vestibule in addition to the large lesion of the lower lip.

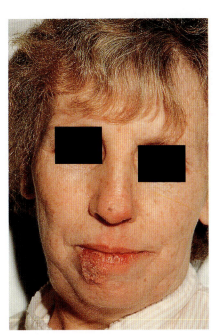

Figure 3.21

Herpes labialis (cold sore)

This photograph shows the response of the severe herpes labialis lesion shown in Figure 3.20 to acyclovir.

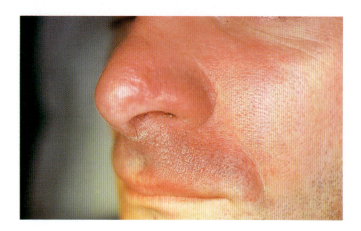

Figure 3.22

Crohn's disease

Swelling of the face and, in particular, the lower lip can develop in oral Crohn's disease and in the related orofacial granulomatosis. Local lymph node obstruction is considered the predisposing pathology. In this atypical example, the red and swollen discolouration of the upper lip shown was caused by Crohn's disease.

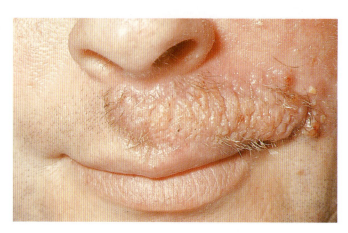

Figure 3.23

Ringworm of the lip

A dermatophytic infection of the skin such as ringworm can affect the lip. The extensive swelling and induration of this upper lip is due to a tinea or ringworm infection.

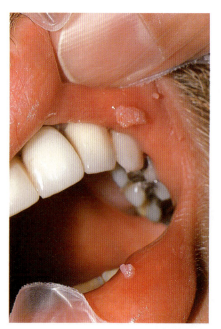

Figure 3.24

Papilloma of the lip

A benign squamous cell papilloma of the lip often has a characteristic warty appearance and is probably of viral origin. The squamous papillomas of these lips were associated with genital warts. (Most papillomas on the lips are not associated with genital warts.)

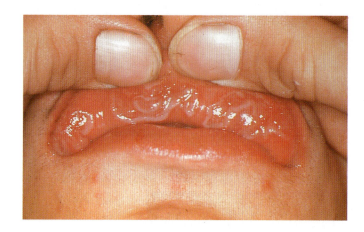

Figure 3.25

Syphilis (secondary mucous patches of the lip)

Oral mucous patches or 'snail track' ulcers are characteristic of secondary syphilis. This patient is everting his own lip to show mucous patches or 'snail tracks' of the upper lip. Such lesions are more commonly seen on the palate.

Teeth

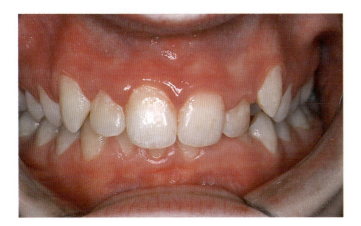

Figure 3.26
Gingivitis

Gingivitis or infection of the gums (gingiva) is common. In this example, marginal gingivitis is shown. The gingival papillae are slightly swollen and have a smooth, shiny, red appearance.

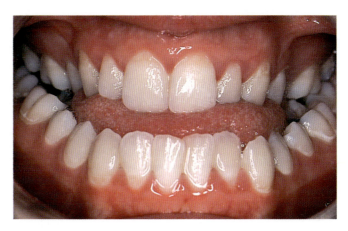

Figure 3.27
Gingivitis

The red, haemorrhagic areas seen in both gums are chronic gingivitis, which resulted from poor oral hygiene in a patient with severe malocclusion. There is marked class III malocclusion, which is caused by a discrepancy in the anteroposterior position of the upper and the lower jaws.

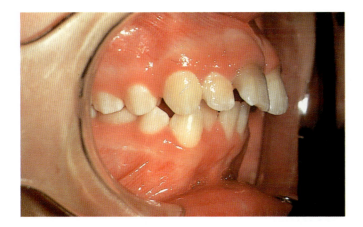

Figure 3.28
Dental malocclusion

This patient with severe nasal obstruction as a result of enlarged adenoids has an unsightly dental malocclusion. The establishment of a clear nasal airway is required before dental correction. Marginal gingivitis is also shown.

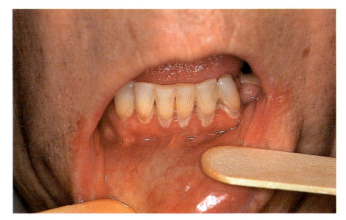

Figure 3.29
Dental caries

Dental caries is the gradual decay and disintegration of a tooth with progressive decalcification of the enamel and dentine. Moderate caries in this adult is visible around the roots of the teeth.

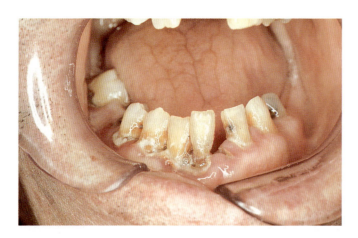

Figure 3.30
Dental calculus

The accumulation of scale or dental calculus around the roots of the teeth is a characteristic feature of poor dental hygiene. Note the associated gingivitis.

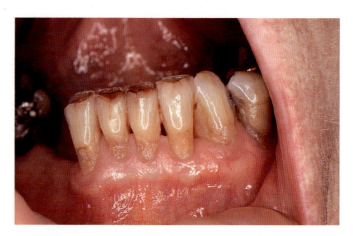

Figure 3.31
Exposed tooth roots

Poor dental hygiene and chronic gingivitis may cause significant erosion of the gingiva. The bone around the roots of this patient's lower teeth has resorbed and as a result the roots are exposed. The result is devitalization and instability of the affected teeth.

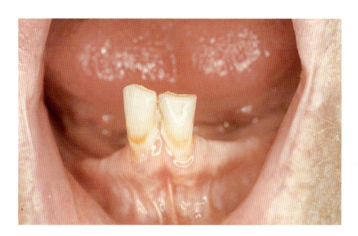

Figure 3.32
Mandibular resorption

The mandible and its teeth appear to have a symbiotic relationship. Note the severe resorption of the mandible that has developed in those areas where there are no longer any teeth.

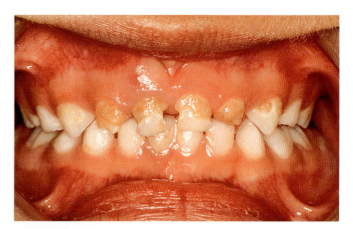

Figure 3.33
Dental caries

This 5-year-old child has widespread decay (caries) of her deciduous dentition caused by frequent ingestion of sugary drinks at night from a feeding bottle (bottle mouth). Dental extraction of the decayed teeth under general anaesthetic was required.

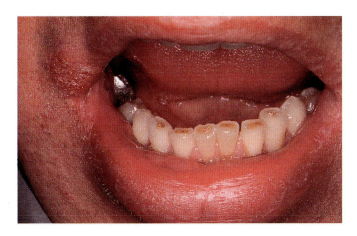

Figure 3.34

Dental abrasion

Dental abrasion is the term used when loss of teeth substance has resulted from extrinsic, usually chronic, trauma. This man always held his pipe in the right-hand side of his mouth and this has worn down the crowns of those teeth that gripped his pipe.

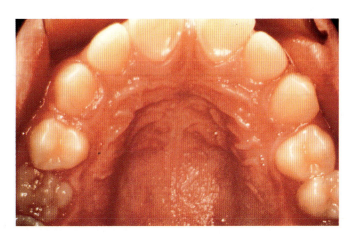

Figure 3.35

Dental erosion

This patient regularly drank large quantities of a well-known 'fizzy' drink, the acid content of which caused erosion of the palatal aspect of her upper front teeth. The hollowing-out of these teeth is pathognomonic.

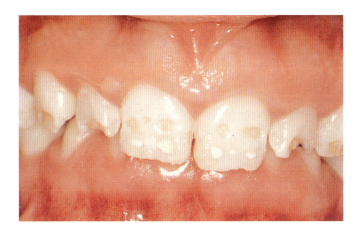

Figure 3.36

Dental hypoplasia

This 14-year-old girl suffered measles as an infant. The rubella infection interfered with the formation of that portion of her permanent teeth that was actively being developed at the time of the illness. Thus the earlier-forming upper central incisors are affected halfway down the crown, whereas the later-forming lateral incisors are affected at the tip. Veneers (porcelain facings) are required to improve the appearance of these teeth.

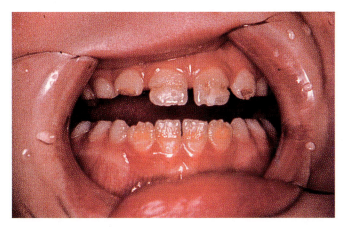

Figure 3.37

Enamel hypoplasia

Marked enamel hypoplasia gives rise to the pitting and the poor cosmetic appearance of these teeth.

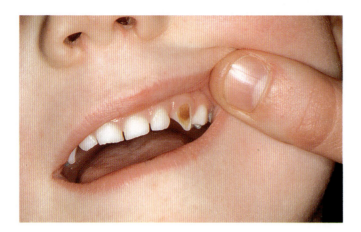

Figure 3.38
Discoloured teeth

Local trauma such as a fall onto or a blow to a tooth can result in devitalization and an alteration in colour. Trauma to this child's left upper incisor has resulted in local discolouration.

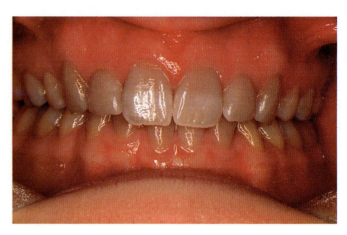

Figure 3.39
Tetracycline staining

This patient was prescribed systemic tetracycline during the period when her tooth buds were forming. This has resulted in discolouration of the permanent teeth. The tetracycline antibiotic group should be avoided in children under 10 years of age.

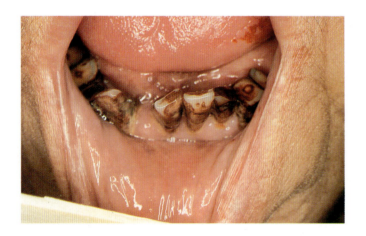

Figure 3.40
Betel nut stain

In some countries the chewing of a mixture composed of betel nuts, tobacco and slaked lime is a popular pastime. The black staining of the lower teeth in this photograph has arisen from that habit. Betel nuts are carcinogenic to the oral mucous membranes.

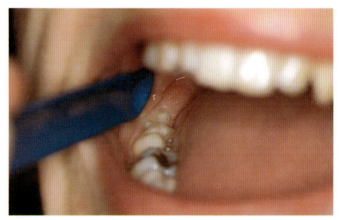

Figure 3.41
Molar tooth eruption

As a molar tooth erupts, the overlying mucosa can be seen to thin and retreat. The third lower molar or wisdom tooth can be seen erupting from the lower jaw of this patient.

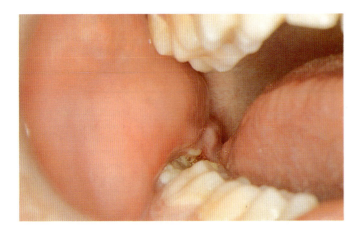

Figure 3.42

Pericornitis: lower third molar

The thinning mucosal flap overlying an erupting third molar tooth has been traumatized recurrently by an upper molar tooth. This is termed 'pericornitis'. Treatment may require the removal of the upper tooth.

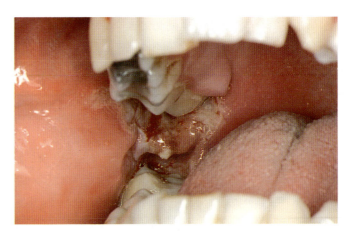

Figure 3.43

Pericornitis: upper molar

Pericornitis can also affect an upper molar. This example shows severe trauma to the mucosa of the upper molar, and the cusp of the tooth can be seen protruding through the damaged mucosa.

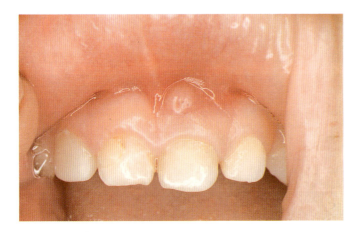

Figure 3.44

Dental abscess

A pyogenic abscess can develop in relation to the root of a tooth. Where such a dental abscess presents depends on the local anatomy. In this example the swelling overlying the root of the upper incisor tooth is characteristic of a periapical abscess of that tooth.

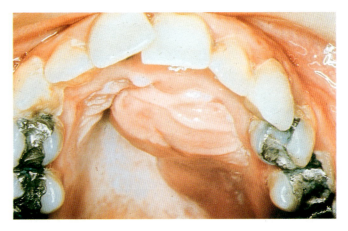

Figure 3.45

Dental abscess

An abscess of the left upper lateral incisor has tracked posteriorly and presented as a swelling of the palate. The most characteristic place for such an abscess to present is at the junction between the soft and hard palate.

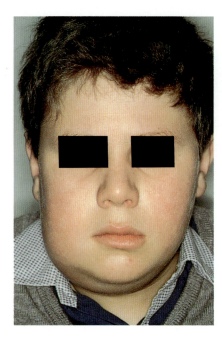

Figure 3.46
Dental abscess (molar tooth abscess)

The swelling of the lower right-hand side of this young man's face is pathognomonic of a molar tooth abscess.

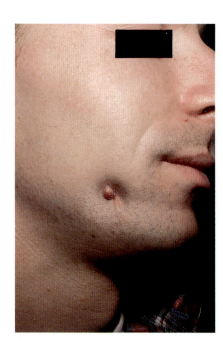

Figure 3.47
Dental abscess (facial sinus)

When infection from a dental abscess localizes either as a result of antibiotic therapy or spontaneously, an external sinus can develop. Such a sinus, when established, can be a source of misdiagnosis. The nodule on the cheek of this man could be mistaken for a cutaneous tumour.

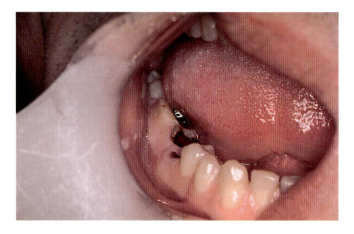

Figure 3.48
Dental abscess (facial sinus)

This is the intraoral picture of the patient with the facial sinus shown in Figure 3.47. There is an abscess of the root of the first lower molar, which tracked out into the cheek.

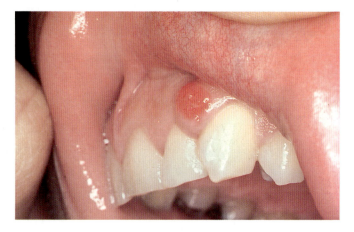

Figure 3.49
Epulides (pyogenic granuloma)

The gingival tissues are very prone to develop exuberant inflammatory overgrowths (epulides). These overgrowths are often found to contain immature, vascular granulation tissue. The type of epulis is named according to a combination of its histological and aetiological factors. Pregnancy increases the predisposition to form an epulis. In this example an infective aetiology is proposed and the lesion is termed a pyogenic granuloma. The smooth pink swelling with the central area of protruding granulation tissue is the pyogenic granuloma.

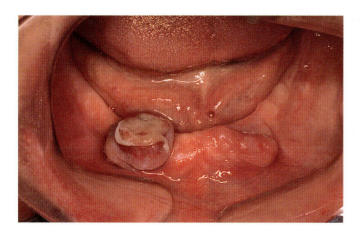

Figure 3.50
Epulides (pyogenic granuloma)

This pyogenic granuloma has a larger and more purple appearance. The histology showed immature, vascular granulation tissue.

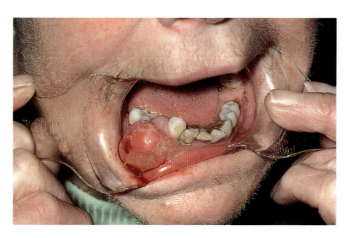

Figure 3.51
Epulides (fibrous)

The differentiation of the name of this purple, swollen lesion arising from the gingivae is based on its histology. The granulation tissue in this case was less vascular and the lesion contained more fibrous tissue than that of the pyogenic granulomas shown in Figures 3.49 and 3.50.

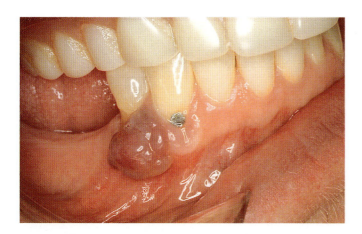

Figure 3.52
Epulides (peripheral giant cell granuloma)

The red-to-purplish swelling on the lower gingivae was diagnosed as a peripheral giant cell granuloma by the demonstration of osteoclast-like giant cells on histological examination. The exclusion of hyperparathyroidism in this situation is required.

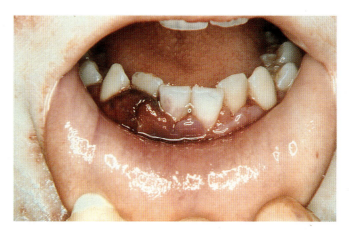

Figure 3.53
Gingival infiltration (leukaemia)

Enlargement and inflammation of the gingivae can occur during the hormonal changes of puberty or pregnancy. Drugs such as phenytoin, cyclosporin and nifedipine can all produce gingival hypertrophy. Arguably the most important diagnosis to recognize, however, is that which occurs when a leukaemia infiltrates the gingivae (leukaemic infiltration). The bluish haemorrhagic infiltration of these lower gingivae is due to an acute myelomonocytic leukaemia.

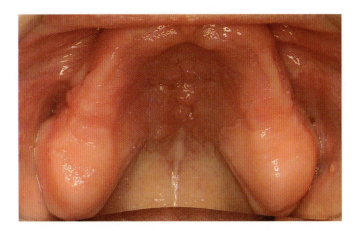

Figure 3.54
Denture granuloma

An ill-fitting denture can cause recurrent local trauma and irritation of the mucosa of the mouth. This chronic irritation can incite a connective tissue response to the trauma producing a local overgrowth of tissue. In this first example, there is a polypoid thickening of the upper gingival soft tissue combined with an excess of tissue in the midline of the palate. This patient also has very large maxillary tuberosities.

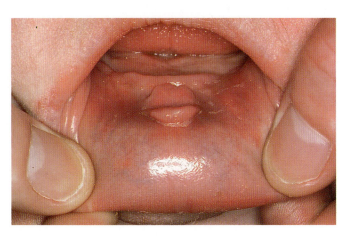

Figure 3.55
Denture granuloma

The flange of organized granulation tissue protruding from the middle of the base of the lower lip/gingival margin was caused by a loose-fitting denture. Removal of the granulation tissue combined with a refit of the dentures is required.

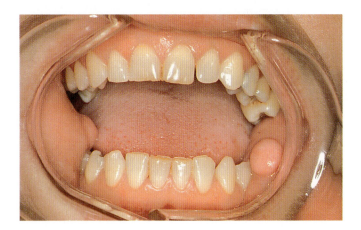

Figure 3.56
Fibroepithelial polyp

The smooth, pink, sessile, benign polyps at each corner of this patient's mouth (commissure) are fibroepithelial polyps. They have arisen because of chronic, mild frictional trauma from the teeth. Fibroepithelial polyps sometimes have a white surface.

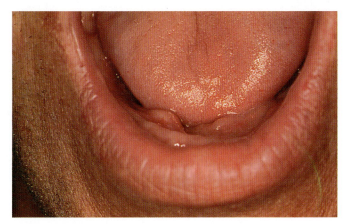

Figure 3.57
Torus mandibularis

A torus mandibularis is a smooth, hard, bony swelling that protrudes characteristically from the lingual surface of the mandible in the premolar region. A torus mandibularis is composed of compact lamellar bone. The two smooth, bony protuberances arising from the mandible and pointed to by the tip of the tongue are tori. The edentulous lower mandible can also be seen.

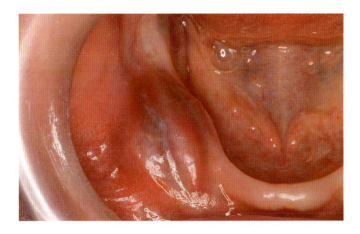

Figure 3.58

Odontogenic keratocyst

An odontogenic keratocyst is a keratin-containing cyst that most commonly occurs at the angle of the mandible. This example shows a characteristic smooth and slightly indentable swelling of the lower mandible. Such cysts, when they occur in the maxilla, are more likely to rupture and discharge keratin.

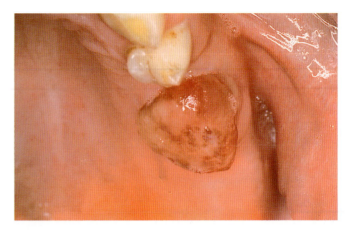

Figure 3.59

Antral mucosal prolapse through a tooth socket

Sometimes after the extraction of an upper tooth, particularly a molar, a fistula can arise between the mouth and the maxillary sinus. Antral mucosa can then prolapse through the fistula producing a smooth, pink, compressible swelling protruding from a tooth socket, as shown in this illustration.

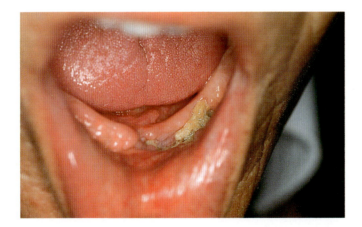

Figure 3.60

Exposed mandible from radiotherapy necrosis

This patient received extensive radiotherapy to treat a squamous cell carcinoma of the left tonsil. The patient developed osteoradionecrosis of the mandible, which was subsequently revealed when the mucosa over the edentulous lower mandible broke down and a piece of necrotic bone was exposed.

Mucosal surfaces

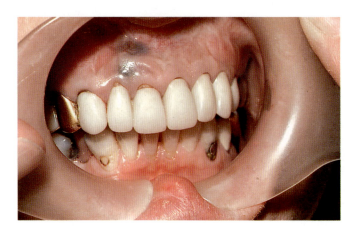

Figure 3.61
Amalgam tattoo

The blue discolouration of the gingiva developed following some recent dental work in which an adjacent tooth was filled with dental amalgam. Occasionally, isolated amalgam spots can be mistaken for an intradermal melanonaevus or even for a small melanoma. A dental radiograph will often demonstrate calcification in an amalgam tattoo.

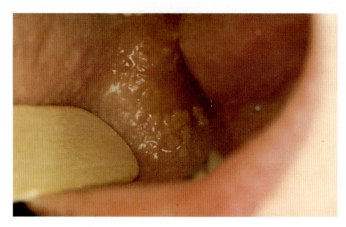

Figure 3.62
Fordyce spots

The yellow, slightly raised spots demonstrated on the inner mucosal surface of the cheek are prominent but normal sebaceous glands known as Fordyce spots. This is a normal finding.

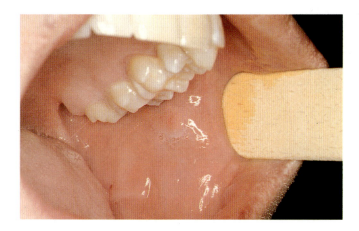

Figure 3.63
Parotid duct papilla

The parotid duct opens into the oral cavity through the buccal mucosa approximately opposite the second upper molar. The raised area with the central red section at the distal end of the wooden spatula is a normal parotid duct papilla.

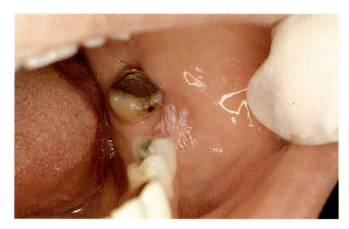

Figure 3.64
Leukoplakia (buccal)

Leukoplakia is the term used for a white patch on the oral mucosa that cannot be wiped off and is not susceptible to any other clinical diagnosis. A biopsy is always required to reach a histological diagnosis and to exclude malignancy. Regular review and often repeated biopsy is required when the initial biopsy is negative for malignancy. A number of examples of leukoplakia will be shown. It is considered that patches of leukoplakia with a slightly speckled appearance, with an associated erythroplasia or with associated candidal hyphae have the greatest premalignant potential. The example above shows an area of leukoplakia on the buccal reflection of the lower jaw. The slightly red appearance surrounding this lesion increases the possibility for malignant transformation.

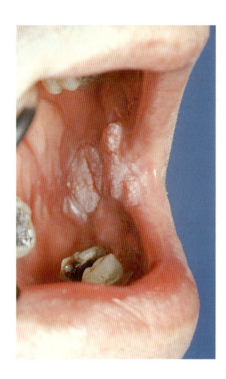

Figure 3.65

Leukoplakia
(speckled)

The two areas of
leukoplakia on the
buccal mucosa of
this patient have a
slightly speckled
appearance, which
increases 'malignant
potential'.

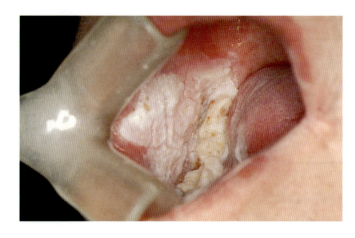

Figure 3.66

Leukoplakia (buccal)

This example shows a fairly extensive plaque of leukoplakia
involving the buccal mucosa.

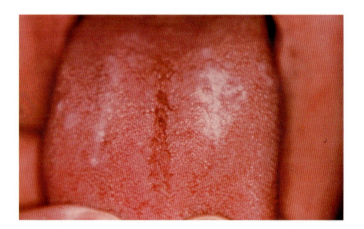

Figure 3.67

Leukoplakia (lingual)

Areas of hyperkeratosis/leukoplakia can be seen on the dorsum of
this tongue. Marked hyperkeratosis was found at histology.

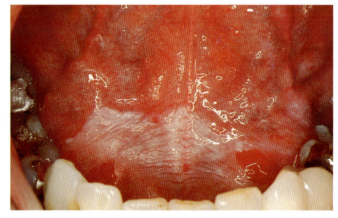

Figure 3.68

Leukoplakia (sublingual)

A large area of sublingual keratosis is visible.

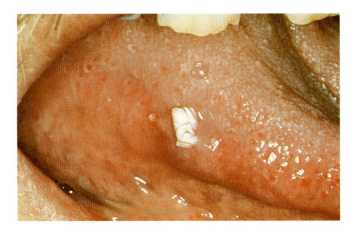

Figure 3.69

Leukoplakia (lingual keratosis)

A small keratotic papilloma can be seen on the lateral border of this tongue. This was shown on histological examination to be a severely dysplastic squamous papilloma.

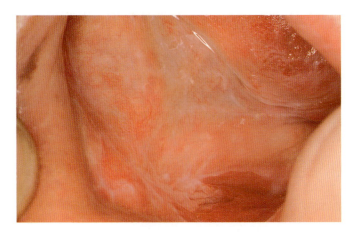

Figure 3.70

Erythroplakia (floor of mouth)

The area of leukoplakia on the left floor of the mouth in this patient has red areas interspersed throughout the lesion. These red areas give rise to the name 'erythroplakia'. The malignant potential of erythroplakia is greater than that of leukoplakia.

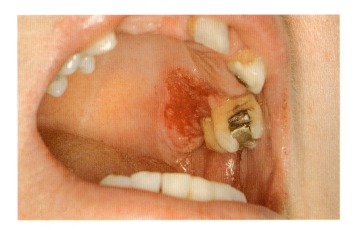

Figure 3.71

Erythroplakia (carcinoma in situ)

This patient had an area of leukoplakia visible on the hard palate, which developed over several years into erythroplakia. The red ulcerative area now seen on the hard palate was found to be a carcinoma in situ at the latest biopsy.

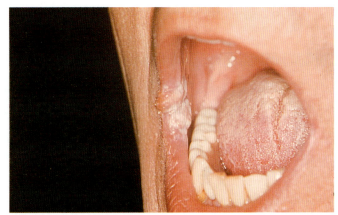

Figure 3.72

Leukoplakia (candidal)

The white heaped-up lesion at the corner of the mouth is an area of chronic hyperplastic epithelium infiltrated with candidal hyphae. The causal relationship between the leukoplakia and the candidal infection is unknown. These lesions are more likely to undergo malignant transformation than leukoplakia without *Candida*.

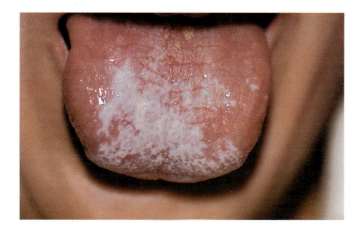

Figure 3.73

Leukoplakia (candidal)

In this patient an area of leukoplakia has developed on the dorsum of the tongue. Candidal hyphae were seen in the histological specimen. There is not a reliable clinical appearance that enables the examiner to differentiate between candidal and non-candidal leukoplakia. Histology, as always, is the critical diagnostic factor. Compare this illustration with Figure 3.67.

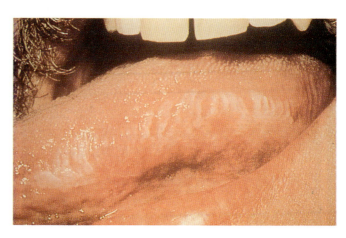

Figure 3.74

Leukoplakia (hairy leukoplakia)

Hairy leukoplakia is characteristically a white, slightly raised lesion with a corrugated surface. The lesion can be found throughout the oral cavity, but is most common along the lateral margins of the tongue and on the buccal surface of the cheek. Hairy leukoplakia is diagnostic of AIDS. The white ridged area shown along the lateral border of this tongue is hairy leukoplakia.

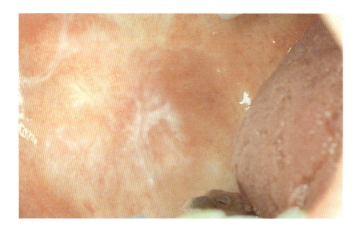

Figure 3.75

Lichen planus (non-erosive, buccal mucosa)

Lichen planus is a relatively common inflammatory disease of the oral mucous membranes, which may result either from local abnormalities of immune function or as a drug reaction. There is a wide range of appearances of lichen planus in the mouth ranging from a non-erosive variety through minor erosive to a major erosive type. The variation in appearance of non-erosive lichen planus with its characteristic white lace-like reticulations can be seen in this illustration as well as in Figures 3.76 and 3.77.

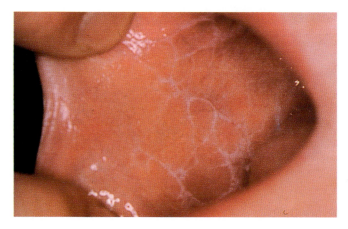

Figure 3.76

Lichen planus (non-erosive, buccal mucosa)

There is an area of non-erosive lichen planus on the buccal mucosa of this patient.

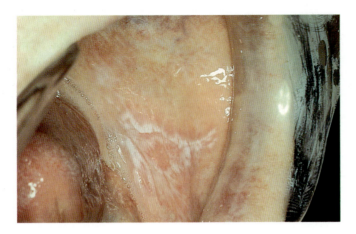

Figure 3.77

Lichen planus (non-erosive, buccal mucosa)

Another area of non-erosive lichen planus on the buccal mucosa of this patient.

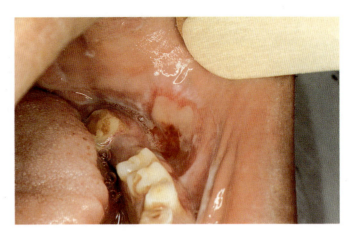

Figure 3.78

Lichen planus (minor erosive)

There has been a loss of the atrophic areas of the epithelium to form a shallow ulcer. The white reticulations can be seen surrounding the ulcer.

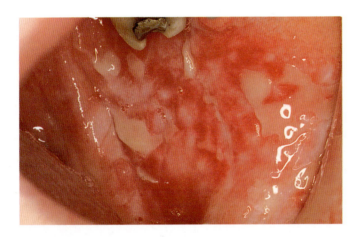

Figure 3.79

Lichen planus (major erosive)

In the major erosive variety of lichen planus, well-defined areas of extensive ulceration of sudden onset are characteristically seen on the buccal mucosa (this illustration) and also along the lateral border of the tongue as shown in Figure 3.80.

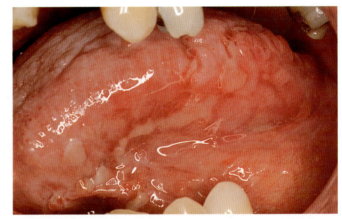

Figure 3.80

Lichen planus (major erosive)

This photograph shows a large ulcer along the lateral border of the tongue, which has arisen from acute-onset lichen planus.

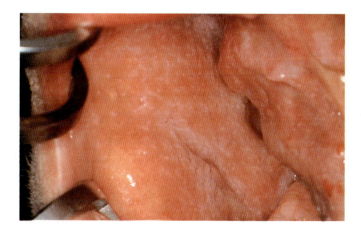

Figure 3.81

Darier's disease

A number of genetically determined disorders can produce white lesions of the oral mucosa. The white cobblestone appearance of the buccal mucosa in this patient is the result of Darier's disease, an inherited disorder of keratinization.

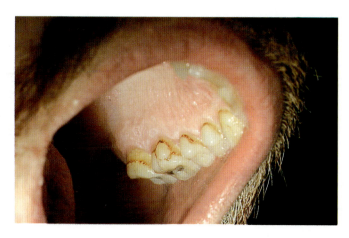

Figure 3.82

Darier's disease

The pale papules on the hard palate and along the gingival margin of this patient are also characteristic of Darier's disease.

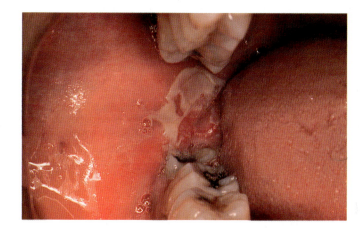

Figure 3.83

Aspirin burn (buccal sulcus)

One white but sometimes misdiagnosed condition of the mouth is an aspirin burn. The patient, as in this example, has pain in a tooth and holds an aspirin tablet next to the tooth in an effort to alleviate the ache. A white slough ulcer results.

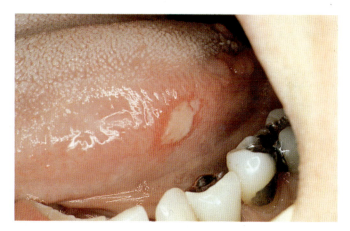

Figure 3.84

Aphthous stomatitis (aphthous ulcers)

Aphthous stomatitis is characterized by recurrent 'crops' of superficial ulcerations of the oral mucosa. The aetiology of this condition is unknown. These acute lesions are well demarcated with a yellow fibrin-covered base surrounded by a red halo. The white and extremely uncomfortable ulcer on the lateral border of this tongue is an aphthous ulcer. The characteristic erythematous surround to the ulcer is demonstrated well in this illustration.

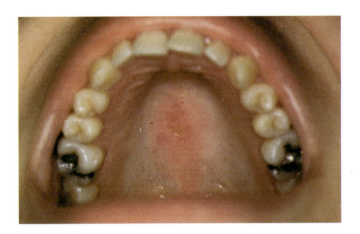

Figure 3.85

Aphthous ulcer (palatal ulcer)

A very painful aphthous ulcer has arisen in the centre of the hard palate. The white fibrinous base is not well shown. Eating was extremely uncomfortable.

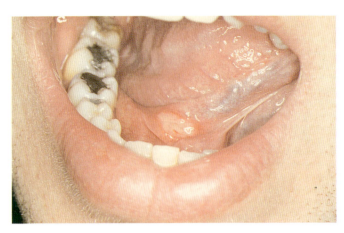

Figure 3.86

Aphthous ulcer (healing)

This sublingual aphthous ulcer is in the healing stage. Small areas of red, where the oral mucosa is regenerating, can be seen through the white slough of the ulcer. At this stage the ulcer is no longer acutely painful.

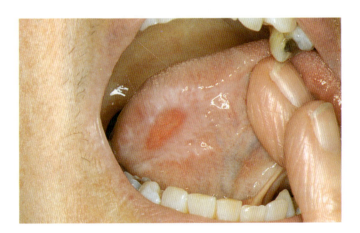

Figure 3.87

Solitary giant aphthous ulcer

The giant aphthous ulcer is usually bigger than the multiple aphthous ulcer and can be greater than 1 cm in diameter. The red and large deep ulcer in the side of this patient's tongue is a giant aphthous ulcer. Pain was not particularly severe; however, this ulcer required several weeks to heal.

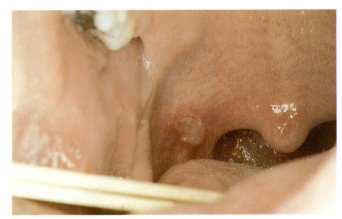

Figure 3.88

Solitary giant aphthous ulcer

The large solitary ulcer visible on the upper part of the right tonsil pillar is a persistent giant aphthous ulcer.

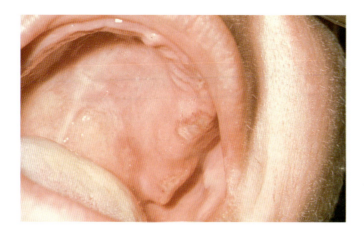

Figure 3.89

Behçet's syndrome

A number of ulcers indistinguishable from aphthous ulcers are visible on the palate (particularly the edentulous upper jaw) of this patient. The patient also had genital ulcers and suffered from Behçet's syndrome. Other associations with this syndrome include arthropathy and vasculitic problems.

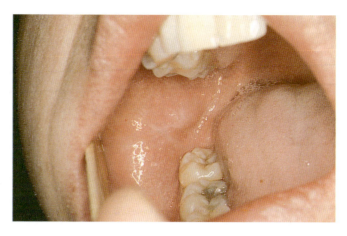

Figure 3.90

Cheek bite (traumatic factitious ulceration)

Some people, particularly those with a nervous disposition, chew the buccal mucosa with their molar teeth. This can result in an ulcer or more commonly a small white frictional area. The white area above the lower molar tooth in this illustration is the result of regular chewing of the buccal mucosa.

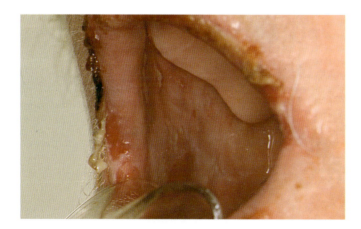

Figure 3.91

Pemphigus

Pemphigus is an autoimmune condition in which widespread fragile bullous lesions can develop in the mouth. Using immunofluorescent studies, IgG class antibodies can be found binding to the intercellular structures and to the cell walls of the stratum spinosum. In this example a large intraoral bulla can be seen. There has been breakdown of a bulla at the corner of the mouth.

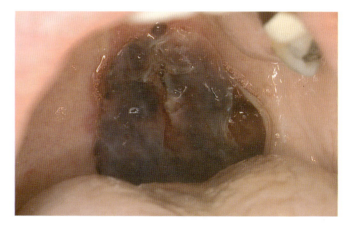

Figure 3.92

Benign mucous membrane pemphigoid

Pemphigoid occurs in two principal forms: a predominantly cutaneous form and a predominantly mucosal form. Subepithelial blisters develop associated with the deposition of IgG class antibodies along the basal zone. These oral bullae break down easily to leave large eroded areas, particularly on the palate. Benign mucous membrane pemphigoid represents a particular form of pemphigoid. The large bullae of benign mucous membrane pemphigoid can be seen on this hard palate.

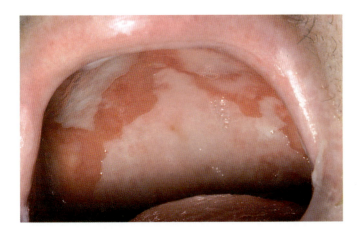

Figure 3.93

Benign mucous membrane pemphigoid

This illustration shows the more typical appearance of benign mucous membrane pemphigoid after the oral bullae have disintegrated leaving, particularly on the palate, large eroded areas. The erythematous areas are the abnormality.

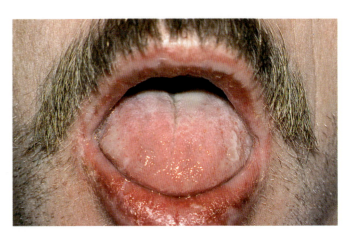

Figure 3.94

Stevens–Johnson syndrome (erythema multiforme)

Stevens–Johnson syndrome is an immunologically mediated syndrome comprising the triad of cutaneous lesions (erythema multiforme), stomatitis and conjunctivitis. This illustration shows the typical crusted, swollen and haemorrhagic appearance of the lips in Stevens–Johnson syndrome. An intact vesicle is visible on the left side of the tongue.

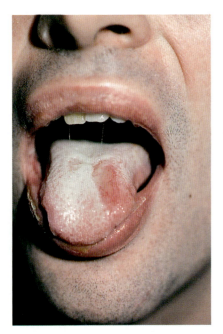

Figure 3.95

Stevens–Johnson syndrome (erythema multiforme)

Within the oral cavity, intact vesicles are unusual and widespread sloughing lesions with poorly defined margins are more commonly seen. A typical tongue ulcer is shown.

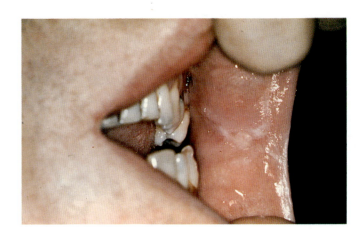

Figure 3.96

Stevens–Johnson syndrome (erythema multiforme)

An example of a developing buccal vesicle in Stevens–Johnson syndrome is shown.

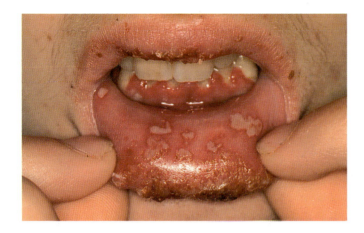

Figure 3.97

Herpetic gingivostomatitis

Herpetic gingivostomatitis is the gingival and oral response to a herpes simplex infection. In this teenage patient the characteristic ulcers on the lips and an intense painful inflammation of the gingivae can be seen.

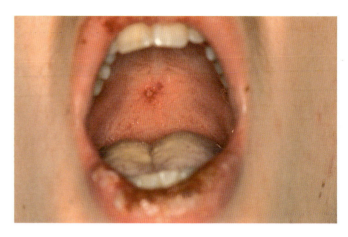

Figure 3.98

Herpetic gingivostomatitis

In herpetic gingivostomatitis, there are often multiple shallow painful ulcers within the oral cavity, particularly on the palate. This illustration is of the same patient as shown in Figure 3.97 and shows an isolated shallow painful ulcer of the palate.

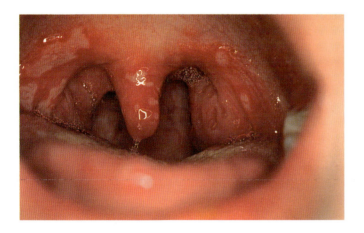

Figure 3.99

Herpetic gingivostomatitis

In this variation of herpetic gingivostomatitis, extensive shallow, confluent, soft palate ulcers can be seen.

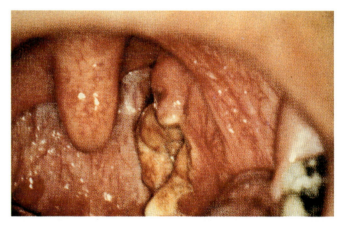

Figure 3.100

Acute necrotizing ulcerative pharyngitis (Vincent's angina)

Acute necrotizing ulcerative pharyngitis is an acute non-communicable inflammatory disease of the pharynx, which results from an infection by Vincent's organisms: *Borrelia vincentii* and *Fusobacterium nucleatum*. A yellow slough can be seen on the surface of the left tonsil, which is characteristic of Vincent's angina.

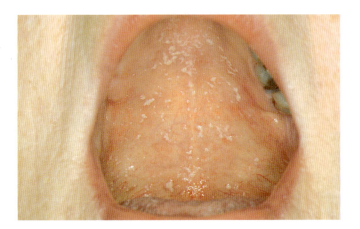

Figure 3.101
Candida

Candida species are effectively a commensal in the normal mouth. Any loss of immunological competence can result in an acute pseudomembranous candidiasis (thrush) of the mouth. There is, however, a wide range of appearances to this condition. In this illustration of mild thrush, a number of small white curds can be seen on the hard palate.

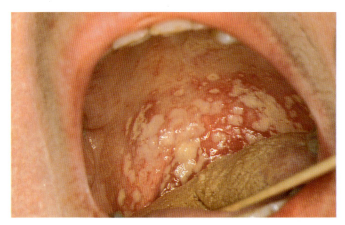

Figure 3.102
Candida

This illustration shows a more aggressive form of thrush with more extensive curd-like patches associated with an underlying painful erythema of the palate.

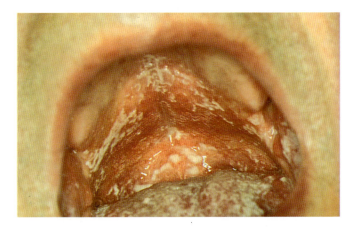

Figure 3.103
Candida

In this example of candidiasis the erythema has become more prominent than the curd-like lesions. In this patient, lymphoma predisposed to the development of candidiasis.

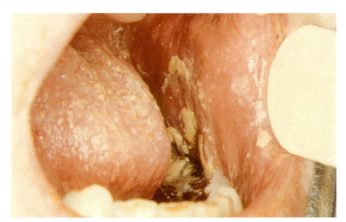

Figure 3.104
Candida

The 'curds' of *Candida* have become heaped up on the buccal mucosa of this patient.

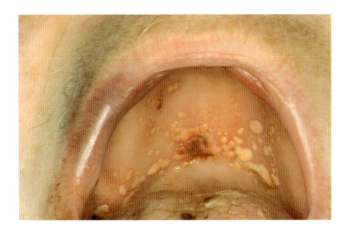

Figure 3.105

Candida (denture candidiasis)

Candida can often develop under a loose-fitting edge of a denture as shown in this illustration. The denture has been removed to reveal the very precise line of demarcation. It is important to use antifungal agents on both the dentures and the mouth to alleviate such oral candidiasis. This patient had acute myeloid leukemia, which predisposed to the candidal infection.

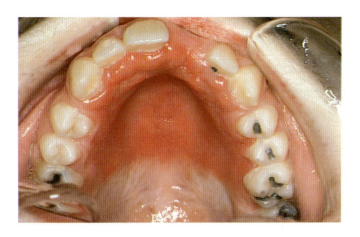

Figure 3.106

Candida (denture sore mouth)

This is a painless condition that develops under dentures that have been worn fairly continuously. The fiery red appearance, as demonstrated in this illustration, gives rise to the other inappropriate name for this condition of 'denture sore mouth'.

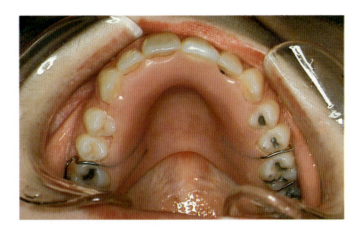

Figure 3.107

Candida (denture sore mouth)

This illustration shows the patient wearing the denture that caused the problem depicted in Figure 3.106.

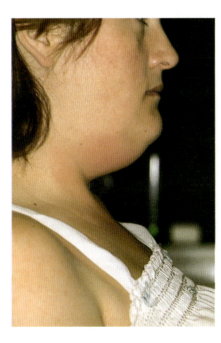

Figure 3.108

Ludwig's angina (floor of mouth cellulitis)

Ludwig's angina is an infection of the floor of the mouth, which results in cellulitis and swelling of the submandibular space. The floor of the mouth is extremely oedematous with posterosuperior elevation of the tongue. In this example the swelling is easily visible in the area under the chin, where there is also erythema that marks the extending cellulitis.

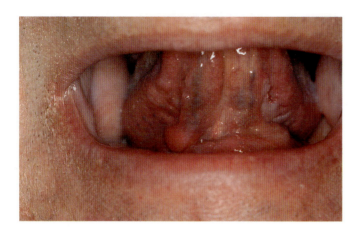

Figure 3.109
Squamous cell carcinoma (sublingual)

Squamous cell carcinoma presents as a number of shapes and sizes within the oral cavity. It may present as an indurated ulcer, as a nodule or arise from an area of leukoplakia or erythroplakia. Any ulcer within the oral cavity that does not heal within 1 month should be biopsied to exclude malignancy. This example shows a sublingual squamous cell carcinoma. The grey area on the left undersurface of the tongue is the tumour. This patient presented with neck nodes and the primary tumour was difficult to identify.

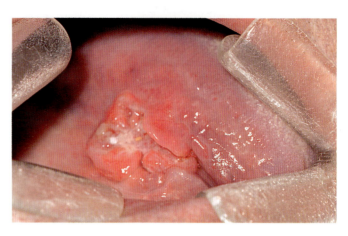

Figure 3.110
Squamous cell carcinoma (sublingual)

This example shows a more characteristic sublingual/floor of mouth squamous carcinoma. Note the typical raised and ulcerated mass.

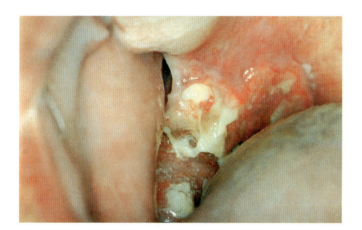

Figure 3.111
Squamous cell carcinoma (coffin corner)

There is an ulcerating and infiltrating squamous cell carcinoma developing behind the last lower molar tooth. This area is known as 'coffin corner' and is a site easily overlooked in clinical examination.

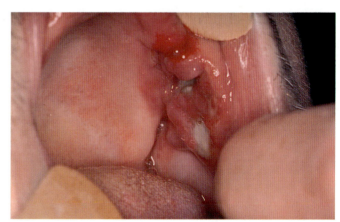

Figure 3.112
Squamous cell carcinoma (buccal mucosa)

This example of a squamous cell carcinoma of the buccal mucosa shows a deep haemorrhagic ulcer of the mucosa. A heaped-up edge is present on this malignant ulcer.

Palate

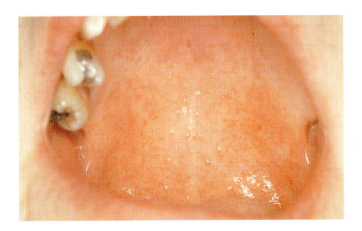

Figure 3.113

Smoker's mouth

There is often a characteristic redness to the mouth of a cigarette smoker. A large number of prominent small blood vessels can sometimes be identified on the hard palate, as shown in this example.

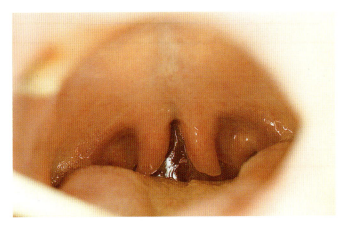

Figure 3.114

Bifid uvula

There is a bifid uvula or cleft uvula. A bifid uvula is a minor congenital abnormality that may be associated with a submucosal separation of the soft palate (a submucosal cleft palate). Palpation is required to confirm the presence of the submucosal cleft.

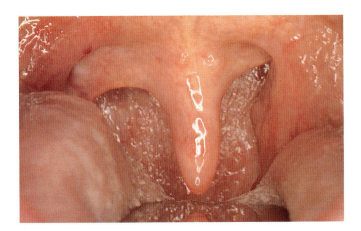

Figure 3.115

Long uvula

The normal length of the uvula is extremely varied. This example shows an elongated but normal uvula. In those rare instances when the uvula becomes so long that it reaches the laryngeal inlet and causes gagging or coughing, it may need to be excised.

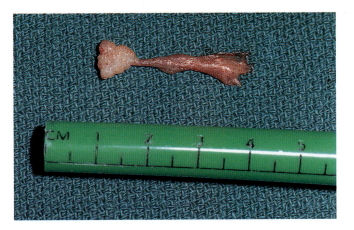

Figure 3.116

Long uvula

This patient had an elongated uvula that caused a sensation of 'something sticking' in the back of her throat. A uvulectomy was performed for symptomatic relief. Note the cauliflower-like squamous papilloma arising from the tip of this 3 cm long specimen.

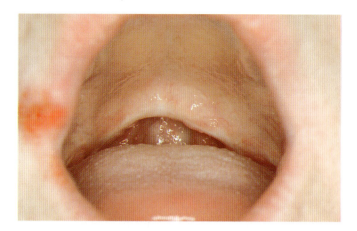

Figure 3.117
Uvulo-palatopharyngoplasty (UVPP)

This patient has had a tonsillectomy combined with excision of the margin of the soft palate and the uvula for the alleviation of snoring. The anterior and posterior tonsil pillars have been sutured together and the raw margin of the soft palate closed. This is one form of uvulo-palatopharyngoplasty (UVPP).

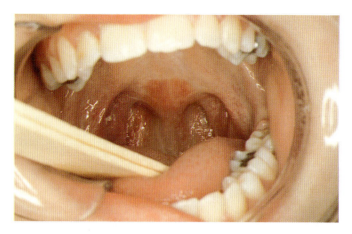

Figure 3.118
Palatoplasty

This patient has undergone a palatoplasty for velopharyngeal incompetence that resulted from a posterior cleft of the palate. Note the flap of pharyngeal mucosa that has been inserted into the free margin of the soft palate.

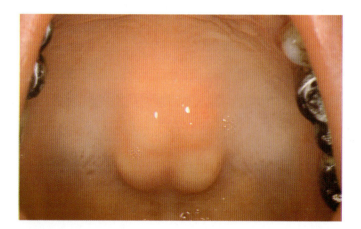

Figure 3.119
Torus palatinus

The discrete, hard, lobulated swelling in the midline of the hard palate of this patient is composed of compact lamellar bone. This is a torus palatinus.

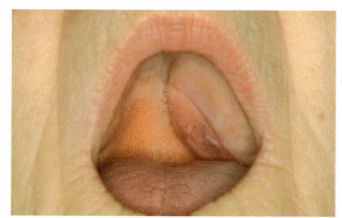

Figure 3.120
Ossifying fibroma

This palatal lesion has been present and unchanged for many years. A recent biopsy site is visible. This is an example of an ossifying fibroma.

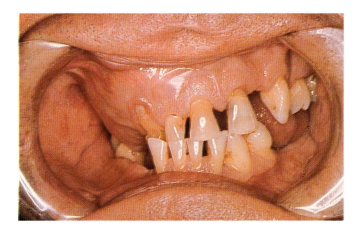

Figure 3.121

Fibrous dysplasia (dental bite alteration)

Fibrous dysplasia is a disease of unknown aetiology in which the medullary cavity of the bone is replaced by fibrous tissue with a potential for metaplastic new bone formation. In this example the fibrous dysplasia has affected the maxilla and a gross abnormality of the dental bite has developed.

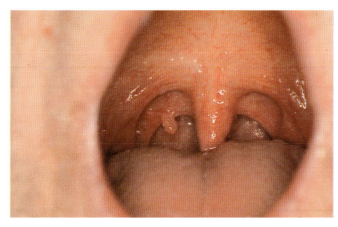

Figure 3.122

Papilloma (soft palate)

Oral papillomas are benign neoplasms derived from squamous epithelium, which can be found in any part of the oral cavity, although the soft palate, uvula and tonsillar regions are the most common. The lesion can be broad based or pedunculated and often, but not always, has a cauliflower-like appearance. In this example the papilloma is in the soft palate.

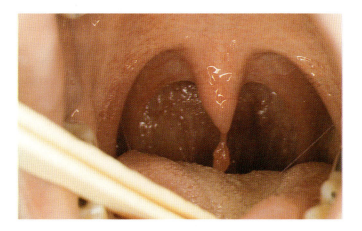

Figure 3.123

Papilloma (uvula)

This papilloma has developed from the tip of the uvula.

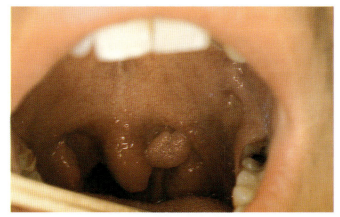

Figure 3.124

Papilloma (tonsillar fossa)

A large squamous papilloma arising from the tonsil is illustrated.

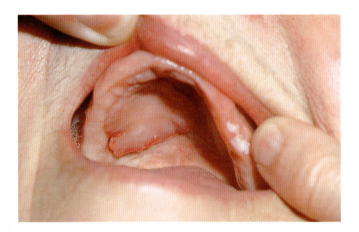

Figure 3.125
Fibroma of the palate

A palatal fibroma or similar lesion can sometimes be 'tucked' under a denture, and a doctor who examines the mouth without removing the dentures could miss significant disease. A smooth, pink fibroma is shown in the 'tucked up' position.

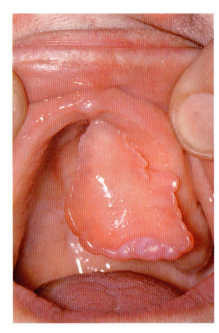

Figure 3.126
Fibroma of the palate

This shows the palatal fibroma shown in Figure 3.125 dangling by its stalk.

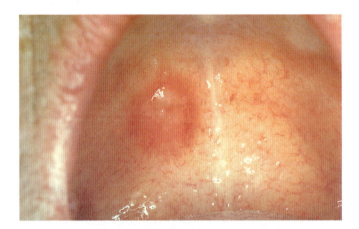

Figure 3.127
Pleomorphic adenoma (minor salivary gland)

A pleomorphic adenoma can arise in any salivary gland. In this example a pleomorphic adenoma has arisen in a minor salivary gland situated in the hard palate. A single lobulated adenoma is more common than a multilobulated tumour on the palate. The red raised lesion on the hard palate is the pleomorphic adenoma. This adenoma has been repeatedly compressed by a denture plate.

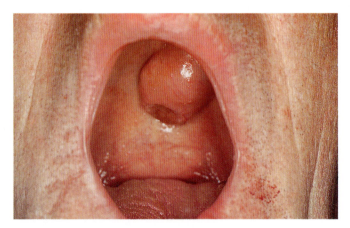

Figure 3.128
Pleomorphic adenoma (minor salivary gland)

This patient presented with a pink expanding mass on the hard palate, which was a pleomorphic adenoma arising from a minor salivary gland. The biopsy site can be seen.

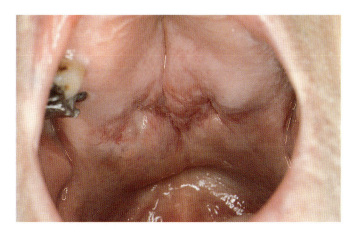

Figure 3.129

Lymphoma

An irregular, enlarging area of the palate raises a suspicion of malignancy. The diffuse, infiltrative but non-ulcerative irregularity of the centre of this hard palate was found to be a lymphoma on biopsy. The tonsil is the most common site of oral lymphoma.

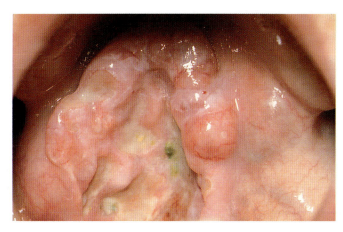

Figure 3.130

Adenoid cystic carcinoma

This irregular, lobulated and infected lesion of the hard palate was shown to be an adenoid cystic tumour at histology.

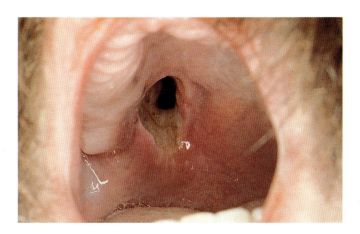

Figure 3.131

Adenocarcinoma

Adenocarcinoma within the oral cavity is a rare lesion, and consequently the possibility that such a lesion is a secondary should always be considered. Both squamous cell carcinoma and adenocarcinoma in the region of the palate can produce a penetrative ulcer and fistula between the mouth and the paranasal cavities at an early stage. Adenocarcinoma created the palatal ulcer shown here.

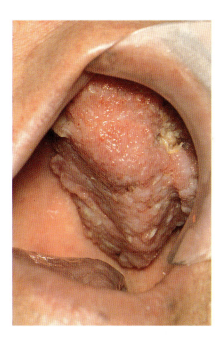

Figure 3.132

Verrucous carcinoma

A verrucous carcinoma typically (and as shown in this illustration) has a pink, warty and non-ulcerated surface. It is a relatively soft tumour that characteristically occurs in those areas of the mouth where a tobacco chewing quid is regularly held. The diagnosis of a verrucous carcinoma is a combined clinical and histological diagnosis. This verrucous tumour extended from the buccal mucosa onto the hard palate.

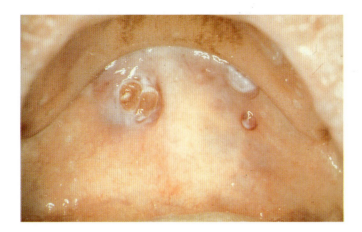

Figure 3.133

Kaposi's sarcoma

The raised, bluish lesions on the hard palate of this patient with AIDS is a Kaposi's sarcoma. The cutaneous lesions have a similar appearance.

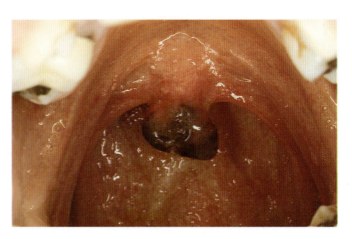

Figure 3.134

Blood blisters (spontaneous haematoma uvula)

Blood blisters (angina bullosa haemorrhagica) can arise within the mouth as a result of trauma, clotting disorders or 'spontaneously'. They often develop when a patient is eating and characteristically occur on the hard or soft palate. In this example a spontaneous haematoma of the uvula is visible. Simple rupture is usually curative.

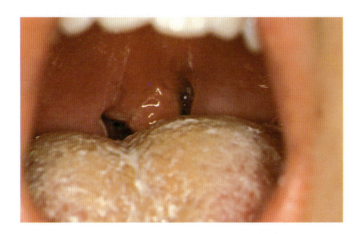

Figure 3.135

Oedematous uvula with acute tonsillitis

Gross enlargement of the uvula may occur in the course of an acute pharyngitis or tonsillitis. In this example the oedematous uvula is visible along with oedematous and inflamed palatine tonsils. This infection was viral in origin.

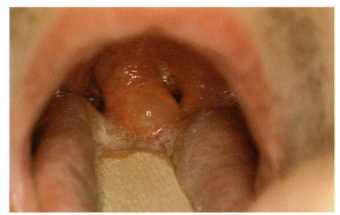

Figure 3.136

Acute oedema of the uvula

Acute swelling of the uvula may arise from trauma, as part of an allergic reaction or as part of an infective process. In this example a clumsy endotracheal intubation resulted in a swollen uvula. The patient had the sensation of a lump in the throat and the swelling resolved within 72 hours.

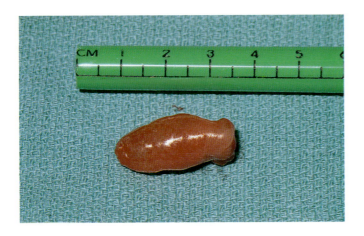

Figure 3.137

Acute infection with oedema of the uvula (uvulitis)

This patient developed an infection of the uvula with oedema and swelling. The oedematous uvula acted like a pharyngeal foreign body, causing the patient to gag constantly. An emergency resection of the swollen uvula was performed for relief of symptoms.

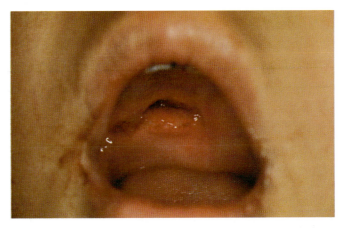

Figure 3.138

Palatal puncture

This unfortunate child fell forwards onto a pen cap. This injury produced a mucosal puncture of the hard palate. No surgery was undertaken and the lesion healed and smoothed such that little abnormality was visible after 1 month.

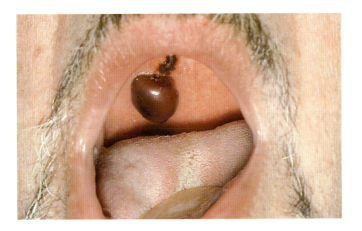

Figure 3.139

Palatal haematoma

The small haematoma or blood blister on this hard palate was the result of minor local trauma.

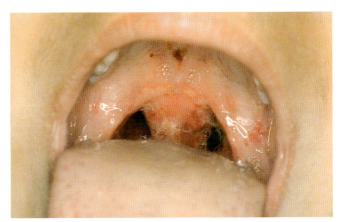

Figure 3.140

Oropharyngeal injury

This young girl fell onto a broom handle with her mouth open. There is considerable swelling of the soft palate and uvula. A 'line can be seen on the soft palate where the broom handle impacted. The lesion was treated conservatively, and healed satisfactorily. There was considerable nasal escape in speech during the first week after the injury.

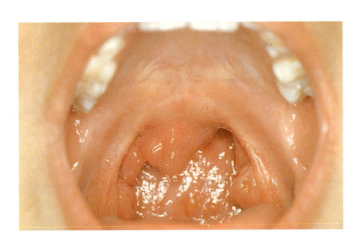

Figure 3.141

Healed oropharyngeal injury

The appearance of the palate of the patient shown in Figure 3.140 after 4 weeks. The speech had returned to normal.

Tongue

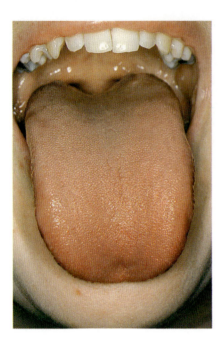

Figure 3.142
Normal tongue

The normal tongue, as it is protruded in the consulting room, has many shapes and sizes. This illustration shows a healthy normal tongue.

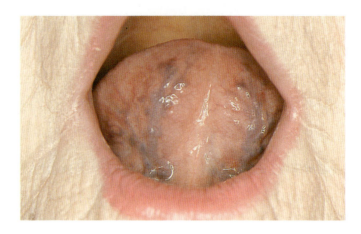

Figure 3.143
Normal tongue (sublingual blood vessels)

Prominent sublingual blood vessels, as shown in this illustration, are a normal finding.

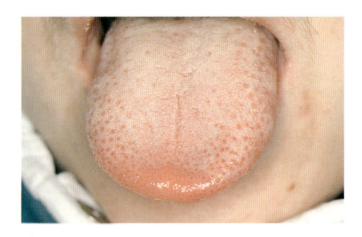

Figure 3.144
Normal tongue (dappled)

This illustration shows a mildly coated tongue with protrusion of papillae through the coating. This is a dappled tongue and also a normal finding.

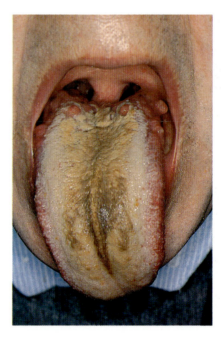

Figure 3.145
Coated tongue

A coated tongue may arise from dehydration, uraemia, prolonged use of oral antibiotics, persistent mouth breathing, poor oral hygiene or for no identifiable reason. This patient was a very heavy cigarette smoker, which was responsible for the thick coating on his tongue. Note the red prominence of the circumvallate papillae appearing through the coated tongue.

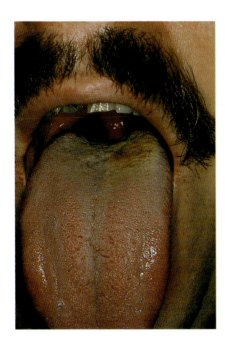

Figure 3.146
Nicotine stain to tongue

This man always smoked with a non-filtered cigarette in the right corner of the mouth. The 'smoking tide' of nicotine has accordingly deposited on the left base of tongue.

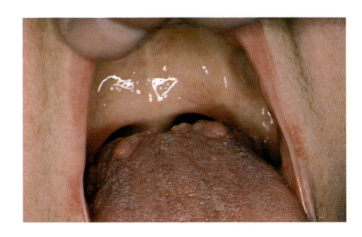

Figure 3.147
Prominent circumvallate papillae

Prominent circumvallate papillae can be a source of concern to a patient if they discover what they think is a suspicious swelling at the base of the tongue. This illustration shows how prominent circumvallate papillae can appear as a small red ridge, raised up on both sides of the base of the tongue. The characteristic apex to the V of the papillae is placed posteriorly on the tongue. Reassurance is all that is required.

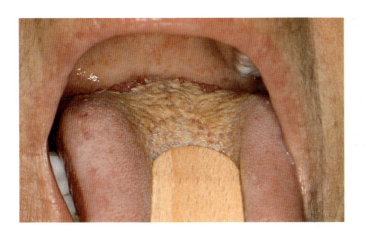

Figure 3.148
Circumvallate papillae prominence

In this example the circumvallate papillae appear to be 'pushing up' through the coated tongue, giving the appearance of an angry and inflamed lesion. Reassurance may be required.

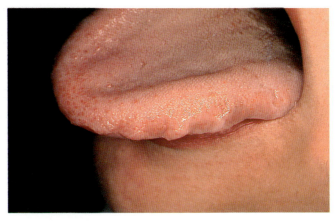

Figure 3.149
Crenellated tongue

The scalloped indentation seen along the lateral border of this individual's relatively large tongue is a normal variant.

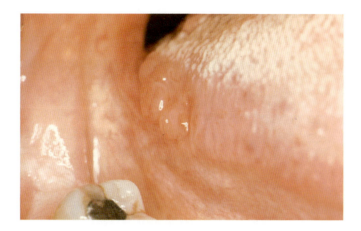

Figure 3.150

Lingual tonsils (lateral lymphoid tissue)

Lymphoid tissue within the base of the tongue is normal but often not easily visible. Rarely, chronic infection may develop in this pad of lingual lymphoid tissue. Prominent lymphoid tissue can sometimes be seen protruding from the lateral base of the tongue. The lymphoid tissue is the lobulated tissue on the lateral border of the tongue. This tissue was a prolongation from the lymphoid tissue at the base of the tongue (lingual tonsils).

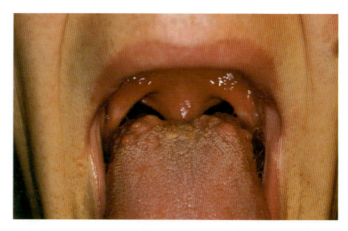

Figure 3.151

Lingual tonsils (lingual lymphoid tonsil)

The more common site to identify lymphoid tissue within the tongue (compared with Figure 3.150) is posterior to the line of the circumvallate papillae. The lingual tonsils can be seen protruding from each lateral base of the tongue as two smooth, red, raised masses behind the prominence of the circumvallate papillae.

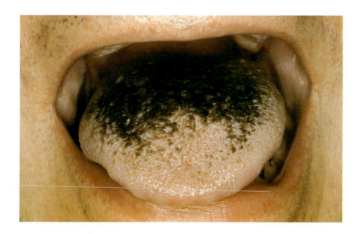

Figure 3.152

Black hairy tongue

This illustration shows a black hairy tongue. Filiform papillae elongate to produce the 'hairy' coating. The true reason for the black colour has never been explained, although antibiotics, tobacco, mouthwashes and chromogenic bacteria have all been suspected.

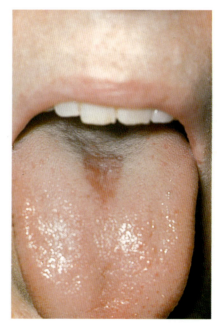

Figure 3.153

Median rhomboid glossitis

Median rhomboid glossitis has been considered a developmental abnormality for a number of years. Recent work suggests that this condition arises from a mild local candidal infection and that 'tongue clicking' against the hard palate may be a significant aetiological factor. In this example, the typically smooth, red, diamond-shaped area located centrally immediately in front of the circumvallate papillae can be seen.

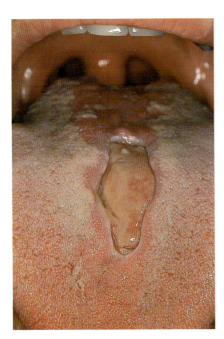

Figure 3.154

Median rhomboid glossitis

This unusual example of median rhomboid glossitis shows a more extensive and almost ulcerated defect located centrally immediately in front of the circumvallate papillae.

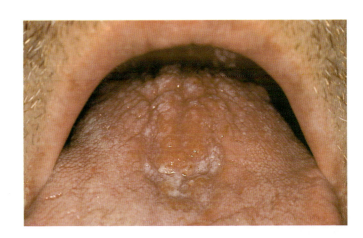

Figure 3.155

Median rhomboid glossitis

This patient has a red, raised area at the base of the tongue, which he thought may be a tumour. This red area has formed at the apex of prominent circumvallate papillae. He protruded his tongue to examine this area in the mirror between 10 and 15 times per day. He developed an ache around his temporomandibular joints, made worse by protruding the tongue!

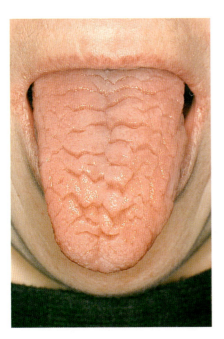

Figure 3.156

Fissured tongue (scrotal tongue)

Almost 5% of the population have a tongue with abnormal fissures and grooves. The fissure pattern is variable. Fissures tend to appear in late childhood and deepen with age. This illustration shows a tongue with transverse fissures and one can understand why the term 'scrotal tongue' is occasionally used.

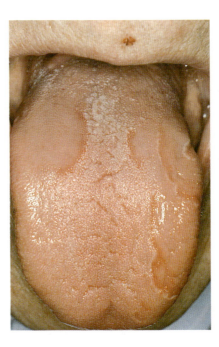

Figure 3.157

Geographic tongue

The filiform papillae disappear from localized areas of the tongue resulting in a patchy red area of depapillation, which is known as 'geographic tongue'. These patches repapillate after a variable time period and new areas of depapillation may occur on the tongue. The two large islands of depapillation on the lateral borders of the tongue are shown in this illustration.

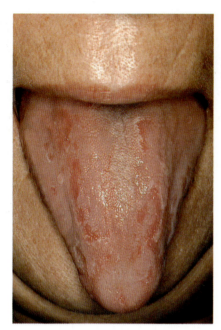

Figure 3.158
Geographic tongue

This tongue has a more linear pattern of geographic tongue.

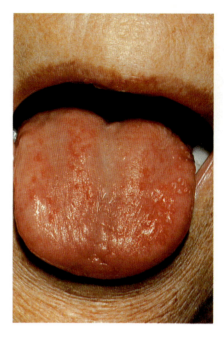

Figure 3.159
Atrophic glossitis

A beefy red glazed tongue of iron deficiency is shown. The smooth red surface develops as a result of the loss of the filiform papillae.

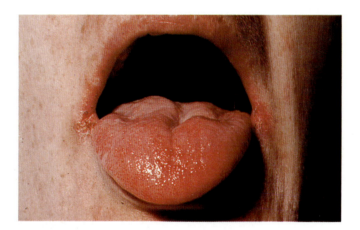

Figure 3.160
Atrophic glossitis

In this example an angular cheilitis can be seen in association with a beefy red glazed tongue of iron deficiency.

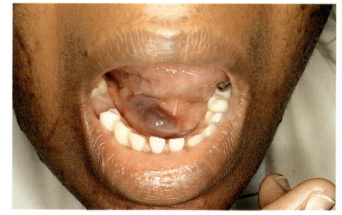

Figure 3.161
Ranula (mucocele of the floor of the mouth)

A ranula is a mucocele of the floor of the mouth, which may arise from obstruction to the duct of one of the minor sublingual salivary glands. This type of mucocele tends to be smaller and more superficially placed. Ranula may also arise from the sublingual glands, and these ranula tend to be larger and more deeply situated. The blue discoloured swelling under the tongue on the floor of this mouth is a ranula.

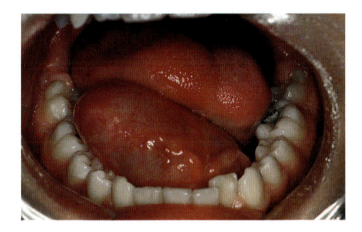

Figure 3.162

Ranula (mucocele of the floor of the mouth)

A large ranula, which is causing difficulty with speech and some mild swallowing difficulty, is shown.

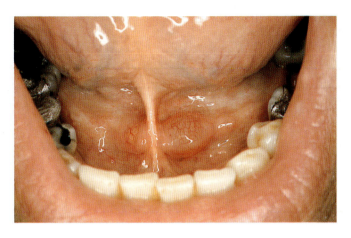

Figure 3.163

Ranula (mucocele of the floor of the mouth)

This illustration shows a terminal swelling around the submandibular ducts on each side of the floor of the mouth. These were small cysts, separate from the submandibular ducts, which contained mucus. This is an example of obstruction to a very minor salivary gland.

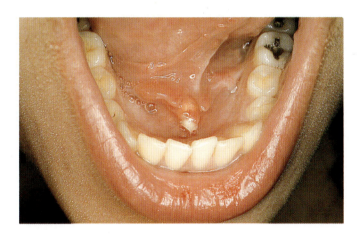

Figure 3.164

Submandibular duct stone

A submandibular duct stone is composed principally of calcium phosphate and develops around debris that collects in the submandibular ducts. In this illustration there is a terminal swelling within the submandibular duct and one can see a stone extruding from the duct.

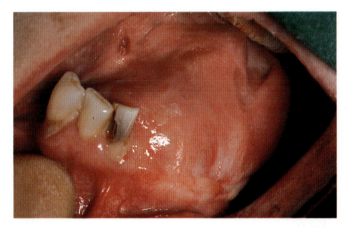

Figure 3.165

Submandibular gland fibroma

This man presented with a progressively enlarging, smooth swelling of the left floor of the mouth, which extended up to the mandibular margin. The mass was mostly intraoral, but the swelling could be identified by bimanual palpation. The lesion was excised through an external approach. Histology showed a submandibular fibroma.

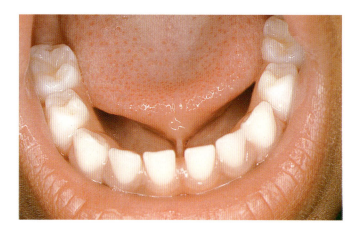

Figure 3.166
Tongue tie (ankyloglossia)

The frenulum of the tongue in this patient is abnormally short, resulting in an inability to protrude the tongue. This is known as a 'tongue tie'.

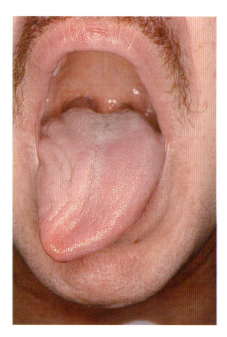

Figure 3.167
Hypoglossal nerve palsy

The right hypoglossal nerve of this patient was damaged in an accident. There is atrophy of the muscle bulk on the right side of the tongue and when the patient protrudes the tongue it deviates to the right (the side of the lesion).

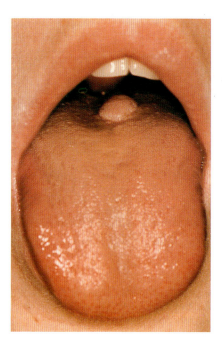

Figure 3.168
Lingual thyroid

The pink raised lesion in the midline of the base of the tongue is a lingual thyroid in a child. A lingual thyroid is more liable to spontaneous internal haemorrhage than the normal thyroid gland. Significant expansion of a lingual thyroid can occur at puberty and in pregnancy.

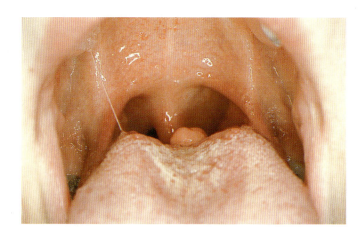

Figure 3.169
Lingual thyroid

The pink dome-shaped mass arising from the posterior surface of this patient's tongue is a lingual thyroid. One surgeon recommended an excisional biopsy. How lucky she was to have sought a second opinion!

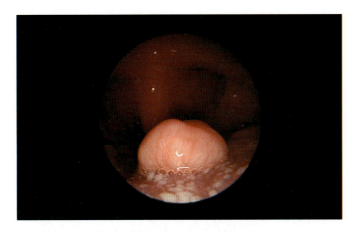

Figure 3.170
Lingual thyroid

This is an endoscopic photograph of the lingual thyroid shown in Figure 3.169.

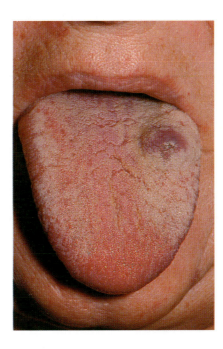

Figure 3.171
Haemangioma of the tongue

The raised, blue, compressible lesion on the dorsum of this tongue has the characteristic features of a benign haemangioma.

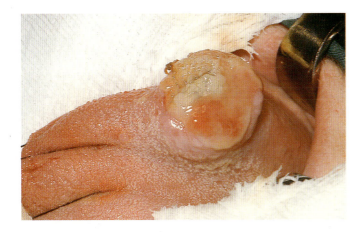

Figure 3.172
Neurilemmoma of the tongue

The smooth, pink, circumscribed lesion on this tongue is a neurilemmoma. The tongue is the most common site of an isolated neurilemmoma. A biopsy site can be seen. CO_2 laser excision of the tumour is about to be performed.

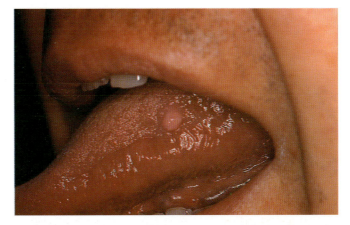

Figure 3.173
Fibroma of the tongue

The smooth, small, painless raised nodule on the side of this tongue was shown to be a fibroma at histological examination.

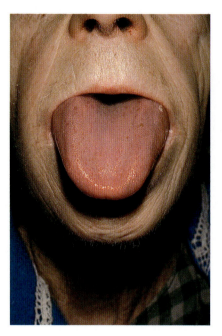

Figure 3.174

Amyloid tongue

This patient has an enlarged and immobile tongue, which caused her difficulty in swallowing. This is due to secondary amyloidosis of the tongue, which developed as a result of severe rheumatoid arthritis.

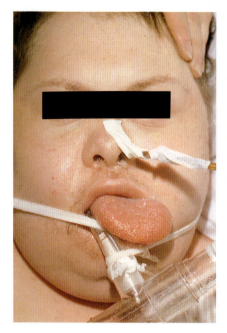

Figure 3.175

Down's enlargement of the tongue

John Langdon Haydon Down, when describing congenital Mongolian idiots, identified the feature of a long, thickened and much roughened tongue as a characteristic feature. This feature has been debated over the years, although the feature of protrusion of the tongue beyond the lips is accepted. This patient with Down's syndrome repeatedly bit his tongue, and a massive swelling with protrusion of the tongue ensued. Intubation was required to control the airway, and with conservative treatment the tongue returned to normal.

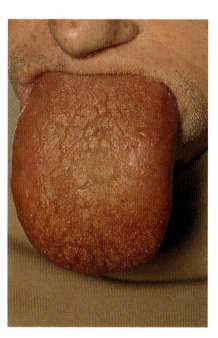

Figure 3.176

Down's enlargement of the tongue

In this patient, also with Down's syndrome, episodic massive enlargement of the tongue occurred. At postmortem examination a congenital lymphangiectasia of the tongue was found. The death was not caused by, or related to, the enlargement of the tongue.

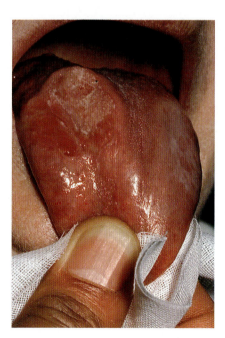

Figure 3.177

Squamous cell carcinoma of the tongue

Squamous cell carcinoma of the tongue can present as an ulcer, a nodule or simply an area of induration of the tongue. This patient presented with swelling on the dorsum of the right side of the tongue, which subsequently ulcerated.

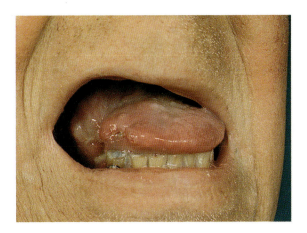

Figure 3.178

Squamous cell carcinoma of the tongue

This is a characteristic ulcerative, infiltrative and advanced squamous cell carcinoma of the lateral border of the tongue, which caused severe limitation of tongue movement.

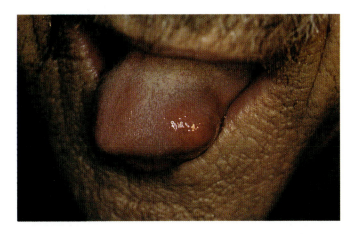

Figure 3.179

Secondary metastatic carcinoma of the tongue

This patient presented with a red, hard, smooth and uncomfortable swelling at the tip of the tongue. This was a secondary deposit from a bronchial carcinoma.

Tonsils

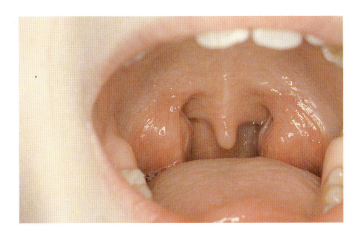

Figure 3.180

Normal tonsils

The appearance of the normal palatine tonsils is extremely varied. The tonsils may appear to protrude so far that they almost meet in the midline or they may be buried in the oropharyngeal wall to such an extent that only the tip of the tonsil is visible. This example shows a pair of normal tonsils placed approximately in the mid range of tonsil protrusion. The extent of protrusion into the oropharynx does not correlate with the overall size of the palatine tonsil.

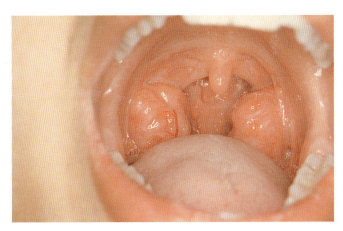

Figure 3.181

Normal tonsils

This illustration shows another pair of normal tonsils in a child.

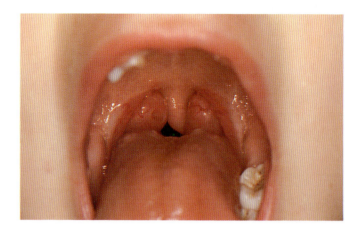

Figure 3.182

Normal tonsils with a prominent blood vessel

This illustration shows a pair of normal tonsils. On each side there is a blood vessel running across the anterior faucial pillar onto the tonsil. This particular blood vessel can sometimes be a source of spontaneous bleeding from the tonsil during an episode of acute tonsillitis.

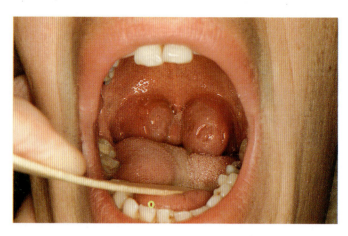

Figure 3.183

Obstructive tonsils

This patient has very large tonsils, which almost meet in the midline. Occasionally the use of a tongue depressor can provoke a gag reflex when examining the palatine tonsils. A gag reflex can cause the palatine tonsils to be pushed towards the midline thus giving a false appearance of 'enlarged tonsils'. This patient did not gag as this picture was taken!

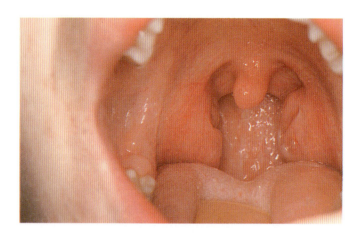

Figure 3.184

Tonsils (recurrent acute tonsillitis/chronic tonsillitis)

There is no characteristic clinical appearance of the palatine tonsils that will either confirm or exclude the diagnosis of recurrent episodes of acute tonsillitis (recurrent acute tonsillitis). To some clinicians the presence of erythema of the anterior pillar is considered of diagnostic significance. A vertical band of erythema can be seen on the anterior pillar of these tonsillar fauces. The child who owned the tonsils seen in this photograph had a very convincing history of acute recurrent tonsillitis.

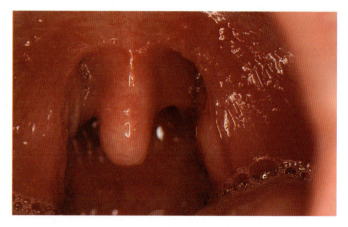

Figure 3.185

Acute tonsillitis (parenchymatous)

This patient has an acute bacterial tonsillitis. The beta-haemolytic streptococcus is the most common bacterium cultured from the throat swab. This is an example of the oedematous or parenchymatous variety of acute tonsillitis.

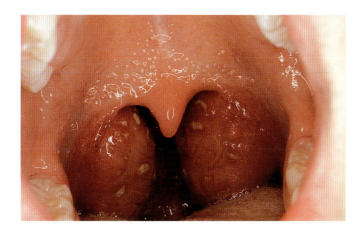

Figure 3.186

Acute tonsillitis (follicular)

This patient also has an acute bacterial tonsillitis. This is the follicular variety of tonsillitis.

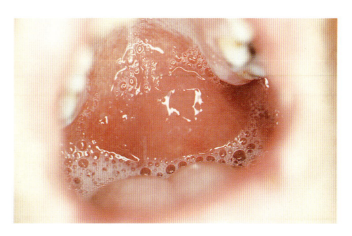

Figure 3.187

Peritonsillar abscess (quinsy)

A peritonsillar abscess is a bacterial abscess located between the tonsillar capsule and the lateral pharyngeal wall. Marked trismus is commonly present. In this illustration, oedema around the affected left tonsil stretches onto the palate and local retention of saliva can be seen. The abscess is not yet 'pointing'. Trismus makes the photography of a peritonsillar abscess difficult.

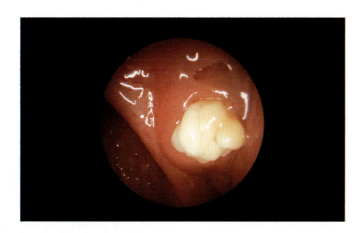

Figure 3.188

Tonsil crypt with debris (chronic cryptic tonsillitis)

Tonsillar crypts can collect debris, as shown in this endoscopically produced illustration. Excessive collection of debris in multiple crypts can result in halitosis. Some patients can become quite adept at manually expressing the debris from their crypts.

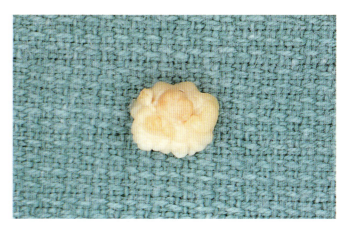

Figure 3.189

Tonsillolith

The ball of accumulating caseous debris within a tonsil may become quite large. When this occurs, the concretion is called a tonsillolith. This tonsillolith measured 1.5 cm in diameter.

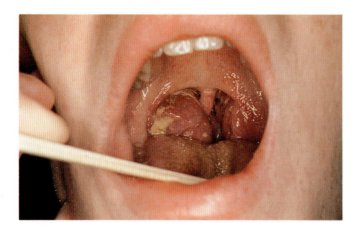

Figure 3.190

Infectious mononucleosis (glandular fever)

The acutely swollen and juicy-looking tonsils covered with yellow debris and associated with palatal petechiae are characteristic of infectious mononucleosis (glandular fever).

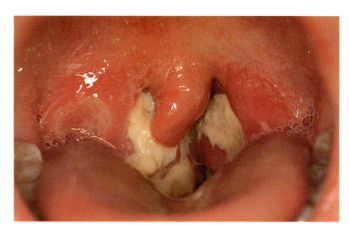

Figure 3.191

Infectious mononucleosis (glandular fever)

These tonsils in a case of infectious mononucleosis again look swollen and juicy, but they are extremely hard and caused considerable discomfort in swallowing. Steroids were used to relieve some of the tonsillar swelling and as a consequence relieve the pain of swallowing.

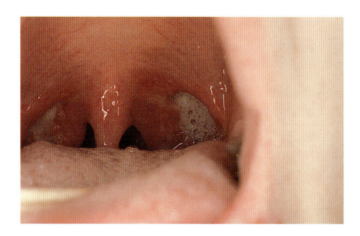

Figure 3.192

Normal postoperative tonsillectomy bed after 1 week

One week after an elective tonsillectomy, some pooling of saliva in the tonsil bed is still present. If the saliva is cleared, the base of the tonsil bed usually contains a grey slough.

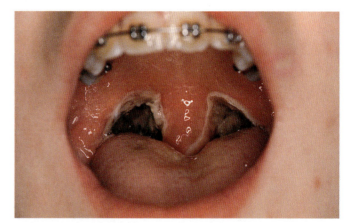

Figure 3.193

Laser tonsillectomy at 1 day

This shows the tonsil beds of a patient who had her tonsils excised using a holmium–YAG laser the previous day. Slough can be seen in the base of the tonsil bed and mild thermal burns of the uvula are visible.

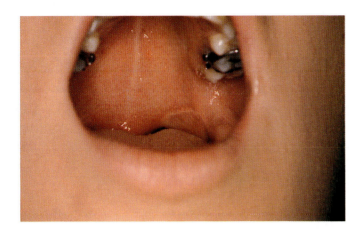

Figure 3.194

Laser tonsillectomy at I month

This shows the small depressed scar that is present I month after a laser tonsillectomy.

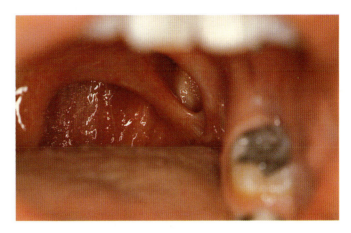

Figure 3.195

Tonsillectomy scar pocket

Occasionally after a traumatic tonsillectomy by dissection, the oropharyngeal healing is not satisfactory. In this example a band has formed across the tonsil bed, which caused the patient problems by forming a pouch that collected food and debris.

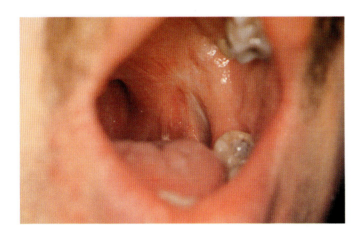

Figure 3.196

Tonsillectomy scar of the faucial pillars

In the area around the anterior pillar and extending into the palate, a considerable amount of scarring as a result of a traumatic tonsillectomy by dissection can be seen.

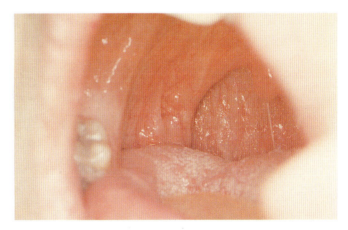

Figure 3.197

Tonsillectomy remnant

It is possible to leave palatine tonsil tissue behind during an untidy tonsillectomy by dissection. Tonsil remnants were even more common following guillotine tonsillectomy. In this illustration the nodule of lymphoid tissue that can be seen protruding through the scarring of the palate and anterior tonsil pillar is a remnant of the palatine tonsil.

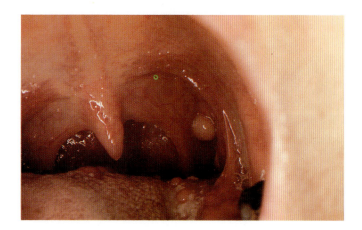

Figure 3.198

Retention cyst of tonsil (mucus retention cyst)

A retention cyst can often be seen in the region of the tonsil. Characteristically such cysts are smooth, creamy white in colour, and can be indented.

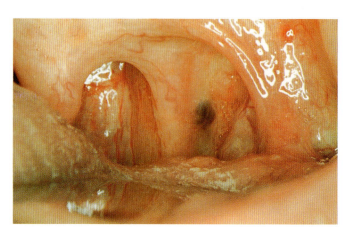

Figure 3.199

Melanonaevus tonsil pillar

This elderly lady presented with a blue discolouration of her tonsillar pillar. The lesion was a simple melanonaevus.

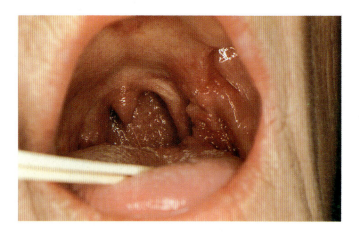

Figure 3.200

Squamous cell carcinoma of the tonsil

The ulcerated and indurated lesion of the left tonsil bed is a squamous cell carcinoma. Such lesions sometimes spread to the tonsil from the retromolar trigone or 'coffin corner'.

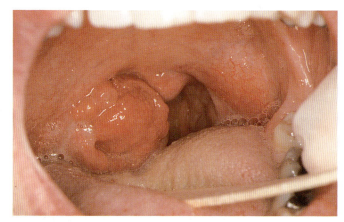

Figure 3.201

Lymphoma of the tonsil

This large fleshy swelling of the right palatine tonsil is characteristic of lymphoma. This was a non-Hodgkin's lymphoma.

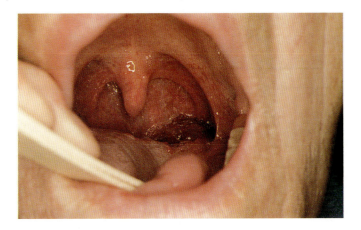

Figure 3.202

Lymphoma of the tonsil

This example of a lymphoma of a tonsil shows a blue discolouration of the tonsil. This feature sometimes occurs in lymphoma.

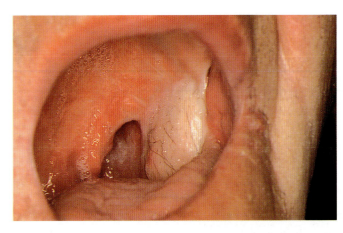

Figure 3.203

Skin of a pectoralis major flap

This patient has undergone an extensive resection to treat a squamous cell carcinoma of the tonsil. Reconstruction was with a pectoralis major flap. The hairs from the chest have been transposed into the mouth!

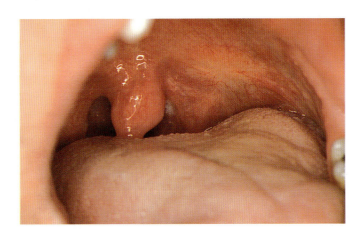

Figure 3.204

Haematoma of tonsil bed (herald bleed carotid artery)

This patient presented with a vague spontaneous discomfort over the left side of his neck. Examination of the mouth revealed a subcutaneous haematoma of the tonsil, particularly visible at the base of the tongue on the left, associated with local oedema and bruising of the oropharynx and soft palate. The discolouration of the haematoma is visible in this illustration. Further investigation identified an aneurysm of the carotid artery. This artery had leaked, giving rise to the clinical sign in the mouth.

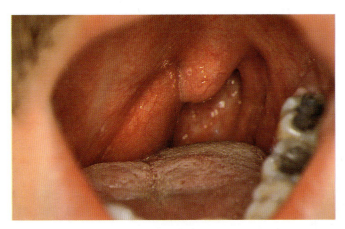

Figure 3.205

Parapharyngeal pleomorphic adenoma

The swelling pushing into the oropharynx is a tumour of the parapharyngeal space. Further investigation determined that the firm, lobulated swelling was a pleomorphic adenoma of the parapharyngeal space (deep lobe parotid gland).

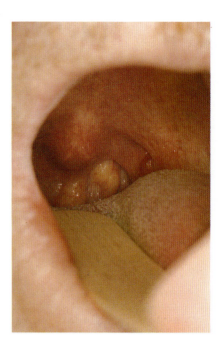

Figure 3.206
Primary amyloidosis (oropharynx and laryngopharynx)

The two yellow, circumscribed, soft lesions on the posterior wall of the oropharynx are deposits of localized primary amyloidosis. Note the blood vessels on the surface of these deposits of amyloid.

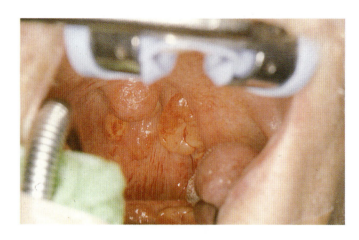

Figure 3.207
Primary amyloidosis (oropharynx and laryngopharynx)

This patient shown in Figure 3.206 had a large deposit of primary amyloid in the pharynx, which obstructed the laryngeal entrance. This illustration provides a clear view of the oropharyngeal amyloid deposit with the patient in position for endoscopic removal of the pharyngeal lesion.

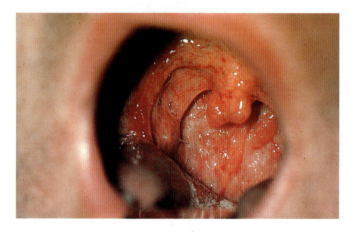

Figure 3.208
Fish bone in tonsil

This patient who ate improperly boned fish presented with a fishbone impacted in the left tonsil.

4
The larynx

Laryngology is the study of the larynx in health and disease, a specialized discipline practised by the laryngologist, broncho-oesophagologist and ear, nose and throat/head and neck surgeon.

Phonosurgical anatomy

The human larynx is a highly developed organ. In primitive animals it was little more than a sphincter mechanism to protect the lower respiratory tract from inhalation but later in evolution the larynx took on the role of phonation, now exquisitely developed in man.

The larynx has a skeletomembranous protective framework consisting of the hyoid bone and the epiglottic, thyroid and cricoid cartilages. This framework, together with the paired arytenoid cartilages and the small corniculate and cuneiform cartilages, is connected by a series of membranes and ligaments. The paired pyramid-shaped arytenoid cartilages articulate with facets on the superior surface of the posterior lamina of the cricoid cartilage; this synovial cricoarytenoid joint is vital in the various complicated movements of the vocal cords which include adduction and abduction during respiration and variations in tension, stiffness and mass of the vocal folds during phonation. The intrinsic muscles of the larynx are innervated by the recurrent laryngeal nerve and serve the various functions of respiration, phonation, stress closure and deglutition.

During phonation, pressure is generated in the subglottic air column by the thoracic respiratory muscles while the vocal cords are adducted and tensed. A critical pressure increase causes the vocal folds to open momentarily but elastic recoil re-establishes glottic adduction, and when the cycle of movement is repeated phonation is initiated. There is a side-to-side vibratory motion of the vocal folds, combined with a slight up-and-down vertical motion of the medial edges, in accordance with the myoelastic-aerodynamic theory of phonation.

Detailed study of the human vocal folds by Hirano has confirmed that the vocal fold is composed of mucosa and muscle. The mucosa has a number of layers, including the superficial epithelial layer, the lamina propria and the vocalis part of the thyroarytenoid muscle. The normal vibration of the vocal folds depends upon normal function of each of the layers.

Several types of epithelium cover the vocal folds: non-keratinized stratified squamous epithelium around the edge of the vocal fold, and typical pseudo-stratified ciliated columnar respiratory epithelium with goblet cells above and below the vibrating vocal fold. The lamina propria contains three layers (superficial, intermediate and deep) beneath the epithelium and superficial to the musculature. They are distinguished from one another because of the difference in elastic and collagen fibres. The superficial layer of the lamina propria is loose and pliable (and referred to as 'Reinke's space') and is the layer that vibrates most significantly. The intermediate layer has mostly branching elastic fibres and the deep layer mostly densely packed collagenous fibres running in bundles parallel to the vocalis muscle from which it is not clearly separated. The intermediate and deep layers of the lamina propria constitute the vocal ligament.

The vocal folds are lubricated by the spread and retention of mucus along microridges in the epithelium, thus keeping the epithelial surfaces moist, mobile and pliant during vibration and phonation.

The vocal fold can thus be thought of functionally as a multi-layered vibrator in three sections – the *cover* (epithelium and superficial layer of the lamina propria), the *transitional layer* (intermediate and deep layers of the lamina propria which make the vocal ligament) and the *body* (vocalis muscle).

Presenting clinical features of voice disorders

Modern laryngology requires a multi-disciplinary approach for the optimum care of a patient with a laryngeal disorder. Sophisticated centres for voice disorders are served not only by a laryngologist but by a speech pathologist and a singing teacher or a specialist concerned with the care of the professional voice.

The history of the patient's complaint and the nature and degree of the voice change, together with other associated symptoms, are carefully elicited. Indirect laryngoscopy is performed using a laryngeal mirror, a flexible fibreoptic pharyngolaryngoscope or a rigid rod lens 70° telescope to assess the appearance and movement of the laryngeal structures and the vocal cords. Occasionally topical anaesthesia is required for patients with a sensitive gag reflex.

Adults

In adults and older children certain methods of study of voice disorders can be used when patients are examined in a fully equipped voice laboratory. These studies include video-laryngoscopy, frequency analysis, spectrography, electroglottography and measurements of airway resistance in the larynx.

However, there is no finer instrument for assessment of the normal or abnormal voice than the human ear. One of the most important elements of the physical examination is evaluation by the laryngologist of the characteristics of the patient's voice. The adult patient may have chronic, persistent, progressive hoarseness (as with vocal nodules or multiple papillomas), a weak voice (as with unilateral vocal cord paralysis), a breathy voice (as with hysterical dysphonia), a strained and choking voice (as with spastic dysphonia) or a dysarthric voice (in neurological disease).

The onset, duration, progression and variability of huskiness are important: haemorrhage into a vocal cord while shouting causes a sudden onset, acute inflammatory laryngitis while an upper respiratory tract infection usually lasts a few days, but huskiness for many years could be due to Reinke's oedema. A persistent, relentless progression of symptoms strongly suggests a neoplastic cause. Variable huskiness can occur with vocal nodules or may be an early manifestation of neurological disease.

Other symptoms important in patients with laryngeal disease include the presence of a lump in the neck, pain referred to the ear, difficulty in swallowing and a feeling of 'something' in the throat.

Children

In contrast to adults, where huskiness of the voice is the paramount symptom of laryngeal disease, stridor is the cardinal feature in infants and children. The stridor is usually inspiratory, sometimes expiratory and occasionally inspiratory and expiratory, and can be heard by listening beside the patient, whereas the expiratory wheeze of asthma is heard by auscultation of the chest with a stethoscope. Observation and examination of an infant with stridor over a period of hours or days may be helpful but the characteristics of the stridor are seldom diagnostic in any particular disease. Although it may be possible to make a preliminary diagnosis before endoscopy, direct examination of the upper airways, including the nasal cavities, pharynx, larynx and tracheobronchial tree, is usually necessary to make an accurate diagnosis.

The mode of presentation of paediatric patients also includes acute airway obstruction in the newborn baby, chronic progressive obstruction, acute obstruction due to inflammation, recurrent or atypical croup, the presence of a husky voice, inhalation of a foreign body, weak or absent cry, repeated aspiration, cyanotic or apnoeic attacks, atypical lower respiratory tract infection and tracheobronchial compression by vascular anomalies or a mediastinal mass.

Indirect laryngoscopy

Owing to their location the laryngopharynx and the larynx cannot be directly visualized during routine physical examination. For this reason examination of these structures in the consulting room, office or clinic relies on a technique of indirect visualization known as indirect laryngoscopy. Indirect laryngoscopy may be performed by three different techniques, which use different instruments: the laryngeal mirror (Figure 4.1), the rigid, rod lens, angled telescope (Figures 4.2 and 4.4), or the flexible fibreoptic laryngoscope (Figure 4.7). While any one of these methods can be used, sometimes in combination with one or even both of the others, one technique is never used to the exclusion of the others. Some patients can be satisfactorily examined only by one technique, e.g. a flexible fibreoptic laryngoscope passed through the nose in those patients who have an active gag reflex or who cannot open their mouth satisfactorily.

The image obtained with the rigid Hopkins rod lens telescopes, either 70° or 90°, with or without a device for focusing or changing the image size, is bright and clear, and the image can be recorded by 35 mm photography (Figure 4.5). An image from a video screen (Figure 4.6) can be transferred to a video recorder or can be used for making an instant hard-copy print. Stroboscopy, to study the phonatory vibration of the edge of the vocal fold in slow motion, can be achieved with either a rigid telescope (Figure 4.4) or a flexible laryngoscope (Figure 4.7).

An excellent view of the base of the tongue, pharynx and larynx for routine diagnostic indirect laryngoscopy can be obtained with a slim 4.0 mm diameter rigid rod lens telescope. The 10 mm diameter laryngeal telescope provides an enlarged image, but usually requires the use of topical anaesthesia.

Documentation and teaching

Photography

For over 100 years, endoscopists have been searching for a better method for the permanent recording of their findings. While many successful methods have been described, the most reliable and versatile modern system uses a 35 mm single-frame, single-lens reflex camera with Hopkins telescopes and a synchronized, automatic-exposure, computer-controlled remote electronic flash generator. This system using 35 mm photography for routine documentation of any area accessible to a telescope is a practical reality, close-up photography is possible and the telescopes have a wide latitude in the depth of focus. This system gives consistently reproducible photographs under all conditions.

Teaching

Teaching of a medical student, Resident, Registrar or Fellow or the nursing staff in the operating room is difficult when using a telescope alone but is facilitated with specially designed optical, photographic and electronic equipment.

The Wittmoser multi-articulated optical arm is a remarkable teaching tool. It has four joints and its dual beam splitter can be set at 50–50 per cent for examiner and observer or 10–90 per cent for documentation using a 35 mm still camera, a cine-camera or a television camera. For teaching the image is split 50–50 so that an observer sees simultaneously exactly the same view as the surgeon; the superb image quality ensures that detail is not lost by transmission through the five Hopkins rigid rod lenses in the Wittmoser arm. The advantage of this system is that there is no interference at any time to the view of the endoscopist.

Other specially designed equipment includes an optical observer arm mounted on one side of the beam splitter of the operating microscope and a closed-circuit television system with a small, high-resolution, low-light-sensitive television camera coupled to any of the rigid telescopes or to the operating microscope during diagnostic endoscopy, microsurgery or laser surgery.

Documentation

It has become increasingly important to have a permanent record for teaching, for documentation of disease, for recording in the patient's history or for the information of another specialist (for example, in radiotherapy or oncology) or for the study of the natural history of disease. A permanent record can be obtained with 35 mm photography but an 'instant print' taken from the monitor of a video system is readily available in a minute or so. The image can be transferred to either a black-and-white or a colour print by a video printer; after the desired image is 'frozen' on the monitor, one or more hard copies can be obtained and these are invaluable for placing in the patient's record, to use for explanation and advice to the patient, to send to another physician involved in the patient's care and for comparison of the disease before and after treatment.

Dynamic changes can be recorded by cinephotography or more usually by a video-recording system. The video recorder should provide a still-frame feature, forward and backward search scanning, playback and programmed access to stored information. Cinephotography is time-consuming and expensive and has largely been replaced by video recordings.

The Kantor–Berci video-microlaryngoscope has been specially designed for documentation and for use with the video camera, which is attached to a telescope, which itself is fixed in a special side-channel in the laryngoscope. Microsurgery can then be performed by viewing the television monitor and it is claimed that this system substitutes for the conventional binocular operating microscope, although its use is limited to the one laryngoscope, which gives a limited view of the glottis. However, the principle of the fixed unchangeable field of view for documentation is good, especially for a series of photographs illustrating a technique (Figures 4.135 and 4.167).

Television

Videographic documentation of the larynx can be obtained in the consulting room or in the operating room using either a rigid telescope or a flexible fibre-optic laryngoscope. While the flexible instruments are versatile and have the great advantage of passing around corners, neither the visual, the photographic nor the video-graphic image is as good as that obtained with rigid telescopes.

In the operating room the equipment should ideally be mounted on a dedicated video trolley. With a two-camera system there is no interruption of the operative procedure: the first camera is used for telescopes and the second camera remains on the C-mount of the microscope, with one video monitor screen serving both cameras. Where video-monitoring is available, the anaesthetist is able to monitor the airway and observe the conditions for anaesthesia, the instrument nurse can anticipate the progress of the procedure and the operating room staff feel more involved in the operation. Recording on ¾ inch or ½ inch video tape through the video monitor gives a clear image with high resolution.

Radiological examination

Various techniques have been used to image the larynx and upper airways, including conventional plain x-ray, xeroradiography, digitized radiography, positive contrast laryngography, coronal tomography, axial computerized tomographic (CT) scan and magnetic resonance imaging (MRI). These studies may show the site and sometimes the nature of tumours, cysts and other abnormalities and are useful in the assessment of soft tissue or pharyngeal space infections, impacted foreign bodies, cysts, laryngoceles and congenital abnormalities. Advanced organ imaging, including examination by CT and MRI, is helpful in defining the pre-epiglottic space, the paralaryngeal spaces and the laryngeal and tracheal framework, which is particularly useful in laryngeal trauma and malignancy.

Anaesthesia for laryngoscopy

General anaesthesia is used for direct laryngoscopy, microlaryngoscopy and microlaryngeal operations including laser surgery. The technique of anaesthesia is critical, as the surgeon and the anaesthesiologist must both safely share the upper airway and at the same time allow diagnostic evaluation and surgical treatment with maximum visual and surgical access, minimum morbidity and optimum safety.

Anaesthesia for laryngeal obstruction

Even when laryngeal obstruction appears not to be severe prior to induction of anaesthesia, all precautions

Techniques of anaesthesia preferred

Infants and children
Spontaneous respiration with inhalational anaesthesia

Adults
A relaxant technique with controlled ventilation using either a jetting system or a modified endotracheal tube

With all techniques, the general anaesthesia is supplemented by the use of a measured amount of local anaesthesia (up to a maximum dose of 5 mg per kg of lignocaine) sprayed on the larynx and upper trachea

should be taken to manage an unexpected airway problem such as might occur in patients with suspected or known glottic or supraglottic pathology such as a large tumour mass or a cyst. Anaesthesia for laryngoscopy and intubation in specific conditions, for example in acute airway obstruction caused by acute epiglottitis, is difficult and when possible should be performed by an experienced anaesthetist.

Anaesthesia and laser surgery

Special precautions to prevent laser ignition of the anaesthesia tube must be followed when performing laser surgery. In adults these include either using a 'laser proof' tube, moving the tube out of the operative field being treated or using a proximal jetting technique with the metal cannula secured within the lumen of the laryngoscope. A moist cottonoid neurosurgical 'patty' can be used to protect the anaesthetic tube. The use of a 40% oxygen : 60% helium gas mixture not only lowers the inspired oxygen concentration, but the conductive qualities of helium rapidly dissipate heat, thus greatly minimizing the likelihood of tube ignition. Care on the part of the endoscopic surgeon during laser use remains the single most important safety factor.

Because spontaneous respiration inhalational anaesthesia in children does not require an endotracheal tube, no special precautions are necessary.

Three-stage laryngoscopy

Stage 1   Hand-held laryngoscopy
Preliminary examination with the naked eye or with telescope

Stage 2   Suspension laryngoscopy
Detailed evaluation with the laryngeal telescopes

Stage 3   Microlaryngoscopy
Microlaryngeal or laser surgery

Direct laryngoscopy technique

A systematic technique of diagnostic endoscopy of the larynx and pharynx requires firstly a preliminary naked eye examination with the hand-held laryngoscope, and secondly a more detailed evaluation under suspension laryngoscopy with rigid telescopes for image magnification, thus providing diagnostic information for the third stage, which depends on use of the microscope.

Although it is possible to perform direct laryngoscopy in adults and some older children with topical and nerve block local anaesthesia, modern general anaesthesia is preferable, especially for extended examination and for surgical or microsurgical procedures. The best conditions for the surgeon and the least discomfort for the patient are achieved with general anaesthesia, which is now used almost universally for direct laryngoscopy, microlaryngoscopy and microlaryngeal operations, including laser surgery.

Adults

In many adults direct laryngoscopy is necessary as a diagnostic examination, for instance when indirect examination has been incomplete, unsatisfactory or impossible because of unduly sensitive reflexes. Other reasons for direct endoscopy include removal of benign conditions such as vocal nodule, vocal polyp, vocal granuloma, treatment of Reinke's oedema or other lesions, laser treatment of papillomas, dysplasia or early malignancy, injection of Teflon or Gelfoam paste, assessment of laryngeal trauma caused by endotracheal intubation, treatment of an acquired web or stenosis and endoscopic arytenoidectomy.

Children

Further investigation including comprehensive, diagnostic endoscopy is indicated in infants and children for severe stridor, progressive stridor, stridor associated with unusual features such an cyanotic or apnoeic attacks, dysphagia, aspiration or failure to thrive, an abnormality found on radiological investigation and stridor where there is undue anxiety on the part of the parents and attending physician.

The *first stage* allows a general survey of the oropharynx and laryngopharynx to be sure that the airway is clear and easily controlled and to localize the site of pathology. The *second stage* requires a laryngoscope, which can be hand-held but is usually suspended for examination with selected rigid telescopes, and is straight ahead and angled for detailed examination of the supraglottic, glottic and subglottic larynx. A laryngoscope in suspension allows use of both hands. In infants and children examination of the larynx is usually combined with naked-eye bronchoscopy followed by bronchoscopy with telescopes, and sometimes with oesophagoscopy. The *third stage* utilizes the operating microscope for microlaryngoscopy, microlaryngeal or laser surgery.

Difficult areas such as the valleculae, the piriform fossae, the laryngeal ventricles, the anterior commissure, the posterior glottic space and the subglottic region are clearly seen with the brightly illuminated magnified view obtained using telescopes. The full extent of malignancies can be accurately evaluated and mapped. Hidden pathology or papillomas in the ventricle can be identified prior to surgery or laser removal. Anatomy not visualized through the microscope can be identified using an angled telescope. During microlaryngoscopy observation is confined to the larynx; there is not the flexibility of endoscopic visualization nor the ease of photographic or tele-video documentation that is available with telescopes which can be so easily passed into the pharynx, larynx, trachea and tracheobronchial tree.

Choice of a laryngoscope to suit the patient's anatomy is vital. The endoscopist may need to change from one laryngoscope to another, sometimes several times during the procedure, to get optimal exposure. Depending upon the circumstances and the individual requirements, one of the standard laryngoscopes or one of the special-purpose laryngoscopes is selected.

The steps in the three stage endoscopic technique in children are shown in Figures 4.38–4.47, and that in adults in Figures 4.49–4.53.

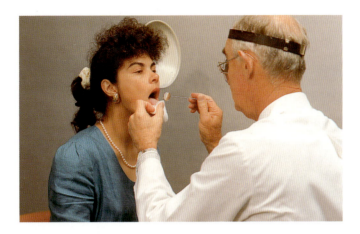

Figure 4.1

The laryngeal mirror

Indirect laryngoscopy using a circular laryngeal mirror and reflected light has been the traditional method of laryngeal examination. Local anaesthesia is seldom required, the equipment is inexpensive and the view is usually satisfactory.

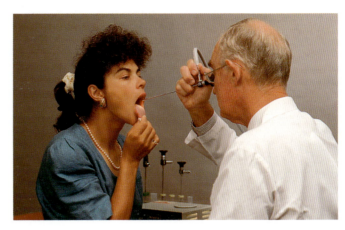

Figure 4.2

The laryngeal telescope

Indirect laryngoscopy using a rigid, 4.0 mm diameter 70° angled Hopkins rod lens laryngeal telescope provides a crystal-clear view of the larynx, laryngopharynx and base of the tongue. The use of this telescope for 'routine laryngoscopy' is highly recommended.

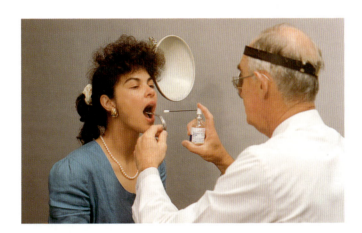

Figure 4.3

Topical anaesthesia

An application of topical anaesthesia may be required for the performance of any one of the techniques of indirect laryngoscopy, especially when using a large diameter (e.g. 10 mm) telescope for stroboscopy, photography or video-recording

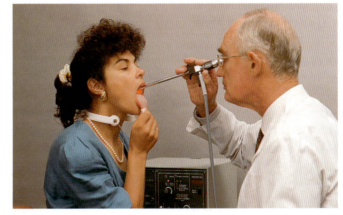

Figure 4.4

Stroboscopic examination of the larynx

A 10 mm diameter, 70° angled laryngeal telescope is being used for stroboscopy. A microphone on the patient's neck synchronizes the flashing stroboscopic light during a period of constant phonation so that the vibrating edges of the vocal folds can be examined in 'slow motion'.

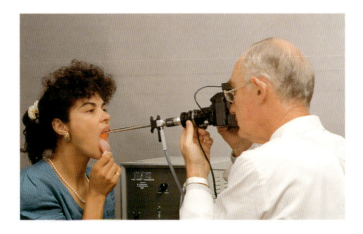

Figure 4.5

Laryngeal photography

Photography of the larynx or pharynx using a 10 mm, 70° telescope with a 35 mm camera, coupled to the Karl Storz 600 computerized light source and flash generator.

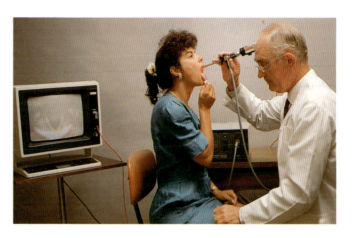

Figure 4.6

Closed-circuit video laryngoscopy

A high quality video camera, with automatic exposure control through the lighting unit, provides an image on the television monitor. Video recording allows replay for later study.

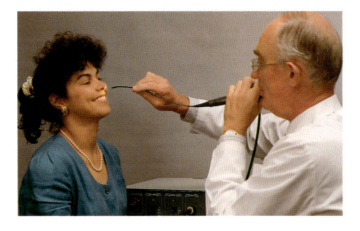

Figure 4.7

The flexible laryngoscope

A flexible nasopharyngolaryngoscope, of 35 mm diameter, is about to be passed through one nasal cavity which has had topical anaesthesia and vasoconstrictor spray applied. The larynx is usually easily visualized but the image is not as sharp and clear as with a mirror or a rigid telescope.

Indirect laryngoscopy

The image seen at indirect laryngoscopy normally shows the epiglottis at the bottom of the picture. To simplify orientation, Figures 4.8–4.27 have been rotated through 180° to position the epiglottis at the top, similar to the view obtained at direct laryngoscopy.

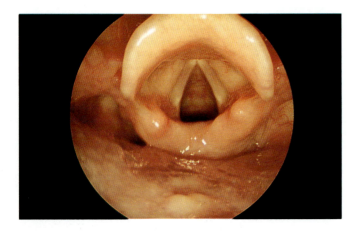

Figure 4.8

Telescopic photograph of a normal larynx

The vocal folds, false vocal cords, arytenoid region, glottis, part of the subglottis and posterior pharyngeal wall are all seen. The piriform fossae are more clearly visualized during phonation (see Figures 4.11, 4.13 and 4.19).

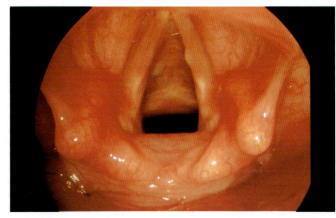

Figure 4.9

Normal larynx

The apparent 'nodule' on the right vocal fold is mucus, which cleared after the patient coughed. Vocal nodules are bilateral.

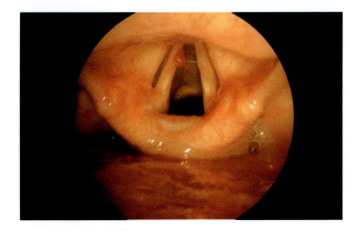

Figure 4.10

Vocal cord polyp

A small haemorrhagic polyp arising from the anterior third of the left vocal fold can be seen during respiration with the cords in abduction. See Figure 4.11.

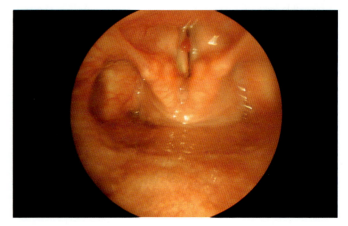

Figure 4.11

Vocal cord polyp

During adduction the polyp interferes with vibration of the edge of the vocal folds, producing a husky voice. This is the same patient as shown in Figure 4.10.

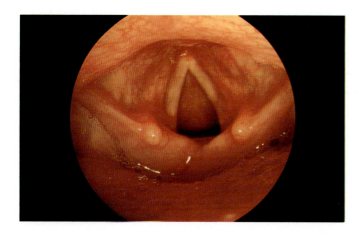

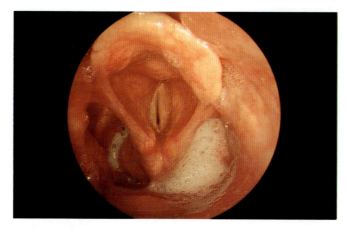

Figure 4.12
Vocal cord paralysis

The immobility of this right vocal cord is the result of a recurrent nerve paralysis. The right vocal cord is paralysed in the paramedian position. During inspiration, the left vocal cord is abducted. See Figure 4.13.

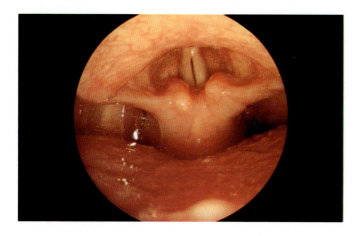

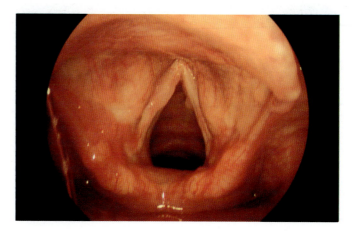

Figure 4.13
Vocal cord paralysis

During phonation, the left vocal fold adducts to attempt approximation with the right. The conversational voice is slightly weak and husky. This is the same patient as shown in Figure 4.12.

Figure 4.14
Ninth and tenth cranial nerve paralysis

This man recently had a vagal paraganglioma removed and has paralysis of the right 9th and 10th cranial nerves. Retained secretions can be seen in both valleculae and in both piriform fossae, more on the right side.

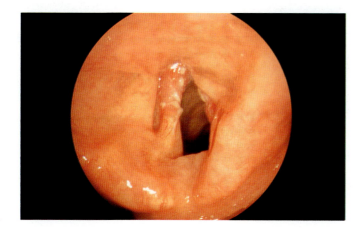

Figure 4.15
Laryngeal dysplasia

Note the irregular areas on both vocal folds. Biopsies showed severe dysplasia but no malignancy.

Figure 4.16
Laryngeal papillomatosis

Multiple respiratory papillomas on the anterior half of the left vocal cord and underneath the anterior part of the right vocal cord.

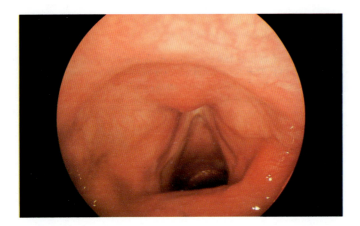

Figure 4.17

Iatrogenic laryngeal web

This patient has had over 40 operations for the removal of laryngeal papillomas and is in remission. The small anterior web shown here is a consequence of the removal of papillomas from the anterior commissure. The voice was slightly husky but strong.

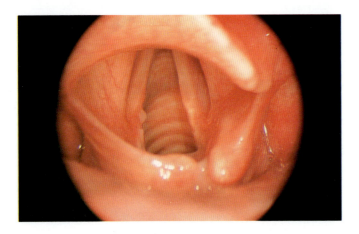

Figure 4.18

Vocal cord granuloma

A small vocal granuloma can be seen arising from the vocal process of the left arytenoid. The vocal cords are in abduction. See Figure 4.19.

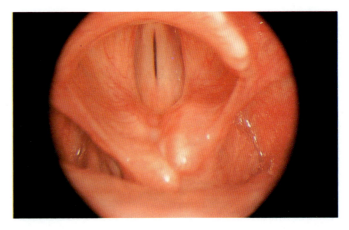

Figure 4.19

Vocal cord granuloma

The same patient as in Figure 4.18 during phonation. The granuloma can no longer be seen. Some patients with vocal granuloma have a near normal voice as the phonatory glottis is relatively unaffected.

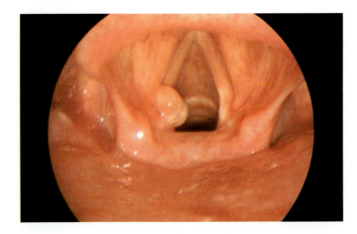

Figure 4.20

Large vocal cord granuloma

A moderately large, irregular, vocal granuloma on the medial surface of the left arytenoid. Removal for histological diagnosis is necessary as very occasionally malignancy or a specific granuloma may present in this area.

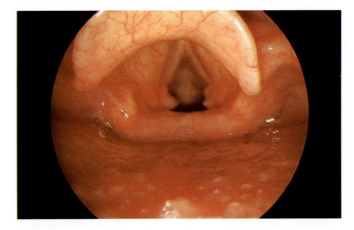

Figure 4.21

Contact ulcers

Bilateral so-called 'contact ulcers'. Contact pachydermia is a better term. There is a saucer-shaped circle of hyperplastic epithelium with a central crater but no actual ulcer. See Figures 4.158 and 4.159.

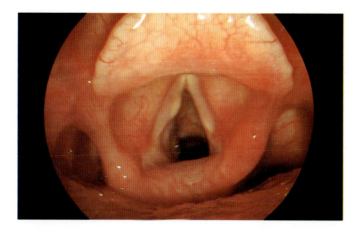

Figure 4.22

Vocal cord cyst

An intracordal cyst in the left vocal fold. Delicate microsurgery is required to remove the cyst from within the vocalis muscle and lamina propria by dissection without damage to the vibrating edge of the membranous vocal fold.

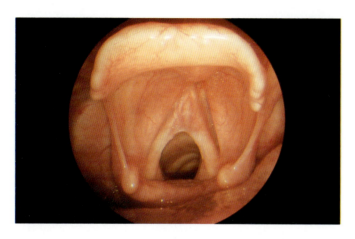

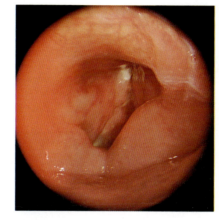

Figure 4.24

Advanced laryngeal carcinoma

Advanced laryngeal squamous cell carcinoma causing severe airway obstruction. The vocal cords cannot be seen. Note the marked oedema of the arytenoids.

Figure 4.23

Acquired laryngeal web

Acquired laryngeal web following repeated biopsy and laser surgery for epithelial dysplasia and intraepithelial carcinoma. There was no invasive carcinoma in repeated biopsies over an 8-year period.

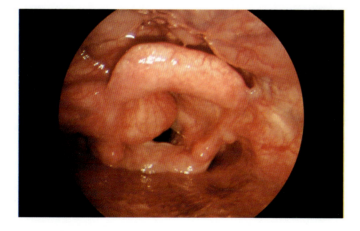

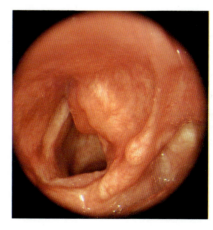

Figure 4.26

Laryngeal amyloid

Large localized deposit of amyloid in the right supraglottic area interfering with vocal fold vibration and causing chronic hoarseness. Treated by endoscopic removal. See Figure 4.290.

Figure 4.25

Supraglottic lateral saccular cyst

Large left-sided supraglottic lateral saccular cyst causing respiratory obstruction especially severe at night. This large cyst was removed successfully using an endoscopic technique. See Figure 4.182.

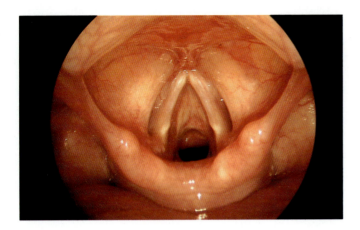

Figure 4.27
Subglottic stenosis: Wegener's granulomatosis

Young woman with proven systemic Wegener's granulomatosis. An irregular subglottic stenosis caused dyspnoea on exertion and required several laser treatments. See Figure 4.295.

Direct laryngoscopy

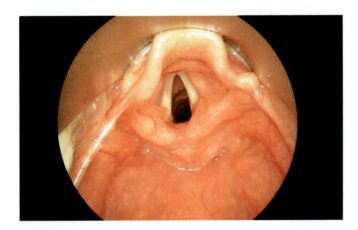

Figure 4.28
Normal infant larynx

Normal infant larynx at direct laryngoscopy using the Lindholm laryngoscope. Anaesthetic gases are insufflated through a cannula in the laryngoscope. (See Figures 4.44 and 4.46.) No endotracheal tube is necessary, thus affording excellent exposure. At the end of the procedure, when anaesthesia is being discontinued, muscle tone returns and vocal cord movements and laryngeal dynamics can be observed.

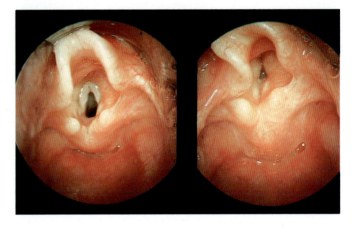

Figure 4.29
Laryngeal spasm

(Left) Normal larynx during spontaneous respiration, and (right) with temporary laryngospasm.

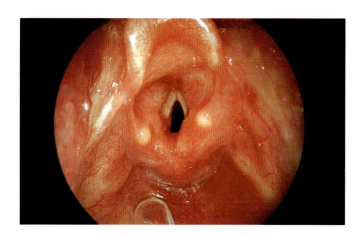

Figure 4.30

Normal infant larynx

Normal infant larynx being observed for vocal cord movement at the conclusion of anaesthesia. A small diameter pernasal endopharyngeal tube, seen at the bottom of the photograph, delivers oxygen. See Figure 4.38.

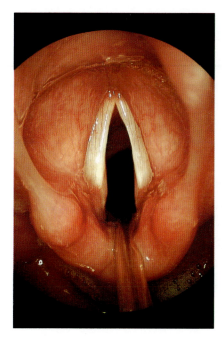

Figure 4.31

Benjet tube

An adult larynx with a Benjet tube for intratracheal jetting (2.8 mm external diameter) sitting unobtrusively in the posterior glottic space. The tube can easily be displaced to the anterior larynx for an unrestricted view of the posterior larynx.

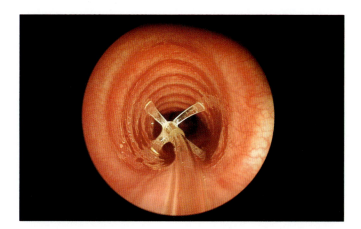

Figure 4.32

Benjet tube

During jet ventilation four soft plastic petals stabilize the Benjet tube in the trachea to prevent the whipping effect of a free-lying tube.

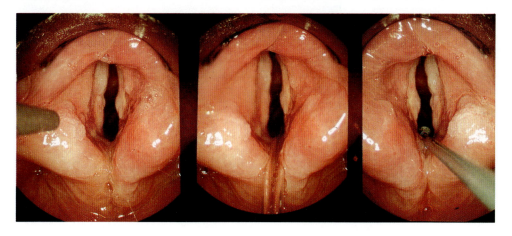

Figure 4.33

Jet anaesthesia

On the left side, fixed to the rim of the laryngoscope, there is a proximal jet metal cannula with a slightly malleable tube adjusted to direct the jet towards the glottic opening. In the centre a Benjet tube is in place for distal jetting in the tracheal lumen. On the right side a longer, distal jet metal cannula has been placed through the glottic opening for jetting in the upper trachea.

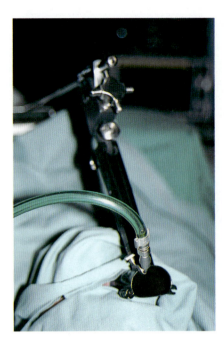

Figure 4.34
Proximal jet anaesthesia

A proximal jet cannula has been fixed to the rim of the laryngoscope by a simple adjustment screw.

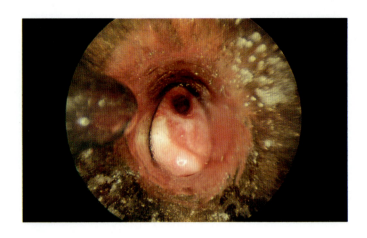

Figure 4.35
Proximal jet anaesthesia

Proximal jet cannula used with a subglottiscope for laser vaporization in a patient with idiopathic subglottic stenosis.

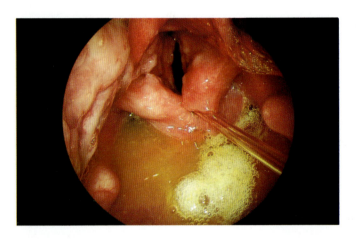

Figure 4.36
Regurgitation of gastric contents

Regurgitation of gastric contents in a paralysed patient having distal jet ventilation for the treatment of laryngeal papillomas. The surgeon must keep the laryngopharynx clear of such secretions.

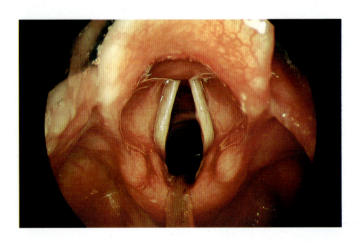

Figure 4.37
Benjet tube vs. endotracheal tube

Comparison of a Benjet tube (left) and a small diameter regular endotracheal tube (right). The larger diameter of the latter obscures the posterior glottic space and the subglottic region.

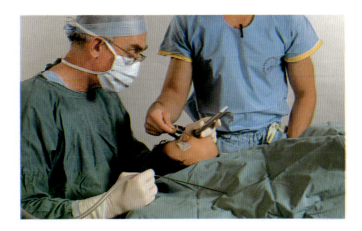

Figure 4.38

Direct laryngoscopy in an infant: stage 1

The preliminary naked eye examination takes place with a hand-held laryngoscope. The anaesthetic gases are insufflated into the laryngopharynx either through a small plastic tube passed through one nasal cavity or through a metal cannula in the side wall of the laryngoscope. The patient is breathing spontaneously.

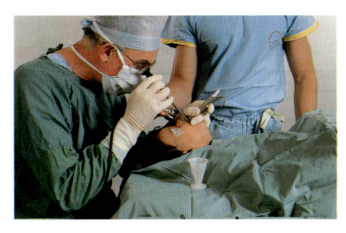

Figure 4.39

Direct laryngoscopy in an infant: stage 2

A more detailed evaluation using a rigid telescope for image magnification is then carried out.

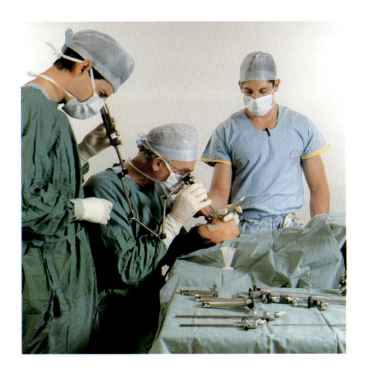

Figure 4.40

Wittmoser articulated teaching arm

The Wittmoser multi-articulated teaching arm is able to split the image from the telescope with the observer seeing exactly the same image as the surgeon.

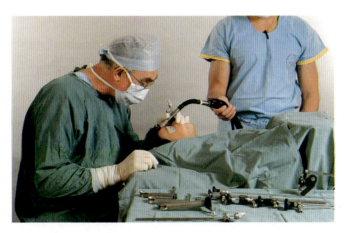

Figure 4.41

Tracheobronchoscopy

Tracheobronchoscopy with the naked eye, using a ventilating bronchoscope. The anaesthetic gases are being delivered through the side channel.

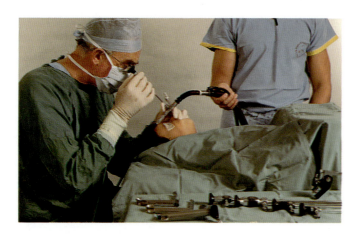

Figure 4.42

Tracheobronchoscopy

Examination of the trachea, main bronchi and segmental openings using 0°, 30° and, if necessary, 70° telescopes of the appropriate size.

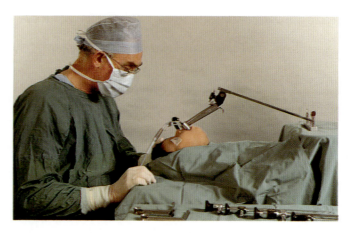

Figure 4.43

Suspension laryngoscopy in an infant

Suspension laryngoscopy and naked eye examination. The self-retaining laryngoscope holder has been positioned so that the examiner's two hands are now available for endolaryngeal manipulation.

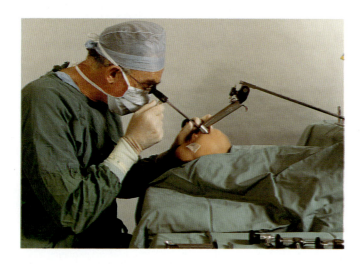

Figure 4.44

Direct laryngoscopy with a telescope in an infant

Examination of the pharynx and larynx with a rigid rod lens telescope. For diagnostic examination of the tracheobronchial tree a longer slimmer telescope with a straight ahead or angled view can be passed into the trachea and main bronchi. Anaesthetic gases are insufflated through a side channel in the laryngoscope.

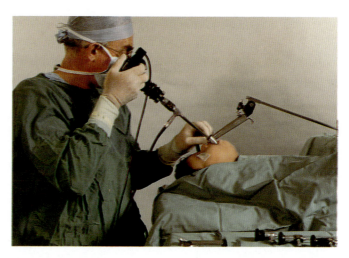

Figure 4.45

Laryngeal photography

Photography using a 35 mm single-frame, single-lens reflex camera with a synchronized, automatic-exposure, computer-controlled, remote electronic flash generator.

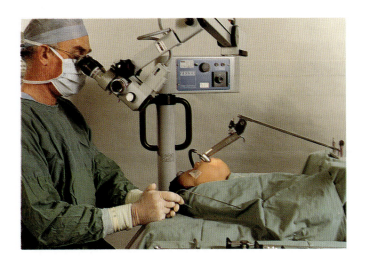

Figure 4.46

Direct laryngoscopy with the microscope in an infant

Microlaryngoscopy is used for a detailed examination, for endolaryngeal microsurgery or for laser surgery.

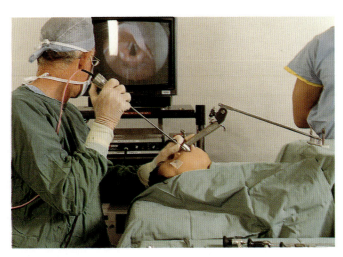

Figure 4.47

Videographic documentation

Videographic documentation can be carried out using a small, high-quality, low light sensitive video camera. The video image can then be either printed in black and white or colour using a video printer or transferred to tape by a video recorder.

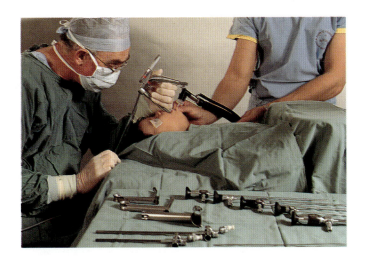

Figure 4.48

Oesophagoscopy

Oesophagoscopy using an open-tube instrument with a round, wide-diameter lumen through which a telescope can be used, a foreign body removed, dilators passed or a biopsy taken.

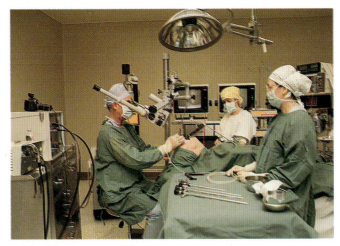

Figure 4.49

Suspension microlaryngoscopy in an adult

Overall view of the arrangements in the operating room showing the endoscopic trolley, photographic equipment, video equipment, anaesthetic and patient monitoring equipment.

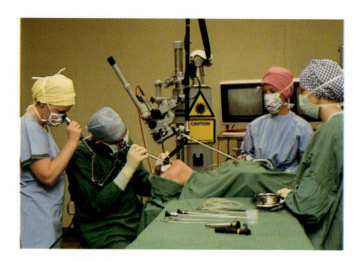

Figure 4.50

Laryngoscopy with a telescope in an adult

Detailed examination with a telescope while an assistant observes through a Wittmoser optical arm. The patient is paralysed and receiving jet ventilation anaesthesia.

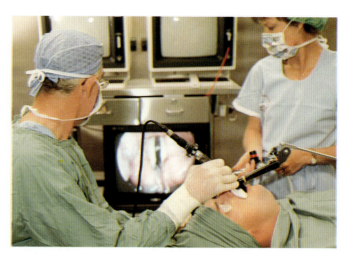

Figure 4.51

Televised examination

The use of a television camera and monitor greatly improves the procedure. The anaesthetist can more accurately monitor the airway and observe the conditions of anaesthesia and the instrument nurses can anticipate the progress of the procedure. The entire operating room staff also feel more involvement in the operation.

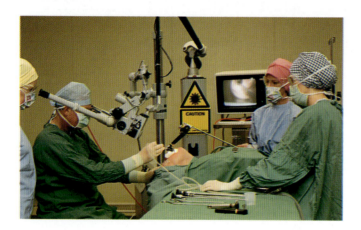

Figure 4.52

Microlaryngoscopy in an adult

Microlaryngoscopy is being performed in this patient in preparation for an endolaryngeal laser procedure.

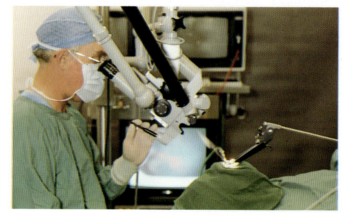

Figure 4.53

Laser surgery

The laser beam is controlled by the surgeon's left hand, using the micromanipulator. The gas mixture for jet ventilation is 60% helium : 40% oxygen.

Normal larynx

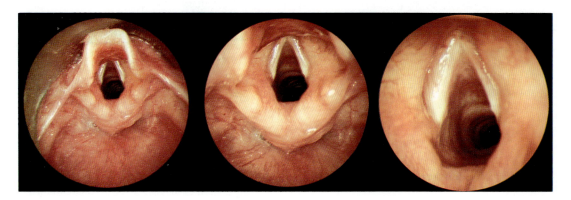

Figure 4.54

Three views of a child's normal larynx

Overall and close-up examination. The first view shows an overall view of the laryngopharynx, the second the supraglottic structures, and third the glottis, subglottis and upper trachea.

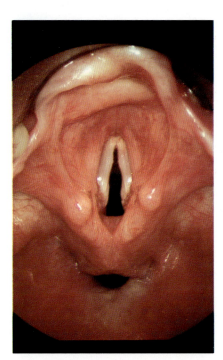

Figure 4.55

Larynx and hypopharynx

The Lindholm laryngoscope gives an excellent panoramic view of the supraglottic and glottic structures and, in this case, the postcricoid region is also widely exposed.

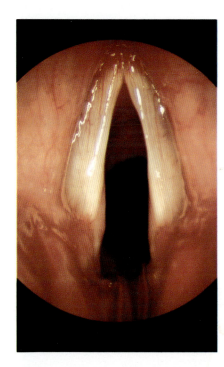

Figure 4.56

Adult glottis

The Benjet tube, which is 2.8 mm in external diameter, sits in the posterior glottic space of this normal larynx.

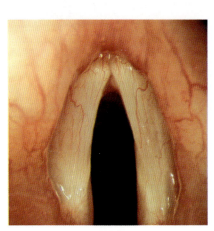

Figure 4.57

Close-up of the vocal folds

The anterior commissure and the false cords in a normal adult.

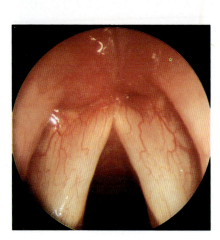

Figure 4.58

Close-up of the anterior commissure

Close-up of the anterior commissure and the 'hidden' area above it, which, in this case, is clearly seen with a 30° laryngeal telescope.

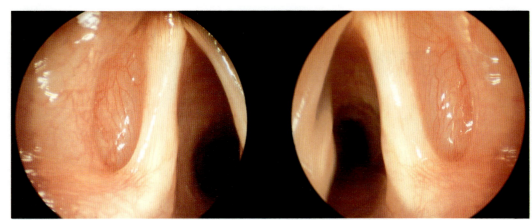

Figure 4.59

Ventricles

Normal ventricles on the left, and on the right seen with a 30° telescope.

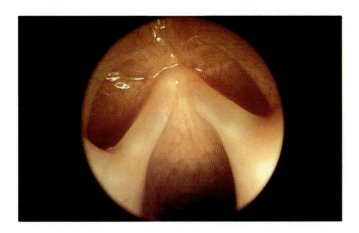

Figure 4.60

Anterior larynx

The anterior subglottic region, the vocal folds and the ventricles seen with a 70° telescope.

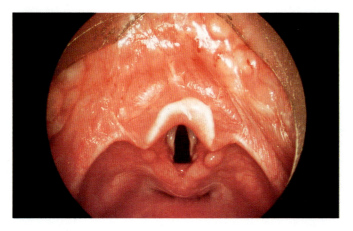

Figure 4.61

Base of tongue

The base of the tongue, valleculae, glosso-epiglottic fold, epiglottis and glossopharyngeal folds with the larynx in the distance. This view was obtained with a Lindholm laryngoscope positioned at the base of the tongue.

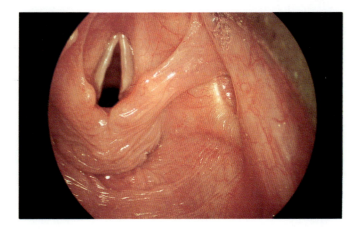

Figure 4.62

Laryngopharynx

By angling the Lindholm laryngoscope, the lateral pharyngeal wall, piriform fossa and part of the postcricoid region are highlighted.

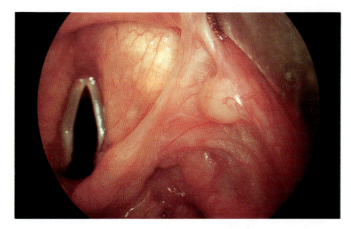

Figure 4.63

Small lymphoid follicle

The small lymphoid follicle just lateral to the right aryepiglottic fold is a normal variant.

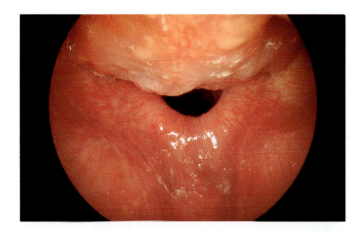

Figure 4.64
Postcricoid region

The postcricoid region and cricopharyngeus muscle have been exposed with the Lindholm laryngoscope.

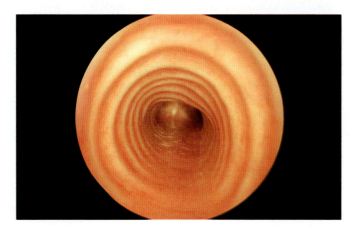

Figure 4.65
Normal trachea

The normal trachea in a child showing the cartilaginous arches and the carina in the distance.

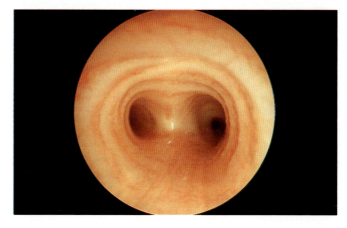

Figure 4.66
Normal trachea

Normal lower trachea, carina and the openings of the left and right main bronchus.

Laryngomalacia

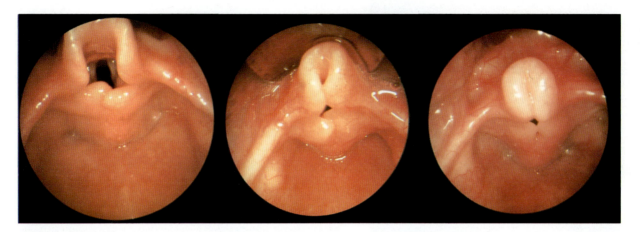

Figure 4.67

Laryngomalacia

Laryngomalacia ('floppy larynx') is the most common cause of laryngeal stridor in infants. Inspiratory stridor usually commences days or weeks before birth. At direct endoscopy it is seen that as inspiration commences there is partial inward collapse of the supraglottic structures, the epiglottis curls upon itself and the cuneiform cartilages are sucked into the glottic opening. At maximum inspiration there is only a small supraglottic laryngeal opening. During expiration the airway is unimpeded.

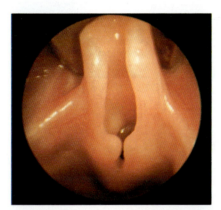

Figure 4.68

Laryngomalacia

Although the low-pitched intermittent inspiratory stridor may be alarming, not only to the parents but to the attending physician, the baby usually has normal general health and development. The epiglottis is often tall, omega-shaped and curled. Most infants become symptom-free within 18–24 months but occasionally the stridor persists for years.

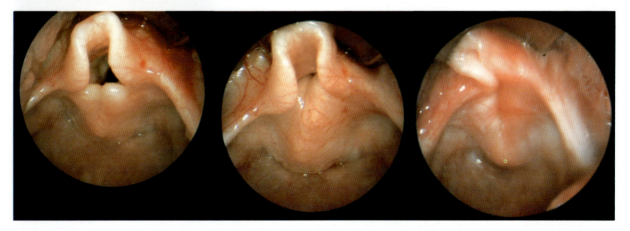

Figure 4.69

Laryngomalacia

These three views show the dynamics of laryngomalacia. Expiration is unimpeded as the supraglottic structures are blown upwards and outwards, but during inspiration the floppy aryepiglottic folds and cuneiform cartilages are sucked into the larynx with accompanying inspiratory stridor. The aryepiglottic folds are short in some cases. The airway obstruction is usually self-correcting with time and further growth, and is very rarely severe enough to warrant surgical treatment.

Other congenital anomalies

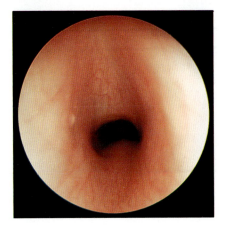

Figure 4.70

Congenital subglottic stenosis

Congenital subglottic stenosis is characterized by a symmetrical, usually circular narrowing of cricoid ring. The internal diameter of the cricoid cartilage can be gauged by comparison with the outside diameter of the bronchoscope, telescope or endotracheal tube that passes through it comfortably. The upper part of the posterior lamina of the normal cricoid cartilage of an infant has a shallow V-configuration, rather than that of a smooth, completely round ring.

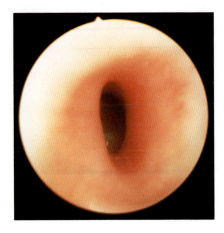

Figure 4.71

Elliptical stenosis of the cricoid

Although the most common abnormality is circumferential stenosis, the lumen may be oval, as in this infant with a congenital elliptical subglottic stenosis. In other cases the abnormal cricoid can be of normal shape but small size, or abnormal shape with a large anterior lamina, or with generalized thickening, or flattened from anterior to posterior.

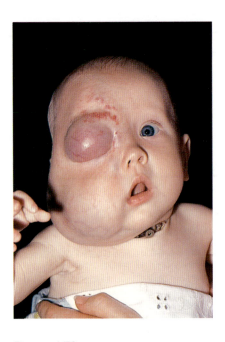

Figure 4.72

Congenital subglottic haemangioma

Congenital subglottic haemangiomas are associated with large or small facial or neck haemangiomas in about 50% of cases. This baby had a tracheotomy to relieve the airway obstruction and allow treatment. A congenital subglottic haemangioma is a hamartoma of blood vessels.

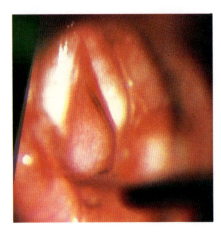

Figure 4.73

Congenital subglottic haemangioma

Note the typical appearance of this large obstructive left subglottic haemangioma which might be amenable to laser treatment. Biopsy is necessary only when the diagnosis is in doubt. They are five times more common in females.

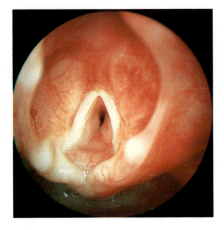

Figure 4.74

Atypical congenital subglottic haemangioma

This congenital laryngeal haemangioma presented in a very unusual fashion as three rounded subglottic masses. There is also submucosal vascular involvement of the supraglottic larynx.

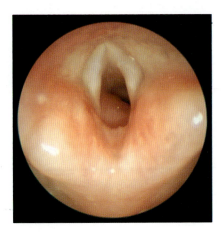

Figure 4.75

Left subglottic haemangioma

This left subglottic haemangioma extends into the posterior subglottic space.

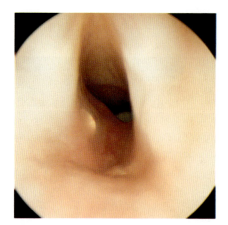

Figure 4.76

Left subglottic haemangioma

Note the remnant of a left subglottic haemangioma 12 weeks after the insertion of a radioactive gold grain, by means of a small platinum coated cylinder 2.5 mm × 0.8 mm, which can be seen just under the mucosa.

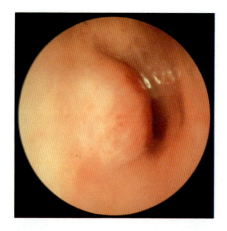

Figure 4.77

Haemangioma of the lateral wall of the upper trachea

This haemangioma of the lateral wall of the upper trachea caused severe airway obstruction. It was removed surgically. The airway was maintained by pernasal intubation for 4 days postoperatively thus avoiding tracheotomy.

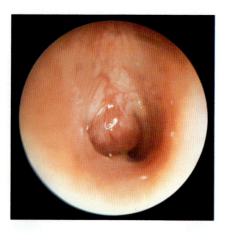

Figure 4.78

Large tracheal haemangioma

This large haemangioma arose from the anterior wall of the upper trachea below the cricoid cartilage. It was removed surgically.

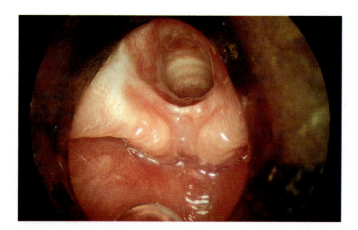

Figure 4.79

Congenital posterior laryngeal cleft

Note the minor cleft extending just below the glottic level. Persistent aspiration during feeding is the cardinal feature. Sometimes a soft tissue mass of lymphangioma occurs near the cleft and contributes to airway obstruction.

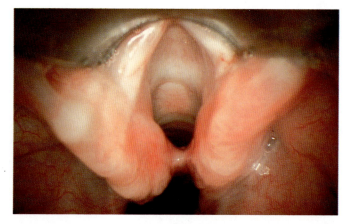

Figure 4.80

Congenital posterior laryngeal cleft

Note the posterior laryngeal cleft extending into the cricoid cartilage. It is typical that, endoscopically, the upper oesophageal lumen can be seen. The cricoid is C-shaped and is open posteriorly in the midline when the posterior cricoid lamina has a complete cleft.

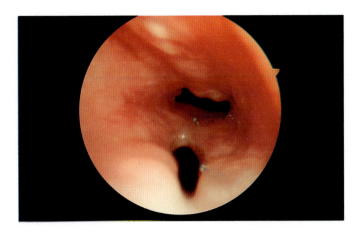

Figure 4.81

Partially repaired congenital posterior laryngeal cleft

The attempted repair of this posterior laryngotracheal cleft was successful superiorly; however, the residual fistula inferiorly requires further surgical repair.

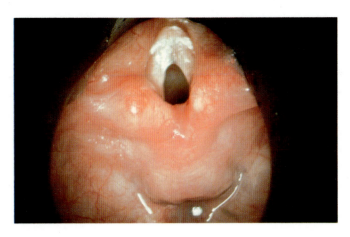

Figure 4.82

Small congenital glottic web

Most congenital webs are anterior. This baby had no cry until the small, thin transparent web was divided with microlaryngoscopy scissors.

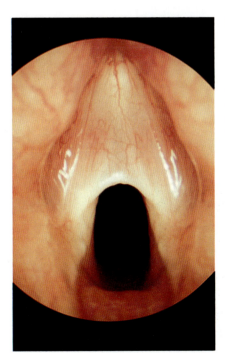

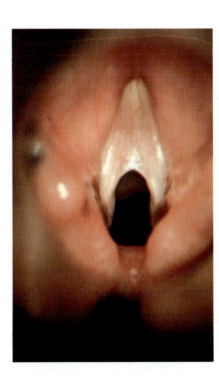

Figure 4.83

Medium congenital glottic web

This is a medium-sized, thicker congenital anterior glottic web. The baby had a husky cry but no airway obstruction.

Figure 4.84

Large congenital glottic web

A larger web in a 12-year-old girl who had always had a 'squeaky' voice. A reasonable result was obtained after laryngofissure, excision of the web and insertion of a keel.

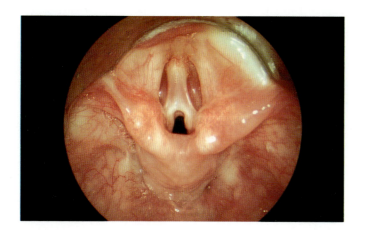

Figure 4.85

Large congenital glottic web

This patient has a large congenital glottic web. The outlines of the vocal ligaments can be seen through the membranous web and the laryngeal ventricles are prominent. There was an associated thick subglottic stenosis about 12–15 mm in length. Severe airway obstruction at birth required a tracheotomy until the lesion was surgically repaired at 4½ years of age.

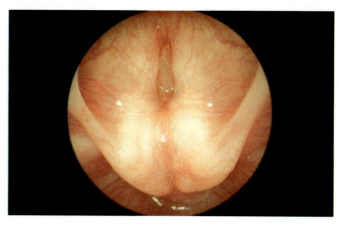

Figure 4.86

Laryngeal atresia

Attempted intubation at birth was unsuccessful in this newborn with laryngeal atresia. Life was maintained for about 20 minutes by positive pressure ventilation via an H-type tracheo-oesophageal fistula until an emergency tracheotomy was performed.

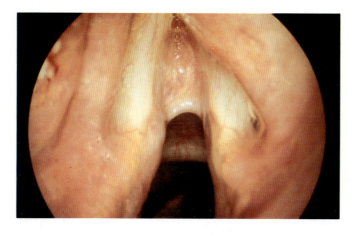

Figure 4.87

Congenital glottic and subglottic web in an adult

This congenital glottic and subglottic web was discovered in a 52-year-old man who had 'always' had a husky voice. Laser treatment produced moderate voice improvement.

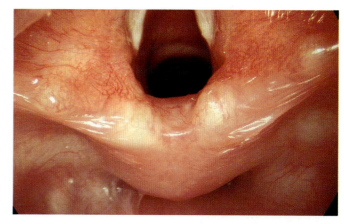

Figure 4.88

Congenital interarytenoid web

A congenital supraglottic interarytenoid web is a rare anomaly in which tissue joins the medial surface of the arytenoids thus restricting abduction of the vocal cords. This anomaly is easily missed or misdiagnosed as bilateral vocal cord paralysis, cricoarytenoid joint fixation or posterior glottic stenosis.

Figure 4.89

Congenital interarytenoid web

Congenital interarytenoid webs often have other associated anomalies including subglottic stenosis, large arytenoids and an abnormal laryngeal position, all of which may make laryngoscopy and airway maintenance difficult during anaesthesia.

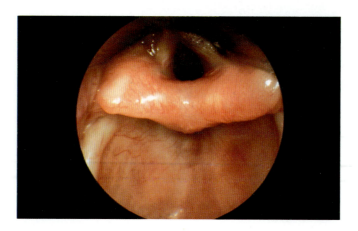

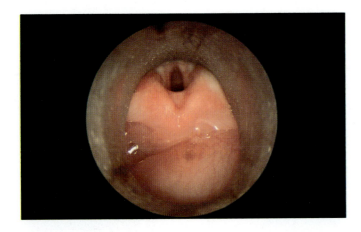

Figure 4.90

Membranous congenital interarytenoid web

Note large arytenoids and the difficulty exposing the larynx using a small Holinger paediatric laryngoscope in this patient with a membranous congenital interarytenoid web.

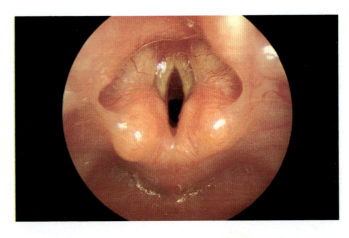

Figure 4.91

Membranous congenital interarytenoid web

This baby with a membranous congenital interarytenoid web presented with unexplained stridor. The arytenoids are very large and possibly contributed to the partial airway obstruction.

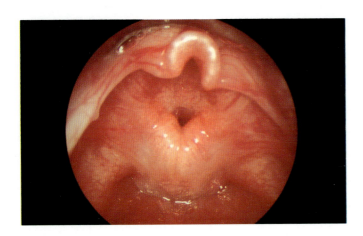

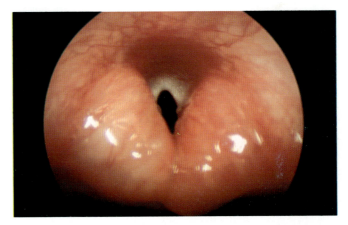

Figure 4.92

Congenital glottic anomalies

This patient has several congenital glottic anomalies. Note the supraglottic narrowing, small epiglottis, large arytenoids, the small glottic opening with anterior webbing and the subglottic stenosis. A tracheotomy was required for repeated cyanotic and apnoeic attacks.

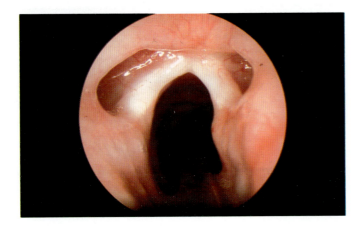

Figure 4.93

Congenital abnormality of the larynx

Congenital abnormality of the larynx in a 16-year-old girl who had a weak and breathy voice. The right vocal cord was short and did not move. There were associated abnormalities of the 9th and 11th cranial nerves on the right side.

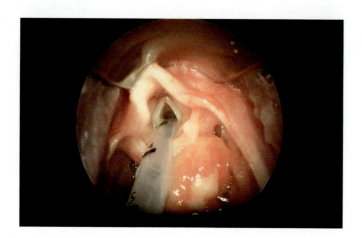

Figure 4.94

Choristoma of the laryngopharynx

The irregular mass on the posterior wall of the laryngopharynx in a baby with stridor, feeding difficulty and failure to thrive was a choristoma consisting of ectopic gastric mucosa. Laser removal was performed.

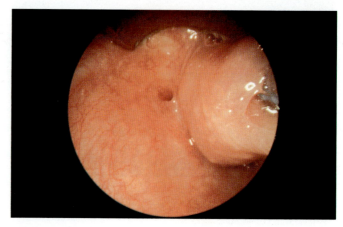

Figure 4.95

Fourth branchial pouch fistula

A fourth branchial pouch fistula can be seen opening in the medial floor of the apex of the left piriform fossa of this 4-month-old infant with severe stridor due to infection and swelling in the pouch in the neck and upper mediastinum.

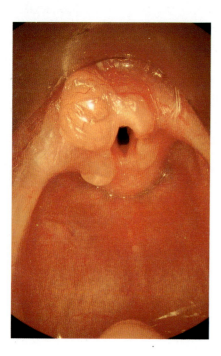

Figure 4.96

Cystic hygroma

Cystic hygroma is a congenital lesion which commonly presents at birth or in the first 12 months of life, usually as a lateral neck mass. It is a painless, diffuse, soft, spongy, single or multiple mass with an ill-defined edge. These abnormalities vary in size from very small to very large masses which cause cosmetic deformities and, in the pharynx and larynx, may cause upper airway obstruction. This oval lymphangioma cyst arises from the left side of the epiglottis with another, smaller, cystic area below it; they were part of a large mass in the left lateral neck.

Vocal nodules

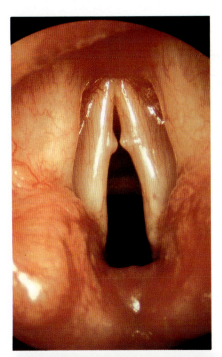

Figure 4.97
Vocal nodules

Vocal nodules are bilateral and occur in both adults and children (mostly boys). They vary in colour, contour and size and are usually similar on each side. These are the vocal nodules of a 12-year-old boy who presented with chronic intermittent huskiness unresponsive to speech therapy.

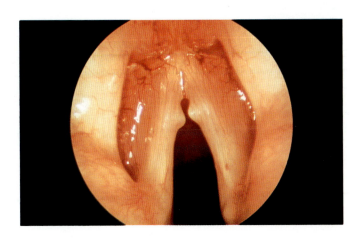

Figure 4.98
Vocal nodules

Chronic vocal nodules seen with a 30° telescope. Vocal nodules form on the edge and undersurface of the centre of the membranous vocal fold. Histological examination of vocal nodules shows thickened epithelium, submucosal oedema, microcystic degeneration and hyalinization in Reinke's space.

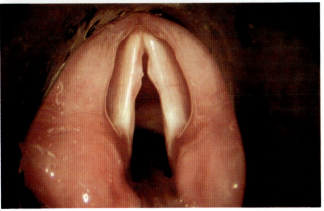

Figure 4.99
Vocal nodules

Voice therapy may be beneficial. However, when the nodules cause troublesome hoarseness for months or years microsurgical removal may be considered. There is nodularity and focal thickening at the junction of the anterior third and the posterior two-thirds of the vocal cords, that is, at the centre of the membranous vocal fold.

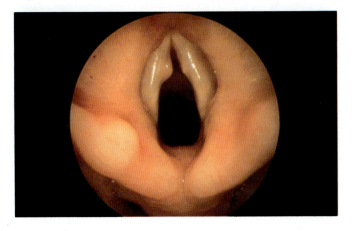

Figure 4.100
Vocal nodules

If the 'nodule' is larger on one side than the other, the possibility of an intracordal cyst should be considered. In this case there was microcystic degeneration in the nodule on the left vocal fold, but no discrete cyst.

Figure 4.101
Vocal nodules

Bilateral vocal nodules, with some haemorrhagic change on the right side.

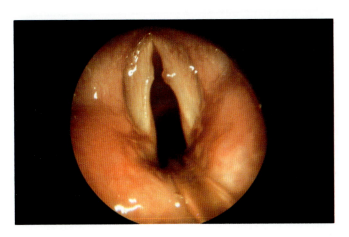

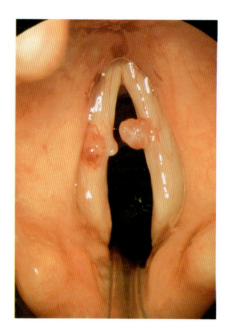

Figure 4.102
Vocal nodules

An unusual appearance, apparently due to degeneration in the vocal nodules of a woman in her thirties who had refused treatment for many years.

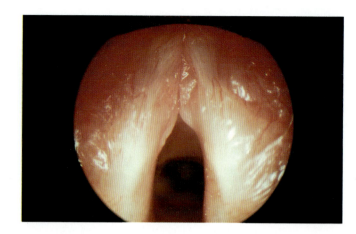

Figure 4.103
Vocal nodules

A baby of only 4 months of age who had always had a husky, weak cry. Removal of these unusual nodules resulted in a near normal cry. Surgical treatment as such an early age is very seldom warranted.

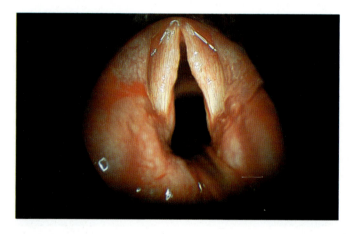

Figure 4.104
Vocal nodules

Vocal nodules with subacute hypertrophic laryngitis and Reinke's oedema. This young woman was a professional singer. Voice rest for 6 weeks resulted in a satisfactory improvement.

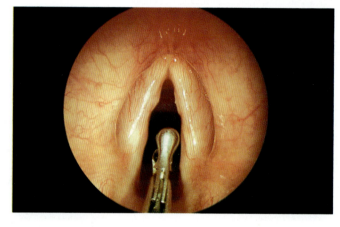

Figure 4.105
Microsurgical removal of vocal nodules

Failure to improve with voice therapy, worsening of the voice or intermittent loss of voice warrant removal of vocal nodules, although rarely before the age of 8 years. The nodule is grasped with upturned cup-shaped forceps, retracted towards the midline to emphasize the wide base and removed with scissors.

Figure 4.106
Chronic laryngitis

Although vocal nodules often have a prominent fusiform longitudinal swelling, in this case there is no focal nodular abnormality and consequently the term 'vocal nodules' would be a misnomer.

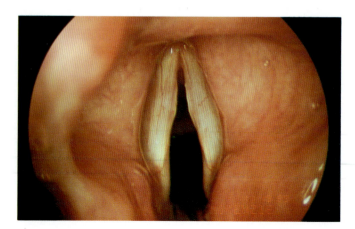

Multiple respiratory papillomatosis

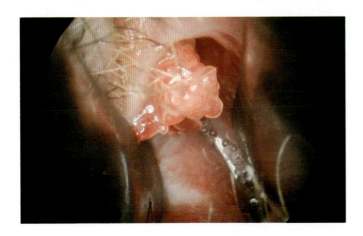

Figure 4.107

Nasal cavity papillomatosis

Papillomas, caused by the human papilloma virus, occur in the upper airway in patients of any age, about two-thirds being younger than 15 years and one-third older than 15 years of age. The highest incidence is before the age of 5 years. Note the mass of papillomas in the vestibule of this patient's nose, probably arising from the squamous epithelium.

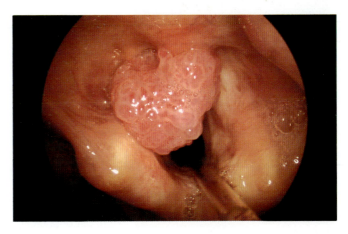

Figure 4.108

Supraglottic papillomatosis

Papillomas occur most commonly in the larynx, but may be found elsewhere in the upper respiratory tract from the nasal mucosa to the lung parenchyma and even in the oesophagus. The large papillomatous mass in the left supraglottic larynx had a relatively small pedicle, which allowed excision of the mass with the carbon dioxide laser.

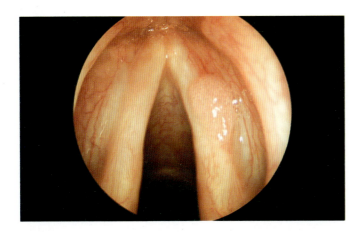

Figure 4.109

Laryngeal papillomatosis

There is no interrelationship between puberty and the age at onset, the rate of control or the rate of recurrence. Consequently, the patient should be treated without regard to his or her age as there is no tendency for regression at puberty. Note the single mass of papillomas on the upper surface of the right vocal fold, extending onto the floor of the ventricle. View with the 30° telescope prior to laser surgery.

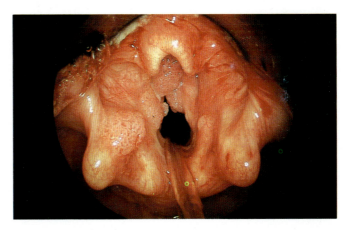

Figure 4.110

Widespread laryngeal papillomatosis

Although unexpected remissions do occur, this disease is notorious for frequent recurrences and multiple sites of involvement. This overall view of the larynx shows many deposits of papilloma. No normal vocal folds can be seen.

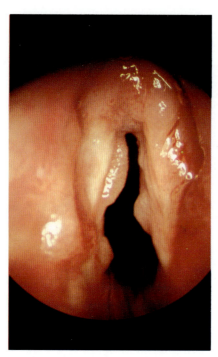

Figure 4.111

Laryngeal papillomatosis: close-up

The growth rate may be irregular and unpredictable with remissions and exacerbations occurring for no apparent reason, and although spontaneous resolution may occur there is usually a tendency for recurrence and progression, in some cases despite all forms of treatment. Note the close-up view of scattered masses mostly affecting the edge of the vocal folds and the anterior commissure.

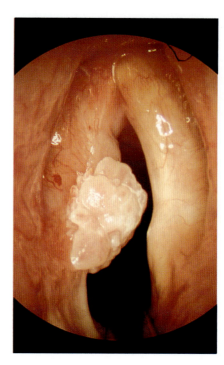

Figure 4.112

Posterior laryngeal papillomatosis

Large mass arising from the area of the vocal process of the left arytenoid. This mass should be differentiated from vocal granuloma. Laryngeal papillomas generally occur in the anterior larynx.

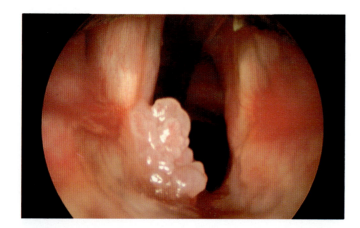

Figure 4.113

Posterior laryngeal papillomatosis

Papillomas in the left posterior glottic space, again producing a similar appearance to vocal granuloma but in this case arising more posteriorly.

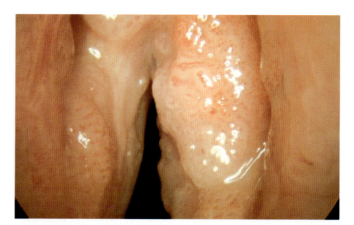

Figure 4.114

Laryngeal papillomatosis: close-up

Close-up view of irregular masses of laryngeal papillomas.

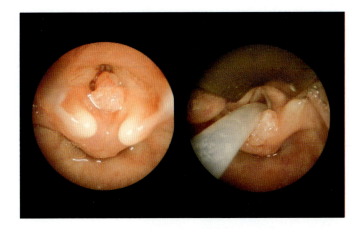

Figure 4.115

Laryngeal papillomatosis in a newborn baby

Neonate with a mass of papillomas in the supraglottis, causing severe intermittent airway obstruction with cyanotic attacks. Endotracheal intubation was required to secure and maintain the airway while most of the papillomas were removed. Subsequent laser surgery was performed for more precise removal of the residual disease.

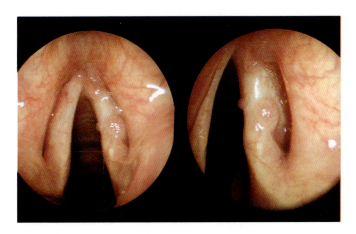

Figure 4.116

Laryngeal papillomatosis

The potential to compromise function of the larynx and cause airway obstruction sometimes makes papillomas of the larynx a serious threat to life. The basis of management is to maintain an adequate airway by removal of the papillomas, usually achieved with the carbon dioxide laser or a combination of laser treatment and removal by cup forceps. Note how the papillomas scattered on the right vocal cord are more clearly delineated, with reference to the laryngeal ventricle, when viewed with the 30° telescope.

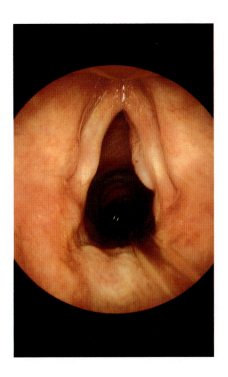
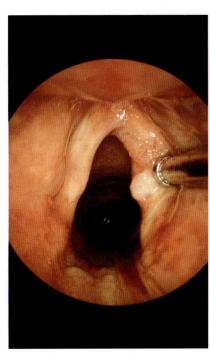

Figure 4.117

Laryngeal papillomatosis and iatrogenic web

Technique of 'rolling' the vocal fold to display papillomas for direct laser treatment. As an alternative the laser beam can be bounced by means of a metal mirror under the vocal fold, into the ventricle or even under an acquired web under which papillomas are forming.

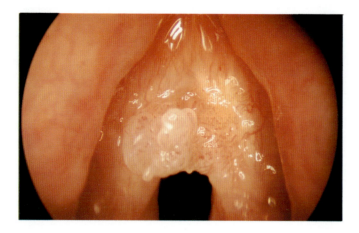

Figure 4.118

Laryngeal papillomatosis, anterior commissure

The anterior commissure is the site of predilection and ultimately, despite careful removal from one side and then the other, it is possible that a web will form after surgical treatment.

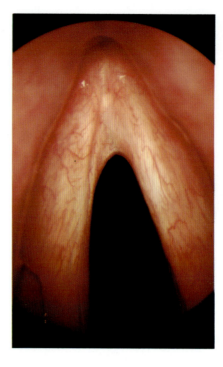

Figure 4.119

Laryngeal papillomatosis and small web

Small acquired anterior glottic web following removal of papillomas. The voice was only marginally affected.

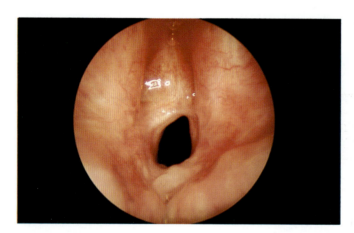

Figure 4.120

Laryngeal papillomatosis and a thick web

This 6-year-old whose laryngeal papillomas had been removed on many occasions at another hospital, presented with an irregular thick web and a very poor voice.

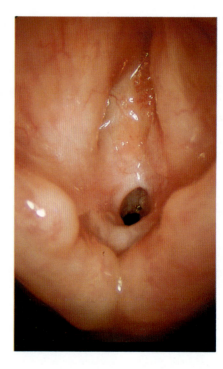

Figure 4.121

Respiratory papillomatosis and thick web

A 12-year-old girl treated in another country by a tracheotomy and multiple operations. There is a large thick web at the glottic level with papillomas underneath it and massive papillomatosis in the upper trachea around the tracheotomy site.

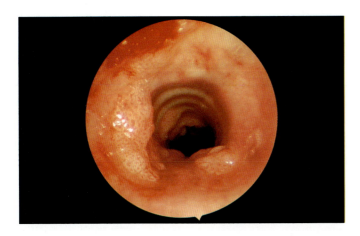

Figure 4.122

Respiratory papillomatosis

Multiple areas of papilloma in the upper and lower trachea. Patients who have aggressively growing lesions in the trachea or bronchi may develop papillomatous nodules in the lung parenchyma. They should have a chest radiograph or CT scan.

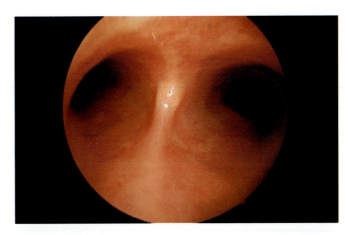

Figure 4.123

Tracheal papillomatosis

This woman had repeated operations for laryngeal papillomas. This single papilloma was found in the trachea. Regular examination of the tracheobronchial tree with a telescope is recommended. It is possible that seeding occurs during surgery, but this is neither proven nor likely.

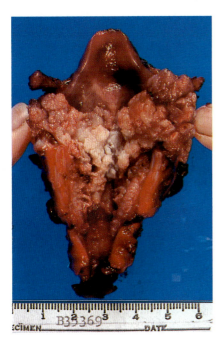

Figure 4.124

Respiratory papillomatosis: verrucous carcinoma

Laryngectomy specimen from a 15-year-old boy who had a tracheotomy at the age of 7 years and was advised to return 'after puberty'. Histological examination showed that a verrucous carcinoma had developed.

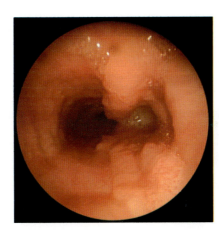

Figure 4.125

Respiratory papillomatosis: oesophageal papillomas

This patient has multiple respiratory papillomas and papillomas in the wall on the right side of the upper oesophagus, an unusual site of occurrence.

Reinke's oedema, vocal polyps and other conditions

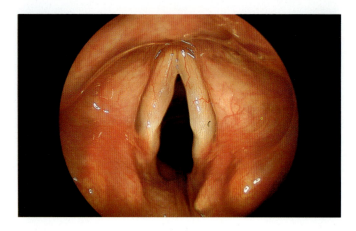

Figure 4.126

Reinke's oedema

Reinke's oedema occurs when excess fluid accumulates in Reinke's space. Chronic oedema in Reinke's space may be unilateral or bilateral and can progress to the formation of large, bilateral vocal cord polyps. Other polyps may be fusiform, pedunculated or generalized. Reinke's oedema results in a hoarse, low-pitched voice, as in hypothyroidism. Note the chronic oedema in Reinke's space in both vocal folds of this middle-aged female who smoked and admitted to excessive talking.

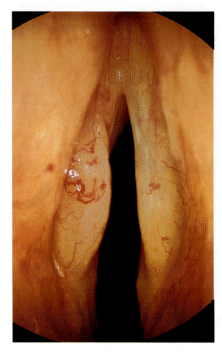

Figure 4.127

Reinke's oedema

Reinke's space is a potential space between the surface mucosa of the vocal fold and the medial thyroarytenoid (vocalis) muscle and vocal ligament. The space stretches from the tip of the vocal process to the anterior commissure, contains loose areolar tissue and allows free movement and vibration of the mucosa of the vocal folds during phonation. The oedema in Reinke's space in this patient has more marked oedema on the left side. The prominent dilated vessels are easily identified.

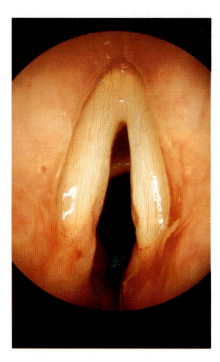

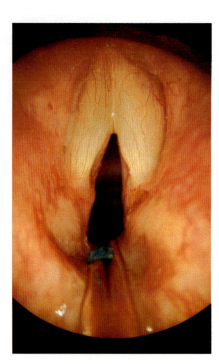

Figure 4.128

Reinke's oedema: difference in appearance

The photograph on the left was taken using a Lindholm laryngoscope placed anterior to the epiglottis. The photograph on the right was taken using a Kleinsasser laryngoscope. The difference in appearance is striking and is related to the different amount of tension put on the vocal ligaments and vocal folds by placement of the laryngoscope.

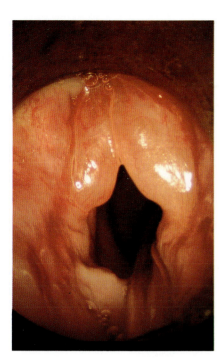

Figure 4.129
Advanced Reinke's oedema

The severe bilateral Reinke's oedema with bilateral generalized polypoidal degeneration in this patient was successfully treated by staged microlaryngeal surgical treatment (first one side and later the other side).

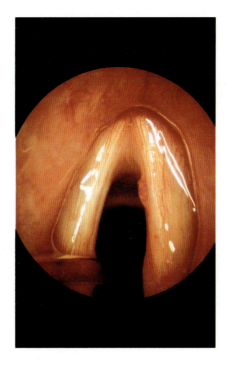

Figure 4.130
Vocal cord polyp

There is a small, slightly irregular polyp on the edge and undersurface of the right vocal fold. Microsurgical removal with cup forceps and scissors gives a better result in this type of polyp than the laser.

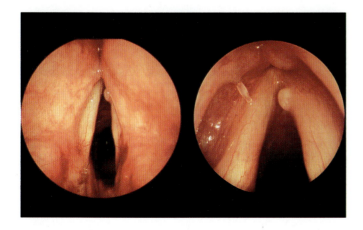

Figure 4.131
Vocal cord polyp

The small polyp on the edge of the anterior third of this right vocal fold can be more clearly seen in the photograph on the right which was taken with a 30° laryngeal telescope. A laryngeal polyp is most likely to form following incomplete resolution of a haematoma caused by rupture of a blood vessel in the laryngeal mucosa.

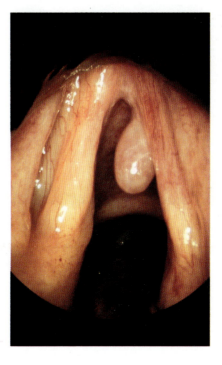

Figure 4.132
Vocal cord polyp

A pedunculated polyp can be seen arising from the undersurface of the right vocal fold. Note the oedema in the anterior subcommissure, which is not an uncommon finding in these patients.

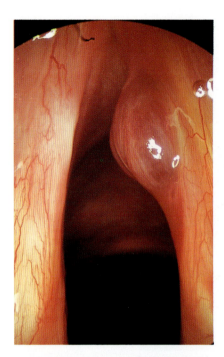

Figure 4.133

Vocal cord polyp: close-up

A close-up photograph of a soft, haemorrhagic polyp on the right side immediately before removal using microsurgical scissors. This type of polyp may be the result of the rupture of a capillary in Reinke's space.

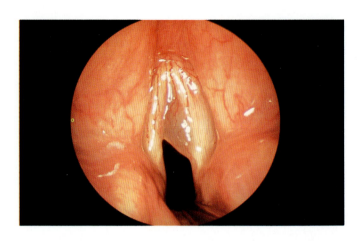

Figure 4.134

Vocal cord polyp

There is a large, thin-walled fusiform polyp of the right vocal fold. The vascular congestion, venous stasis and degree of oedema may vary with voice use.

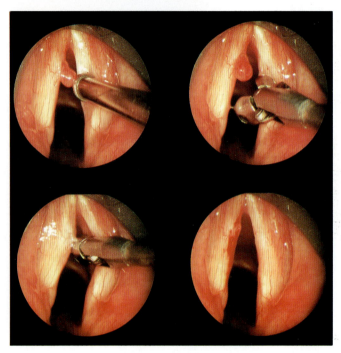

Figure 4.135

Vocal cord polyp: technique of removal

These four views taken using the Kantor–Berci laryngoscope demonstrate the technique used for the removal of a left vocal fold polyp employing cupped forceps and scissors.

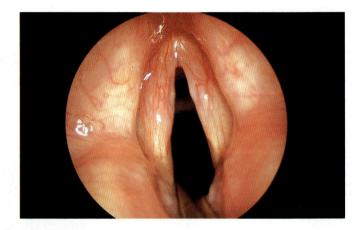

Figure 4.136

Chronic laryngitis

This male patient with chronic laryngitis had a hoarse, low-pitched voice. Note the irregular vocal fold edges, some oedema and the dilated blood vessels.

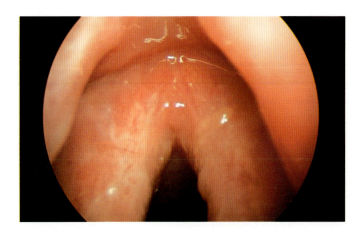

Figure 4.137

Chronic laryngitis

A close-up of the anterior commissure showing a finely granular surface but no focal change. The biopsy showed chronic low-grade inflammation.

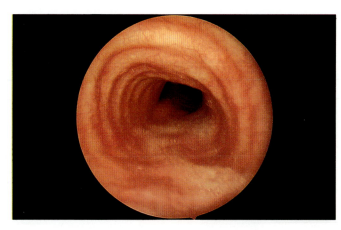

Figure 4.138

Chronic bronchitis

Chronic bronchitis and excessive secretions in a patient with asthma, emphysema and chronic cough.

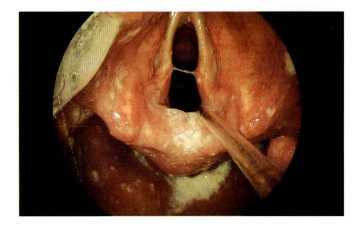

Figure 4.139

Chronic laryngitis: gastro-oesophageal reflux

Chronic laryngitis due to gastro-oesophageal reflux and persistent aspiration.

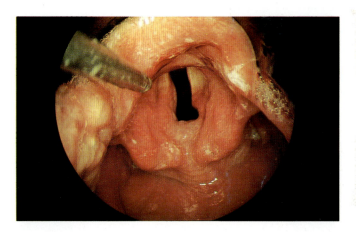

Figure 4.140

Chronic laryngitis

In this patient the chronic laryngitis affects not only the posterior larynx but also the posterior surface of the epiglottis. Photograph taken at direct laryngoscopy using proximal jetting through a metal cannula.

Figure 4.141

Chronic fungal laryngitis

The fungal laryngitis in this teenage boy was the result of the long term inhalation of a metered aerosol synthetic steroid spray for the treatment of asthma.

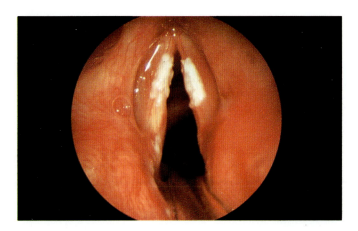

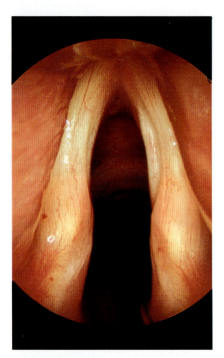

Figure 4.142

Vocal fold sulcus

A vocal fold sulcus is a shallow epithelium lined depression with parallel edges above and below the sulcus. The vocal fold sulcus is often difficult to recognize at indirect examination; each of the lips can be delineated at direct laryngoscopy. A vocal sulcus may be a variant of normal. Some patients have no voice change, whereas others have an abnormal voice and changes seen at stroboscopy.

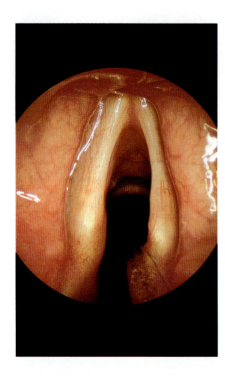

Figure 4.143

Presbyphonia

Presbyphonia is the term used to describe the degeneration that occurs in some patients with age. Presbyphonia is characterized by a visible bowing of the vocal folds with incomplete glottic closure causing a weak, breathy voice that tires with prolonged use. The flaccidity of the vocal folds slowly becomes worse with age.

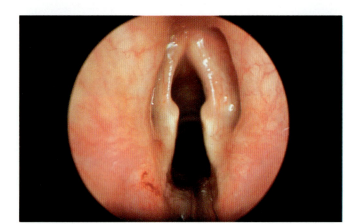

Figure 4.144

Presbyphonia

The advanced bowing of the vocal folds and the 'arrowhead' appearance of presbyphonia. These changes occur more commonly in men. Surgical procedures to increase the tension in the vocal folds appear to have promising short-term results. Careful injection of collagen may improve the voice.

Vocal granulomas and ulceration

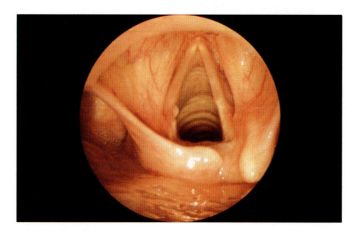

Figure 4.145

Small vocal granuloma: indirect laryngoscopy

Vocal granulomas are uncommon but readily recognized, rounded, sometimes bilobed or even multilobed, yellow, pink or pale red opalescent masses arising from a pedicle on the posterior one-third of the vocal cord adjacent to the vocal process and medial surface of the arytenoid cartilage. This small left-sided vocal granuloma recurred following recent laser surgery. Further follow-up is required to determine whether complete healing will occur or whether the granuloma will recur yet again.

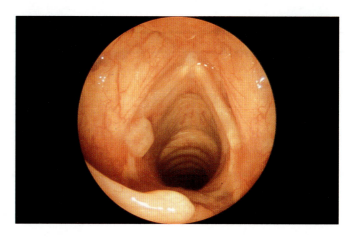

Figure 4.146

Large vocal granuloma: indirect laryngoscopy

There may be inflammation of the surrounding mucosa in the posterior glottic space. Histologically there is a vascular bud from which the granulation tissue arises, sometimes with fibrinous haemorrhagic exudate on the surface. Note the large granuloma arising adjacent to the vocal process of the left arytenoid. This vocal granuloma produced little effect on the voice. Microlaryngoscopy and excision biopsy for histological examination will exclude malignancy or other specific granuloma.

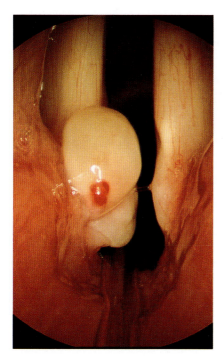

Figure 4.147

Vocal granuloma

Most patients have some degree of hoarseness but in others the voice may be near normal. There is often a feeling of irritation and a desire to clear the throat. Often no causative factors can be found although some patients are said to be aggressive or tense individuals who misuse or overuse their voice. This yellow, multi-lobed, non-specific vocal granuloma shows a prominent haemorrhagic area, probably due to prior trauma from a sucker tip. Gastro-oesophageal acid reflux is said to be a factor in the formation of granuloma.

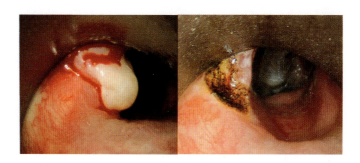

Figure 4.148

Vocal granuloma before and after removal

This right vocal granuloma is shown prior to removal (left) and after laser removal (right). The pedicle was exposed and the granuloma amputated in an attempt to leave the mucoperichondrium intact without exposing the underlying cartilage. Axial CT scans of the larynx show focal or generalized osteosclerosis in the arytenoid adjacent to a vocal granuloma in every patient.

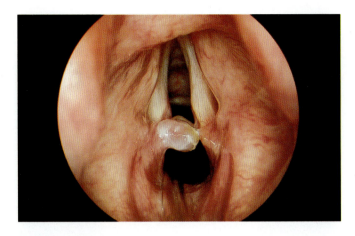

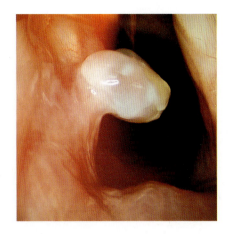

Figure 4.149

Vocal granuloma: close up

Specific granulomas such as tuberculosis, histoplasmosis, coccidioidomycosis, blastomycosis, syphilis, leprosy, sarcoidosis, Wegener's granulomatosis, scleroma and Crohn's disease may occur in the larynx on rare occasions. In these photographs, note the intubation granuloma on the left side following recent endotracheal intubation. The close-up photograph shows the yellow colour of the granuloma with fibrin on the surface and the attachment of the pedicle on the medial surface near the vocal process of the arytenoid.

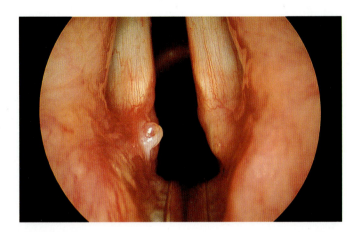

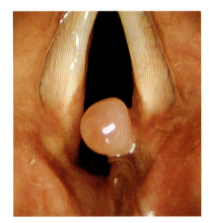

Figure 4.151

Intubation granuloma

Intubation granuloma in an adolescent on the right side prior to removal. There is seldom recurrence after removal of an intubation granuloma.

Figure 4.150

Vocal granuloma: resolution

Small, residual vocal granuloma at direct laryngoscopy. The lesion had been removed several times previously, but on this occasion only a small nubbin of granulomatous tissue was found. Complete resolution occurred within three months.

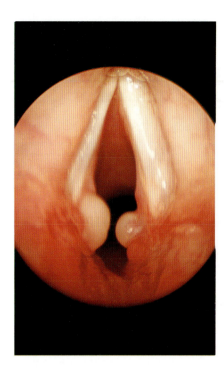

Figure 4.152

Bilateral intubation granulomas

Bilateral intubation granulomas larger on the left side than the right, found only a few weeks after prolonged intubation. The patient has been intubated following inhalation of the products of combustion of a fire.

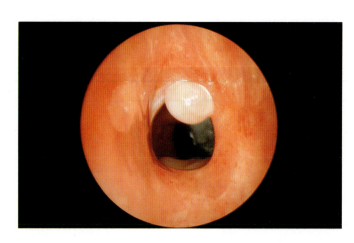

Figure 4.153

Subglottic granuloma and subglottic stenosis

Mature acquired subglottic stenosis with a rounded area of granulation tissue anteriorly. The granulation tissue must be removed and be seen not to recur before definitive treatment of the subglottic stenosis can be undertaken.

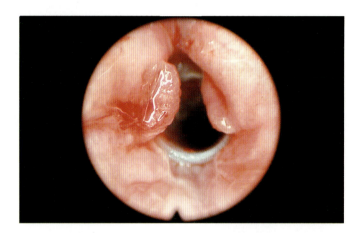

Figure 4.154

Granulation tissue caused by a stent

Bilateral irregular granulation tissue in the glottis caused by irritation and erosion from an indwelling Silastic tube following laryngotracheoplasty.

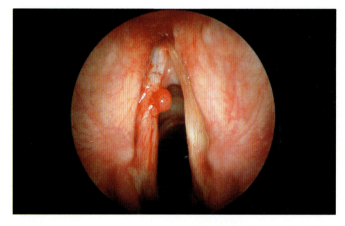

Figure 4.155

Laser granuloma

A laser granuloma may occur when carbon particles act as an irritative focus in the submucosal tissues following laser surgery and promote reactive granulation tissue.

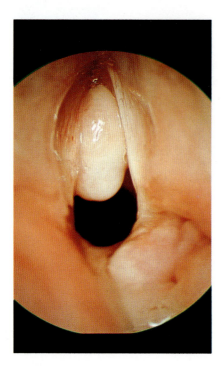

Figure 4.156
Post-laryngofissure granuloma

Large oval granuloma arising from a small pedicle just below the anterior commissure. It was removed without recurrence.

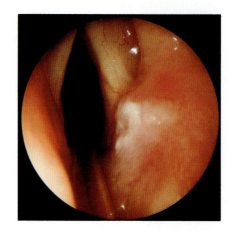

Figure 4.157
Acute ulcer

This idiopathic acute ulcer on the medial surface of the right arytenoid was found incidentally during a direct laryngoscopy for other reasons.

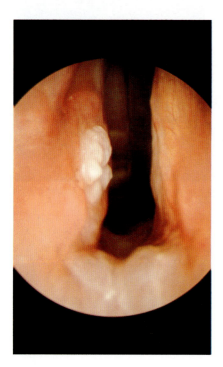

Figure 4.158
Contact pachydermia

A 'contact ulcer' is actually a small saucer-shaped epithelial thickening at the tip of the vocal process, not a true ulcer. Contact pachydermia is a better term. The lesion is a crater, with intact epithelium, in the centre of a circle of hyperplastic epithelium. Note contact pachydermia on the medial surface of the left arytenoid with some reactive thickening of the surface epithelium on the right side.

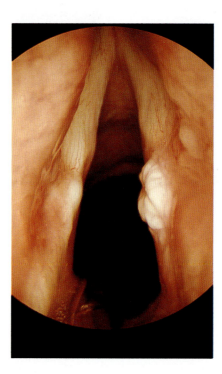

Figure 4.159
Contact pachydermia

Contact pachydermia on the right side with a concentric heaped-up hyperplastic white area and a central depression: a so-called 'contact ulcer'. In the literature reference is often made to vocal granuloma, contact ulcer or to ulcer/granuloma although there is no evidence that this sequence of event occurs or that there is an interrelationship. Stages of the same pathological process may possibly be represented by the granuloma stage and the so-called ulcerated stage.

Vocal cord paralysis and vocal cord augmentation

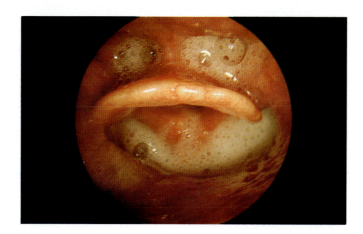

Figure 4.160

Right vocal cord paralysis: indirect laryngoscopy

Most vocal cord paralyses are caused by peripheral lesions with various combinations of paralysis of the superior laryngeal nerve and/or the recurrent laryngeal nerve. The aetiology may be iatrogenic, commonly after thyroidectomy or other neck or cardiac surgery, or malignant, idiopathic or due to external trauma and other miscellaneous reasons. This right vocal cord paralysis developed after the removal of a vagal paraganglioma. Copious secretions caused persistent, troublesome aspiration.

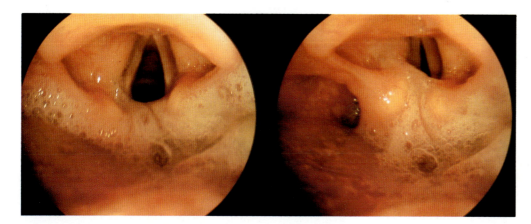

Figure 4.161

Right vocal cord paralysis: indirect laryngoscopy

A small number of vocal cord paralyses have a central cause i.e. a massive lesion of the cerebral cortex, or more commonly a lesion in the brain stem, or an insult to the area around the nucleus ambiguus, whilst others have an infranuclear aetiology such as lesions at or near the jugular foramen. This right vocal cord paralysis is shown at indirect laryngoscopy during quiet respiration and during attempted phonation. Note the pooling of secretions mainly on the right.

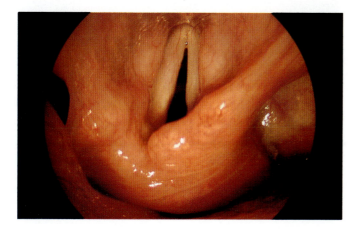

Figure 4.162

Left vocal cord paralysis: indirect laryngoscopy

It is important to distinguish between vocal cord paralysis and vocal cord immobility resulting from fixation of the cricoarytenoid joint; this can be achieved only at direct laryngoscopy by testing passive movement of the arytenoid on the cricoid joint surface. Appearance at indirect laryngoscopy using a 70° angled rigid rod lens telescope. The paralysed vocal cord is in the paramedian position.

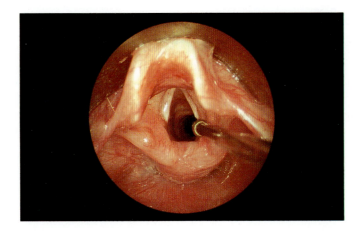

Figure 4.163

Vocal cord paralysis

Direct laryngoscopy immediately prior to injection of paste. Cricoarytenoid joint mobility must be proven to be normal before injection. Teflon is not an ideal material, but when carefully placed using a standardized technique, it gives satisfactory results for most patients. It is particularly suited to those with malignancy or a poor prognosis for survival. Younger patients and those with a good prognosis with long standing vocal cord paralysis may be better treated by vocal cord medialization or one of the techniques of phonosurgery that are now available to produce satisfactory rehabilitation of the voice without introduction of a foreign substance into the laryngeal tissues.

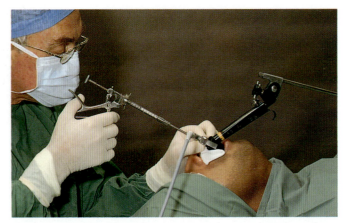

Figure 4.164

Injection for vocal cord paralysis

Injection of Teflon paste using the special high-pressure gun. Suspension laryngoscopy and naked eye visualization.

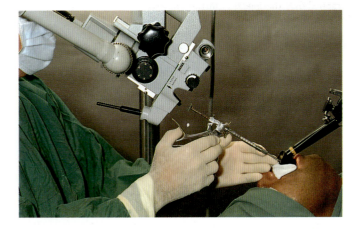

Figure 4.165

Injection for vocal cord paralysis

Injection technique with visualization using the operating microscope. It is a matter of individual preference which technique is used.

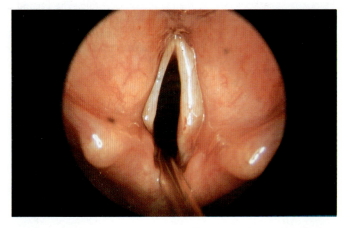

Figure 4.166

Vocal cord paralysis and·atrophy

Long-standing left vocal cord paralysis leading to atrophy and shortening of the left vocal cord.

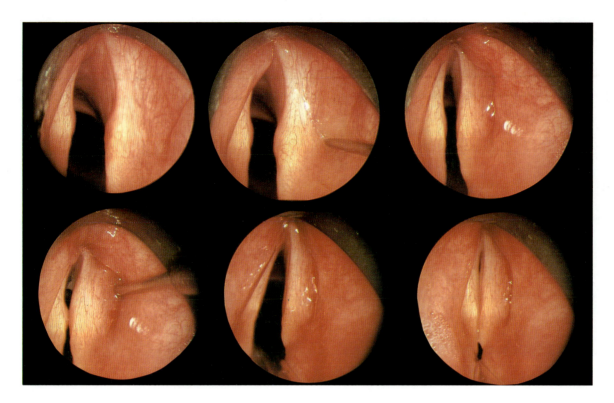

Figure 4.167

Injection technique for vocal cord paralysis

The steps during the injection of Gelfoam or Teflon paste under general anaesthesia. Although referred to as 'vocal cord injection' or 'intracordal injection' both terms are inaccurate. The injection is 'paracordal' to augment and medialize the paralysed hemilarynx so that vibration of the vocal folds becomes more effective. The paste must not be placed superficially in the membranous vocal fold. The second photograph shows the injection in the postero-lateral hemilarynx in the lateral part of the thyroarytenoid muscle, medial to the lamina of the thyroid cartilage and lateral to the vocal process of the arytenoid; the first and often the only site of injection. Sometimes, as in the fourth photograph, a second smaller supplementary injection anterior to the first is needed to achieve adequate medialization. In the fifth and sixth photographs sufficient paste appears to have been injected, and as anaesthesia is discontinued, brisk vocal cord movement returns in the contralateral side allowing a judgment to be made about whether further injection is necessary.

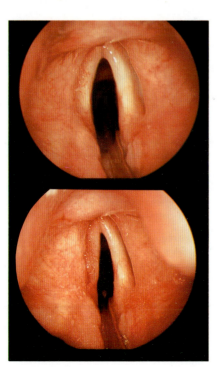

Figure 4.168

Injection for vocal cord paralysis

Photographs at direct laryngoscopy before and after injection of Gelfoam paste in the left hemilarynx. The left vocal fold has been satisfactorily medialized to the midline and the voice was much improved.

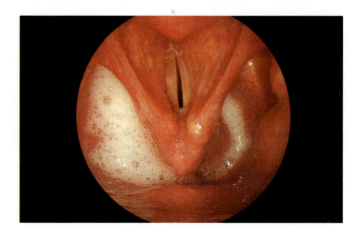

Figure 4.169

Right vocal cord paralysis after injection of Teflon paste: indirect laryngoscopy

Photographed in the office with 70° telescope. The voice was good, but pooled secretions can still be seen.

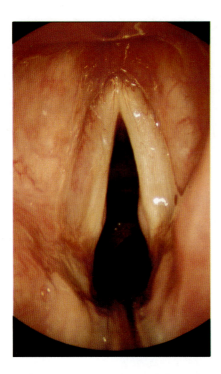

Figure 4.170

Long term result of injection of Teflon paste.

This left hemilarynx was injected with Teflon 10 years previously. The patient has maintained a consistently good voice.

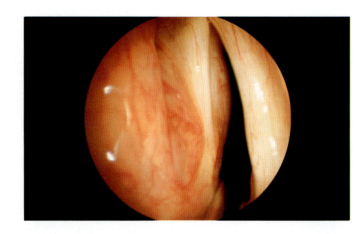

Figure 4.171

Excessive injection of Teflon paste

There has been an ill-judged, excessive injection of Teflon in the left hemilarynx causing the voice to be worse than it was before injection. In such a situation consideration must be given to removal of the Teflon and the surrounding granulomatous tissue.

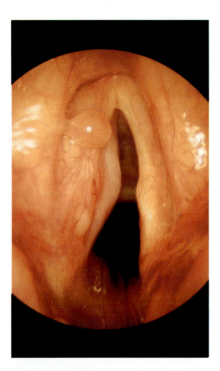

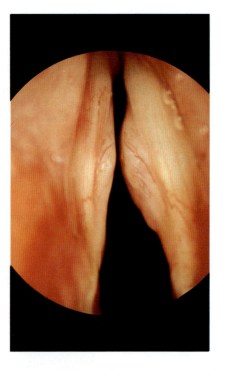

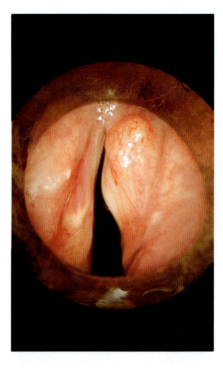

Figure 4.172

Complications after injection of Teflon paste

Excessive injection in the vocal fold itself with a polypoidal mucosal reaction in the anterior ventricle. At the time of the photograph some movement had returned in the left hemilarynx. In retrospect the injection should not have been undertaken.

Figure 4.173

Injection of Teflon paste: contraindication

Bilateral subglottic swellings in a patient after bilateral injection. The injection is far too superficial on each side, and the result was a very poor voice. Bilateral injection is absolutely contraindicated.

Figure 4.174

Teflon granuloma after injection of Teflon paste

This irregular mass was caused by overfilling on the right side, producing a rounded protrusion in the anterior ventricle.

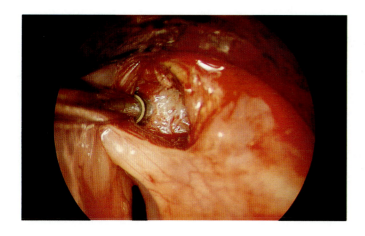

Figure 4.175

Removal of Teflon granuloma

Direct laryngoscopy and removal of Teflon granuloma from the right hemilarynx. A sucker retracts the intact vocal fold edge and displays a greyish-white mass of Teflon granuloma. Troublesome granuloma formation is more likely to occur when too much paste is used or it is injected too superficially. Inappropriate placement, overinjection and granuloma formation may worsen an already compromised voice. Removal of the Teflon is difficult, but may be indicated in selected cases.

Cystic disease of the larynx and pharynx

Classification of cysts of the larynx and pharynx

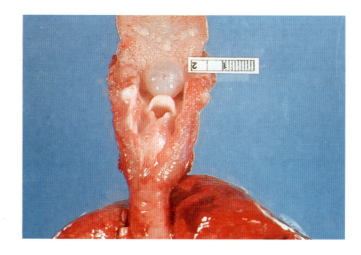

Figure 4.176

Ductal cyst causing death

Ductal cysts are also known as mucus retention cysts. They may be found in the valleculae, within the larynx or most often in the subglottic region and result from retention of mucus in dilated collecting ducts of the submucosal glands. This is the postmortem specimen of an infant with persistent noisy breathing, treated as 'asthma'. Death was by asphyxia.

- *Ductal retention cysts,* which may develop anywhere a mucus producing gland exists

- *Thyroglossal duct cysts,* which occur at the tongue base at the foramen caecum

- *Saccular cysts,* either lateral or (less commonly) anterior

- *Cystic hygroma* (or lymphangioma): a multilocular cystic developmental abnormality arising from lymph vessels

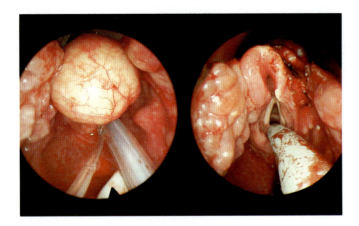

Figure 4.177

Ductal cyst in the base of the tongue

Ductal cysts often occur in premature infants who have undergone prolonged intubation. The irritation and swelling of the mucosa from the endotracheal tube appears to obstruct the mucous gland ducts. The large distended vallecular cyst is shown before and after removal using the carbon dioxide laser. Note the laser-shielded tube in the second photograph.

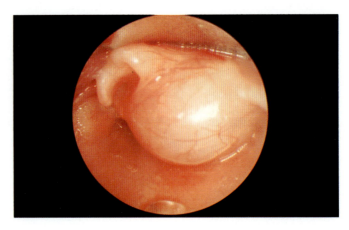

Figure 4.178

Ductal cyst

This large ductal retention cyst in a newborn baby caused severe stridor.

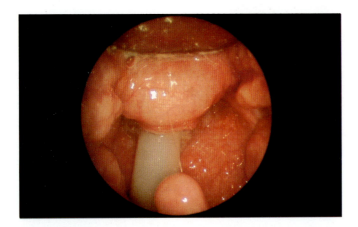

Figure 4.179

Thyroglossal duct cyst

A thyroglossal duct cyst at the base of the tongue. Thyroglossal duct cysts usually present in the anterior neck but can develop anywhere from the foramen caecum to the thyroid gland along the line of the thyroglossal duct. A large cyst, by pushing the epiglottis backwards and downwards, can produce severe upper airway obstruction. Airway obstruction as with any large cyst in the laryngopharynx may become much worse during the induction of anaesthesia and preparation must be made for an immediate incision of the cyst or aspiration of its contents through a wide-bore needle.

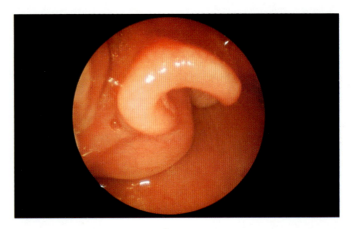

Figure 4.180

Laryngocele

A laryngocele is an air-filled distended saccule. This laryngocele is located in the left supraglottic region. The patient had laryngeal papillomas in the anterior ventricle which caused a valve-like obstruction of the neck of the saccule.

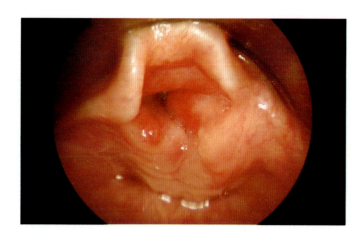

Figure 4.181

Lateral saccular cyst

Right lateral saccular cyst causing severe supraglottic obstruction in an infant who had undergone prolonged endotracheal intubation.

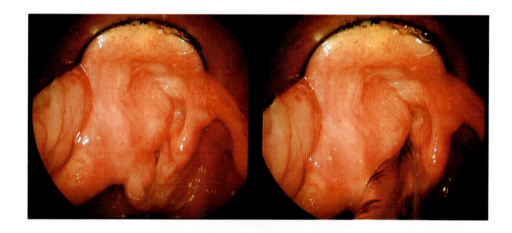

Figure 4.182

Lateral saccular cyst

Large left lateral saccular cyst in a 45-year-old woman. The airway obstruction became progressively worse during induction of anaesthesia and an endotracheal tube has been positioned.

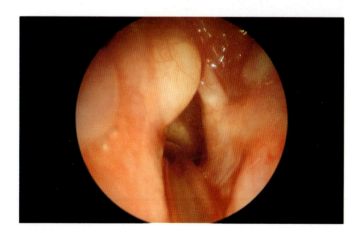

Figure 4.183

Anterior saccular cyst

Anterior saccular cyst on the left side in a 10-year-old girl. This internal laryngocele arises from the saccule at the anterior aspect of the laryngeal ventricle.

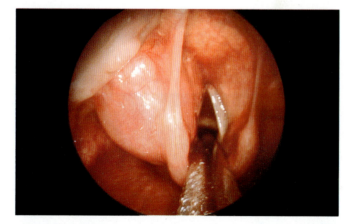

Figure 4.184

Supraglottic cyst

A large left supraglottic cyst seen at direct laryngoscopy before laser removal. It proved to be a rare developmental cyst whose origin was from the internal perichondrium lining the thyroid cartilage.

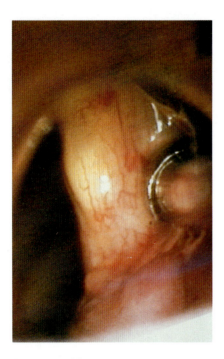

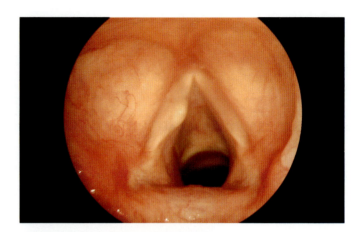

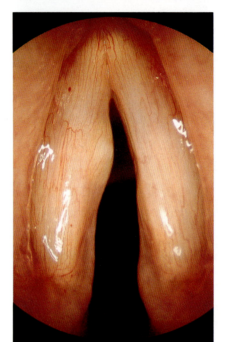

Figure 4.185
Intracordal cyst

A small, rounded, yellow intracordal inclusion cyst within the right vocal fold immediately prior to microsurgical dissection and removal. An intracordal cyst is unilateral but there may be some oedematous reaction in the contralateral vocal fold.

Figure 4.186
Intracordal cyst

(Top) A large, oval, yellow intracordal cyst taken at indirect laryngoscopy. Some minor oedematous changes can be seen in the adjacent vocal fold. (Side) Same cyst seen close-up at direct laryngoscopy before removal (see Figure 4.187).

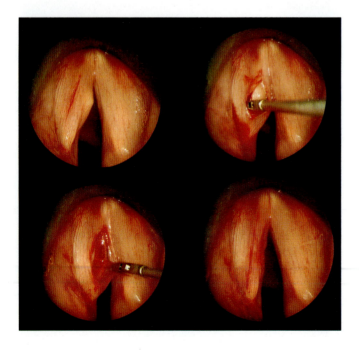

Figure 4.187
Microdissection and removal of an intracordal cyst

This is the same patient as shown in Figure 4.186. A sharp incision is made 2 or 3 mm lateral to the vocal fold edge, and blunt dissection exposes the cyst with vocal ligament and vocalis muscle on the lateral side. The edge of the vocal fold has been preserved.

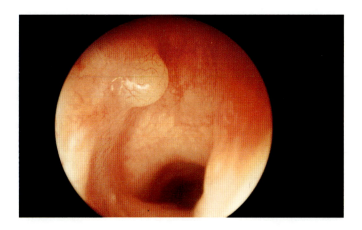

Figure 4.188

Subglottic ductal retention cyst

A subglottic ductal retention cyst on the left side in a small preterm infant treated by prolonged endotracheal tube intubation for hyaline membrane disease.

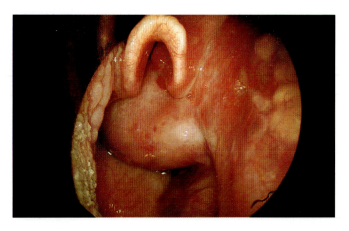

Figure 4.189

Cystic hygroma

A cystic hygroma in the lateral pharyngeal wall and supraglottic larynx of a 16-year-old boy who, as an infant, had surgical removal of a cystic hygroma from the neck. He developed slowly progressive upper airway obstruction. This photograph was taken prior to removal of the pharyngeal cystic hygroma mass in stages, using the carbon dioxide laser.

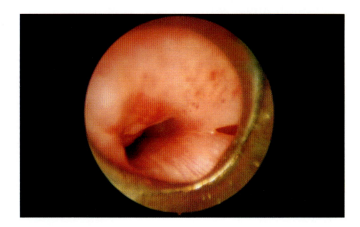

Figure 4.190

Tracheal duplication cyst

The slit-like opening in the right subglottic region of this 3-month-old infant with intermittent stridor leads to a duplication cyst of the upper trachea in the region of the cricoid cartilage. The cyst was seen on CT scan and removed at the age of 12 months via a neck incision.

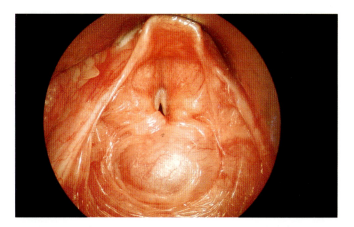

Figure 4.191

Hypopharyngeal duplication cyst

This duplication cyst of the hypopharyngeal region caused intermittent dysphagia and minor stridor in a 10-year-old girl. Laser removal of the roof and partial removal of the lining epithelium was performed.

Prolonged intubation injuries of the larynx

Laryngeal damage from prolonged endotracheal intubation occurs in patients of all ages, but most injuries heal rapidly leaving a normal or near normal larynx. The degree of damage differs from patient to patient; some individuals incur minimal injury while others, intubated for the same time, develop severe changes. Early non-specific changes can be categorized into oedema, granulation tissue, ulceration and miscellaneous injuries.

The endotracheal tube always lies in, and exerts pressure on, the posterior larynx affecting the medial surfaces of the arytenoid cartilages, the cricoarytenoid joints, vocal processes, posterior glottis, interarytenoid region and the subglottis, where it affects the inner surface of the cricoid cartilage. The subglottic space is especially vulnerable in infants. The most important factors contributing to the severity of intubation damage are the duration of intubation and the size of the endotracheal tube.

Predisposing factors for intubation injury of the larynx

- Infants with pre-existing congenital subglottic stenosis

- Prolonged or repeated intubation of very low birth weight premature infants

- Intubation of paediatric patients for airway obstruction due to acute laryngotracheitis

- An abnormal larynx rather than a normal larynx, e.g. crushed larynx or upper airway burns

- Inappropriately large or cuffed tube in infants or children cared for in an adult hospital

- Unconscious patients with a head injury who remain intubated for a long time

- Prolonged intubation followed by tracheotomy in an unconscious patient

- Multiple systemic problems, including poor cardiac output or major organ failure, e.g. renal failure, liver failure

- A larynx that is difficult to intubate, causing pressure in the posterior glottis to be greater

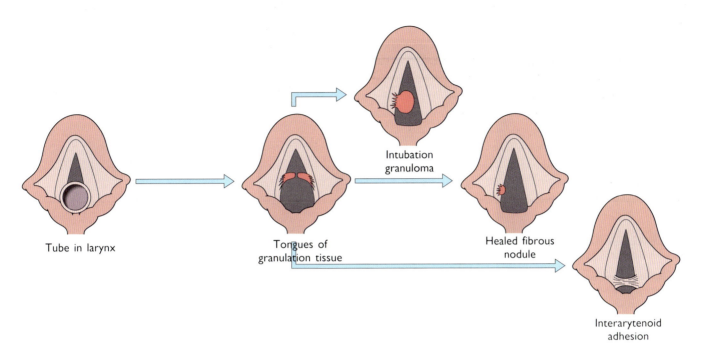

Figure 4.192

Chronic end results of granulation tissue forming during prolonged intubation: intubation granuloma, healed fibrous nodule and interarytenoid adhesion

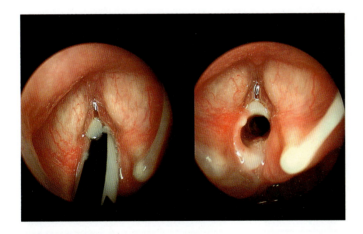

Figure 4.193

Acute intubation injury: assessment without endotracheal tube

While the endotracheal tube is in place, neither the posterior glottis nor the subglottis can be seen. Removal of the tube gives a good view of the glottis and the intubation injury can be appreciated more fully. The nature and degree of laryngeal trauma during prolonged intubation can be assessed precisely using rigid telescopes under general anaesthesia after temporary removal of the endotracheal tube to allow examination, which must include the posterior glottis and subglottic region for complete evaluation. The long-term consequences of both granulation tissue and ulceration into the perichondrium can be illustrated by photographs taken at direct laryngoscopy.

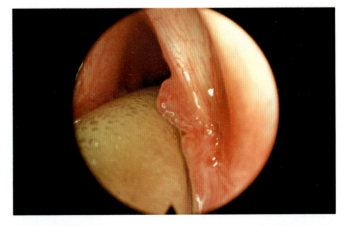

Figure 4.194

Acute intubation injury: granulation tissue formation

Note the granulation tissue beginning to form at the right vocal process in response to irritation from an endotracheal tube. If the endotracheal tube can be removed at this stage the granulation tissue readily resolves.

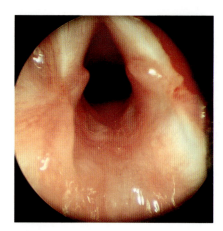

Figure 4.195

Acute intubation injury: tongues of granulation tissue

Note the small tongues of granulation tissue on each vocal process after removal of the tube. There is no ulceration and removal of the tube at this stage allows complete resolution. Some patients, however, may have hoarseness, tiring of the voice, inability to sing or other subtle changes.

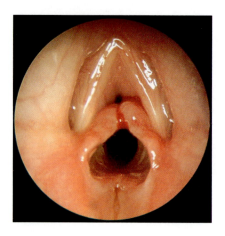

Figure 4.196

Tongues of granulation tissue

Large tongues of granulation tissue, which form around the endotracheal tube as it lies in the posterior glottis. This is a typical appearance seen in many larynges during prolonged intubation.

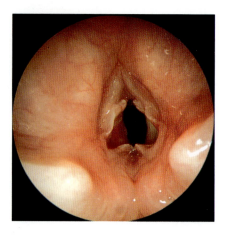

Figure 4.197

Intubation causing granulation tissue in the posterior larynx

Granulation tissue not only forms at the vocal processes of the arytenoids but in some cases encircles the tube as it lies in the posterior larynx.

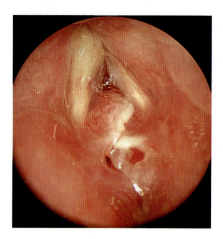

Figure 4.198

Obstructive tongues of granulation tissue

In this patient, exuberant proliferative granulation tissue has formed flap-like obstructions when the tube is removed. Either immediate reintubation or a tracheotomy is necessary.

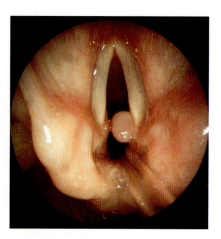

Figure 4.199

Postintubation granuloma

Typical round, mature, pink granuloma arising from the vocal process on the right side. This type of granuloma usually presents some weeks after extubation because the tongues of granulation tissue fail to resolve.

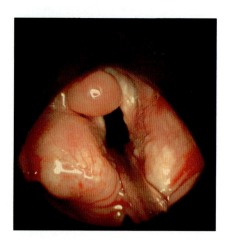

Figure 4.200

Postintubation granuloma

A round granuloma arising from an atypical site anteriorly on the left side, probably caused by laceration from the endotracheal tube or an introducer in the tube.

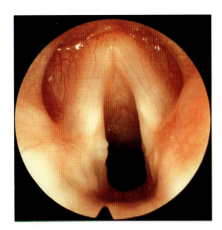

Figure 4.201

Postintubation healed fibrous nodules

The two small healed fibrous nodules just posterior to the vocal process of the arytenoid on the left are the result of incomplete resolution of granulation tissue.

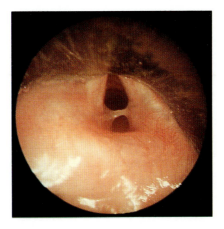

Figure 4.202

Postintubation interarytenoid adhesion

This interarytenoid adhesion in an infant was the result of prolonged intubation. Note the thin transverse fibrous bridge with a triangular anterior opening and a smaller round posterior opening.

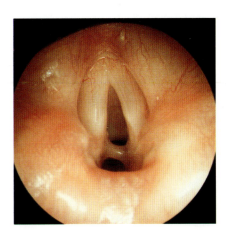

Figure 4.203

Postintubation adhesion

An interarytenoid adhesion in an older child. The vocal cords are tethered to one another causing partial airway obstruction, leading to an erroneous diagnosis of bilateral vocal cord paralysis. The anterior, tall, triangular opening is often mistaken for the glottis.

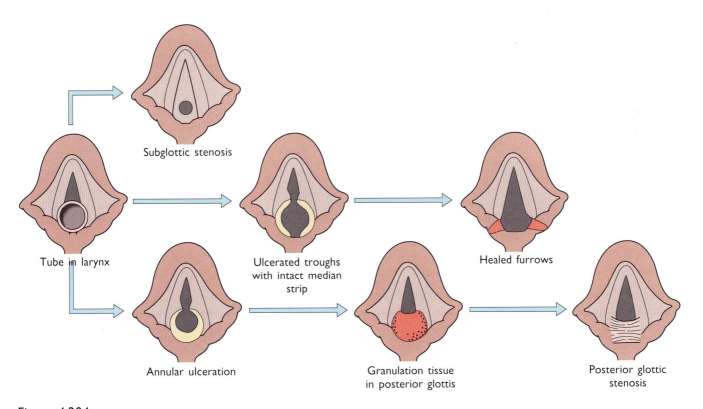

Figure 4.204

Ulceration occurring during prolonged intubation

The three chronic end results of ulceration during prolonged intubation include: subglottic stenosis, healed furrows and posterior glottic stenosis.

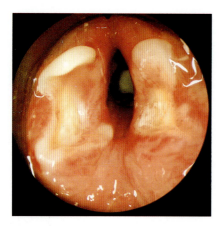

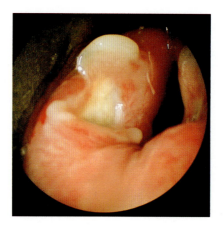

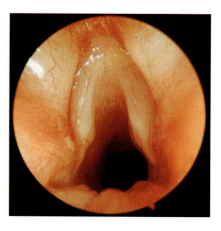

Figure 4.205

Intubation causing ulceration and granuloma

Bilateral ulcerated troughs surrounded by granulation tissue. Note the intact median strip implying that the later development of a posterior glottic stenosis is unlikely.

Figure 4.206

Ulcerated trough

A deep ulcerated trough on the left side, with surrounding granulation tissue. The line of the cricoarytenoid joint can be seen.

Figure 4.207

Bilateral healed furrows

There is a concave deficit posteriorly in each vocal cord. These healed furrows develop from incompletely healed ulcerated troughs and are usually bilateral.

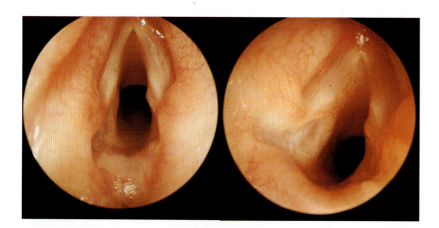

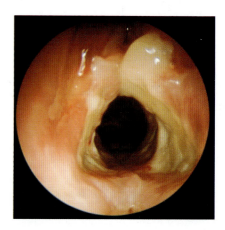

Figure 4.208

Bilateral healed furrows: close-up

The photograph on the left shows healed furrows, more clearly seen on the left than the right. Healed furrows may be difficult to identify (right photograph) but they can be recognized as a scarred depression running craniocaudally. The close-up with a 30° telescope shows the line of the cricoarytenoid joint below the medial surface of the arytenoid cartilage.

Figure 4.209

Circumferential ulceration

There is a circumferential ulceration involving the posterior glottis with some granulation tissue at the vocal processes. There is no intact median strip of mucosa and, consequently, later development of a posterior glottic stenosis is likely.

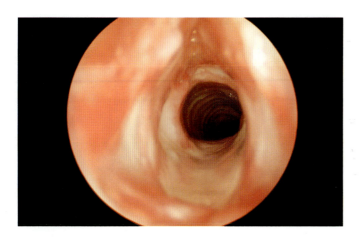

Figure 4.210

Concentric subglottic ulceration

This concentric subglottic ulceration may ultimately lead to the formation of a subglottic stenosis.

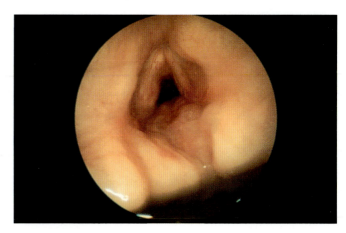

Figure 4.211

Posterior glottic granulation tissue

Note the proliferative granulation tissue in the posterior glottis several weeks after prolonged intubation. This proliferative granulation tissue forms at the site of ulceration in the posterior glottis and matures to form a posterior glottic stenosis.

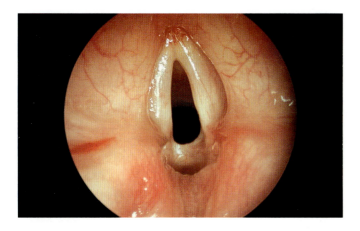

Figure 4.212

Posterior glottic stenosis

There is a mature posterior glottic stenosis with a crescentic anterior edge and the typical appearance of a small depression posteriorly.

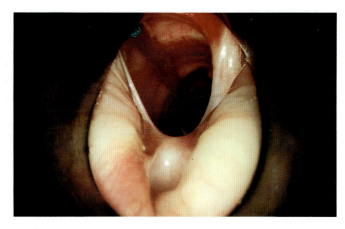

Figure 4.213

Posterior glottic stenosis

This firm unyielding posterior glottic stenosis has been stretched by forceable abduction of the arytenoids with the tip of a laryngoscope. In severe cases the cricoarytenoid joints may be partly or completely fixed.

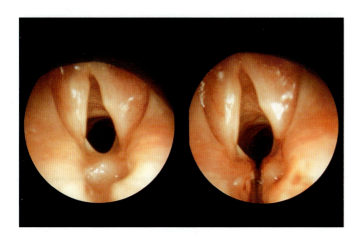

Figure 4.214

Division of posterior glottic stenosis

The mature posterior glottic stenosis (left) caused moderate airway obstruction. The thick transverse scar has been divided with a scalpel blade leaving a deep V-shaped defect where the stenosis has been 'released' (right). This may alleviate the symptoms in some cases; however, subsequent re-stenosis is likely and may require repeated division or other more extensive procedures.

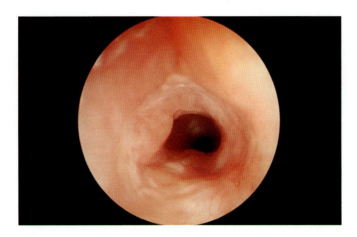

Figure 4.215

Postintubation subglottic stenosis

This so-called 'soft' acquired subglottic stenosis was caused by prolonged intubation for 120 days in a premature infant born at 28 weeks. There is submucosal fibrosis, hyperplasia and dilatation of seromucinous glands and several flat ductal retention cysts.

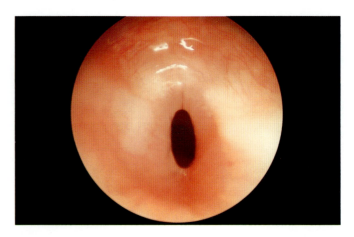

Figure 4.216

Congenital subglottic stenosis

The oval subglottic area is due to an abnormality of the cricoid cartilage. Infants with a relatively minor congenital cartilaginous subglottic stenosis may become symptomatic if endotracheal intubation causes oedema, granulation tissue or subsequent fibrosis.

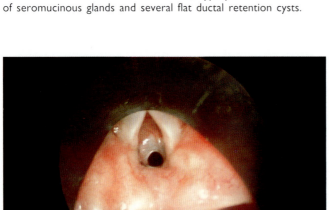

Figure 4.217

Postintubation subglottic stenosis

This acquired subglottic stenosis followed prolonged intubation in a child. The thin web-like stenosis was vaporized by two carbon dioxide laser treatments with complete resolution of symptoms.

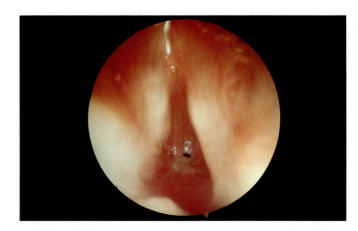

Figure 4.218

Postintubation subglottic stenosis

A mature subglottic stenosis with a tiny pinhole lumen. In this infant, an augmentation laryngotracheoplasty will be required.

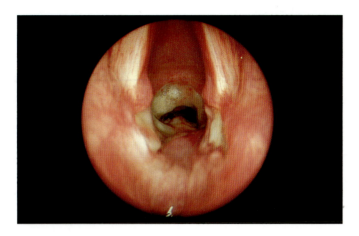

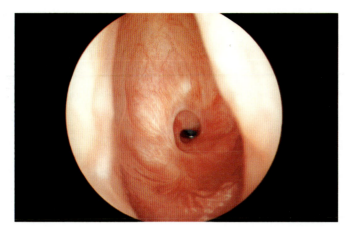

Figure 4.219
Development of subglottic stenosis

The acute circular ulceration in the subglottic region of this adult male developed from intubation with an oversized tube for 8 days (left). Several months later, a mature subglottic stenosis with a residual lumen of only 1 or 2 mm had developed (right). Tracheal resection was required.

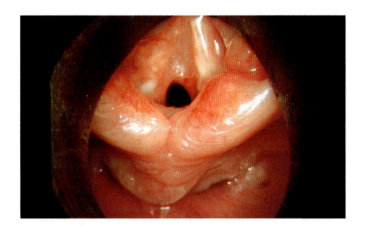

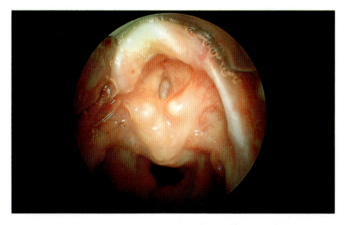

Figure 4.220
Glottic and subglottic stenosis

Severe glottic and subglottic stenosis following trauma from prolonged intubation. Scar tissue replaces the left vocal cord and there is severe stenosis of the glottic and subglottic regions.

Figure 4.221
Total glottic stenosis

This total glottic obstruction following prolonged intubation was worsened by injudicious repeated laser treatments.

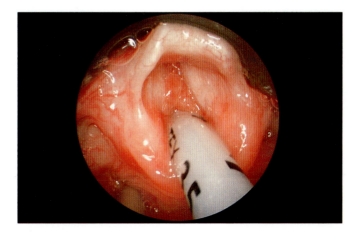

Figure 4.222
Protrusion of oedematous ventricular mucosa

Protrusion of oedematous mucosa from the laryngeal ventricles. Diffuse swelling in this area is a common and prominent change during intubation which subsides quickly once the endotracheal tube is removed.

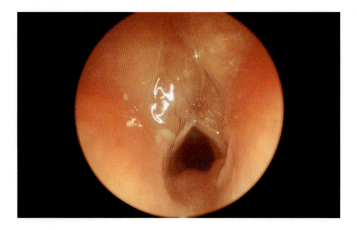

Figure 4.223

Protrusion of oedematous ventricular mucosa

Protrusion of the ventricular mucosa in a premature baby born at 28 weeks and intubated for 4½ weeks. The tube has been removed temporarily to allow observation.

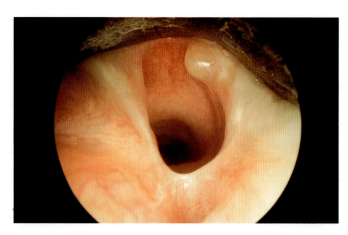

Figure 4.224

Posterior glottic stenosis and ductal retention cyst

Subglottic ductal retention cyst and minor posterior glottic stenosis in an infant. Simple laser vaporization of the cyst was followed by the discharge of thick viscid fluid.

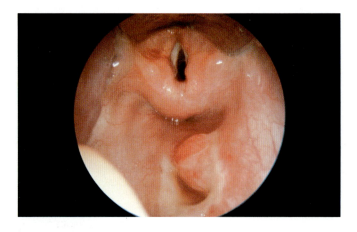

Figure 4.225

Intubation trauma of the pharynx

Trauma of the posterior pharyngeal wall in an infant following attempted pernasal intubation. The tube tip lacerated the posterior pharyngeal wall and burrowed down the posterior wall behind the upper oesophagus. Uneventful resolution followed conservative treatment.

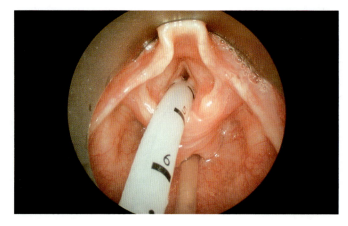

Figure 4.226

Nasogastric tube injury

Nasogastric tubes can cause ulceration of the postcricoid region. Note the small tongues of granulation tissue seen in the larynx from the endotracheal tube.

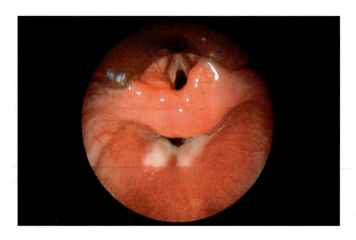

Figure 4.227

Nasogastric tube injury

Ulceration in the postcricoid region from an indwelling nasogastric tube, a change that often goes unrecognized. Removal of the tube usually allows complete resolution.

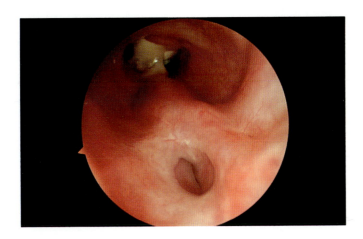

Figure 4.228

Postintubation laryngeal fistula

The fistula passing through the cricoid cartilage between the posterior subglottic region and the anterior wall of the upper oesophagus was caused by infection of opposed ulcerated areas between an endotracheal tube and a nasogastric tube. This is a rare complication of prolonged intubation.

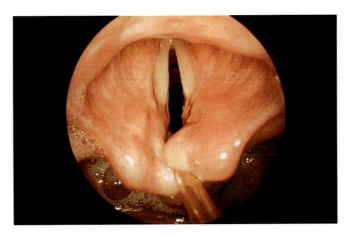

Figure 4.229

Postintubation arytenoid dislocation

Dislocated right arytenoid cartilage caused either by the endotracheal tube or the introducer after a difficult intubation. This type of dislocation occurs more often on the left than the right side, since most anaesthetists intubate from right to left.

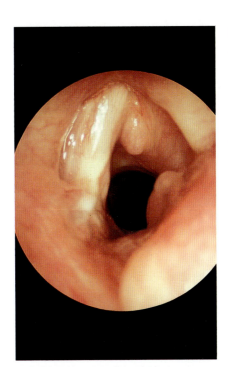

Figure 4.230

Postintubation vocal cord trauma

The large defect of the right vocal cord in this child was the result of a difficult neonatal intubation. The voice was poor and breathy.

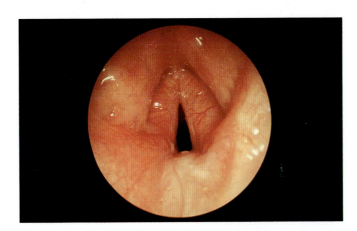

Figure 4.231

Postintubation chronic vocal cord changes

The chronic oedema, dilated vessels, congestion and diffuse scarring of both vocal cords in this child with a weak, hoarse voice was caused by prolonged intubation as a premature infant.

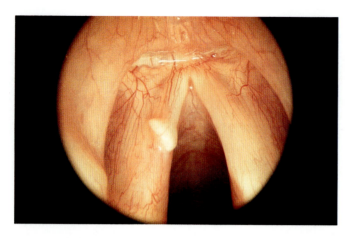

Figure 4.232

Postintubation vocal cord trauma

The irregular scarred tag in the central part of the left vocal cord caused a persistently husky voice following endotracheal intubation for 1 hour. This injury is probably the result of a laceration during intubation.

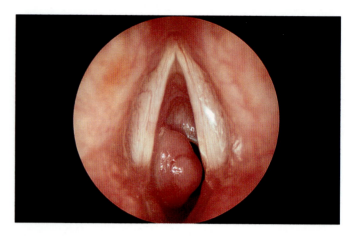

Figure 4.233

Postintubation granuloma and subglottic stenosis

This large left subglottic intubation granuloma and the anterior acquired subglottic stenosis followed prolonged intubation in a 10-year-old boy with a head injury. Laser treatment for each lesion was followed by the establishment of a normally functioning airway.

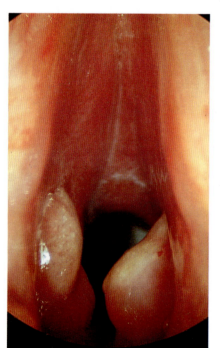

Figure 4.234

Postintubation granulations and perichondritis

These subglottic granulations, persisting 4 weeks after removal of the endotracheal tube, are probably due to perichondritis of the posterior cricoid lamina.

Laryngeal trauma

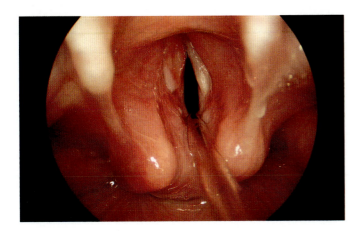

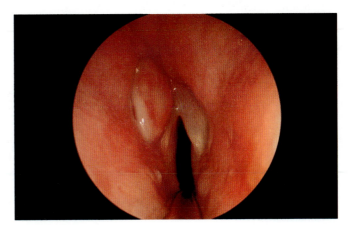

Figure 4.235

Laryngeal trauma: ruptured airway

Laryngeal trauma can be caused by blunt, crushing, strangulating or penetrating injuries, or by inhalation of caustic acid or flames. Iatrogenic laryngeal injury is usually related to long term endotracheal intubation (see previous section) and sometimes to endoscopic microsurgical or laser procedures. This ruptured laryngeal airway occurred in a teenage girl who was kicked in the neck by a horse. Surgical emphysema extended from the skull base to the mediastinum. The first photograph shows submucosal haemorrhage and swelling of the left hemilarynx and the second shows granulations covering the site of rupture at the left false cord.

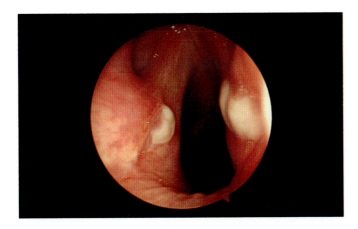

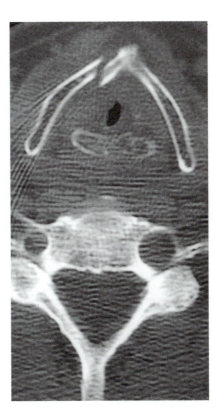

Figure 4.237

Laryngeal trauma: thyroid cartilage fracture

This CT scan shows a fracture of the thyroid lamina on the right side caused by a direct injury from a karate chop to the neck.

Figure 4.236

Laryngeal trauma: blunt neck injury

Direct laryngeal trauma in a 40-year-old man. A heavy piece of wood fell on his neck. There was little stridor but almost complete loss of voice. Note the granulation tissue at both right and left vocal processes with congestion and swelling in each hemilarynx.

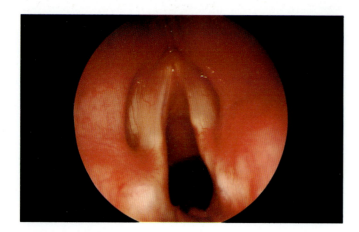

Figure 4.238

Laryngeal trauma: fixed cricoarytenoid joint

This patient sustained an injury to the neck some weeks before resulting in persistent dysphonia. At direct laryngoscopy there was loss of tension and shortening of the right vocal fold. Palpation proved that this was due to a fixation of the right cricoarytenoid joint.

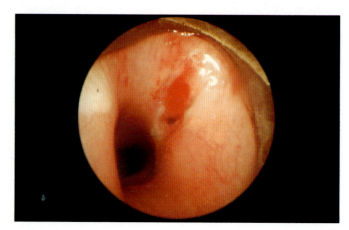

Figure 4.239

Laryngeal trauma: dog bite

Penetrating external injury from a dog bite of the neck. The internal laceration is in the upper trachea just below the cricoid cartilage.

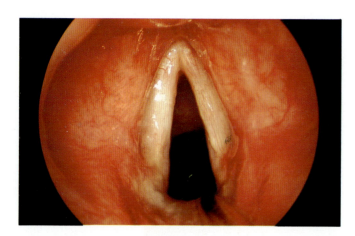

Figure 4.240

Larynx after laser treatment: minimal scarring

Note the appearance of this larynx following eight laser treatments for papillomas in 2 years. There is only a slight irregularity of the left vocal fold but no webbing. The voice was good and the stroboscopic appearance near normal.

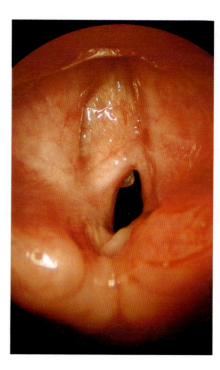

Figure 4.241

Glottic web after removal of papillomas

This severe glottic web followed repeated traumatic removal of papillomas. There are papillomas under the web and in the upper trachea at the site of a long-term tracheotomy.

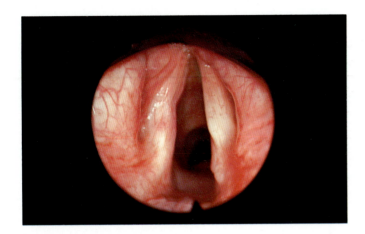

Figure 4.242

Iatrogenic laryngeal trauma

The deficiency of this left vocal fold followed the removal of a vocal cord polyp and resulted in a poor voice. Augmentation with collagen might be beneficial.

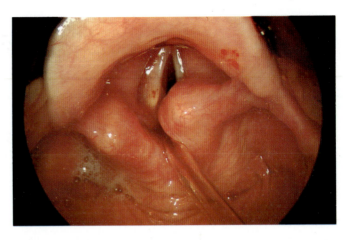

Figure 4.243

Laryngeal trauma: dislocated arytenoid

This dislocation of the right arytenoid was caused by a difficult intubation for anaesthesia and abdominal surgery.

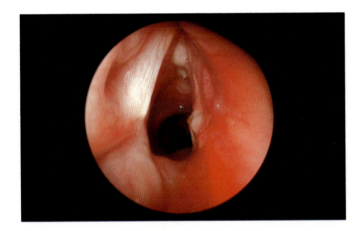

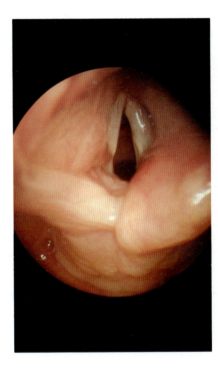

Figure 4.245

Normal appearance after arytenoidectomy

Laryngeal appearance many years after previous left arytenoidectomy for bilateral vocal cord paralysis.

Figure 4.244

Granulation tissue after laryngofissure

The granulations at the anterior commissure and at the site of the arytenoidectomy 10 days after laryngofissure and right arytenoidectomy are part of the normal healing process. Subsequent satisfactory healing occurred by the fourth postoperative week.

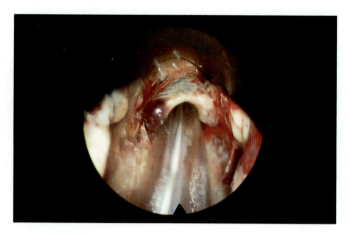

Figure 4.246

Acid burns of the laryngopharynx

Acid burns of the larynx and pharynx. The base of the tongue, the epiglottis and the pharyngeal walls are almost unrecognizable owing to acute ulceration and necrosis of the epithelium.

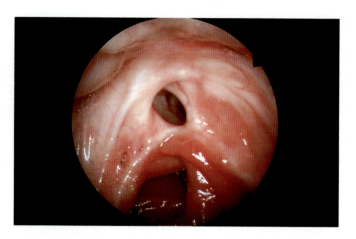

Figure 4.247

Acid burns of the larynx

Caustic ingestion in a child some years before with laryngeal and pharyngeal burns required oesophageal replacement with colon. The epiglottis has been removed. The severe stricture at the site of the colonic anastomosis required two operations for endoscopic reconstruction before the tracheotomy tube was removed.

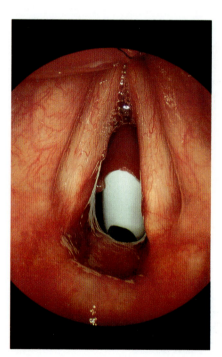

Figure 4.248

Percutaneous tracheotomy: too high

Percutaneous tracheotomy performed in the Intensive Care Unit. The tube is through the cricothyroid membrane. It was replaced by a tracheotomy at the third and fourth tracheal arches.

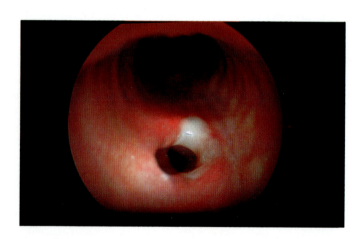

Figure 4.249

Traumatic perforation of the trachea

The traumatic perforation of the posterior membranous tracheal wall was caused by forceable, inexpert introduction of a tracheotomy tube with a hard plastic introducer.

Acute inflammatory airway obstruction

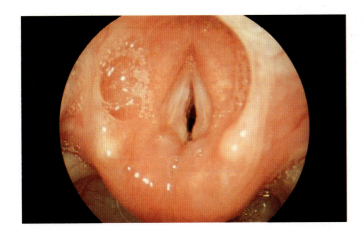

Figure 4.250
Acute laryngotracheitis

Acute laryngotracheitis in a 12-month-old child with symptoms for 2 days with inspiratory stridor worse in the evenings and at night. Note the marked narrowing of the subglottic airway. Acute viral laryngotracheitis, commonly known as croup, is much more common than acute epiglottitis, and much less likely to cause severe airway obstruction. Croup and epiglottitis are usually easy to distinguish.

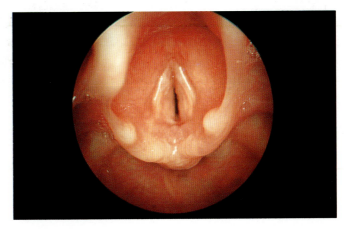

Figure 4.251
Acute laryngotracheitis

Acute laryngotracheitis with severe obstruction due to subglottic inflammation and oedematous swelling. Note the absence of supraglottic changes. Croup is usually caused by parainfluenza type I or respiratory syncytial virus.

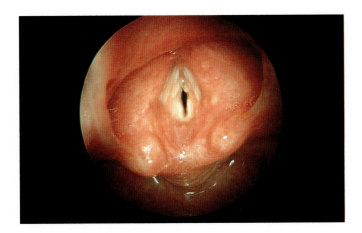

Figure 4.252
Acute laryngotracheitis

Acute laryngotracheitis with severe subglottic obstruction with an irregular surface. A lateral radiograph confirmed a subglottic swelling. Other causes of acute inflammatory airway obstruction include peritonsillar abscess (quinsy), parapharyngeal abscess and diphtheria.

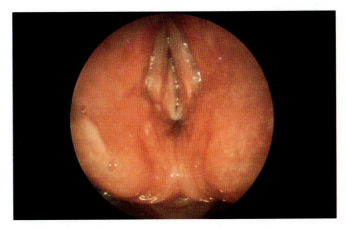

Figure 4.253
Acute laryngotracheitis

Acute laryngotracheitis associated with an attack of measles. There appears to be no subglottic airway during the phase of respiration when this photograph was taken. Pernasal endotracheal intubation relieved the obstruction.

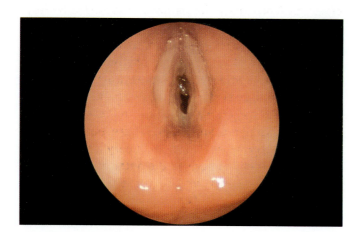

Figure 4.254

Pseudomembranous bacterial tracheitis

Pseudomembranous bacterial tracheitis with membranes and crusts in the tracheal lumen causing inspiratory and expiratory stridor. There was a rapid onset of airway obstruction. Bronchoscopy was required for removal of the crusts and intubation for an artificial airway. Pseudomembranous bacterial tracheitis is an uncommon, atypical, potentially lethal form of croup where infection, usually by *Staph. aureus*, causes formation of crust-like membranes in the tracheobronchial tree.

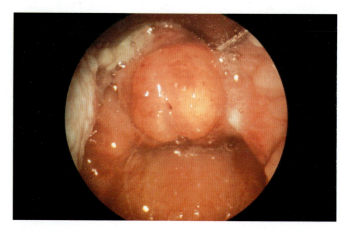

Figure 4.255

Acute epiglottitis

Acute epiglottitis with dramatic obstructive swelling of the epiglottis which has a mottled yellow and red appearance. Intubation of the narrow airway in this type of patient requires experience and skill as it is made difficult by the severe obstruction and the distorted swelling of the supraglottic structures. Acute epiglottitis is usually caused by *Haemophilus influenzae B*.

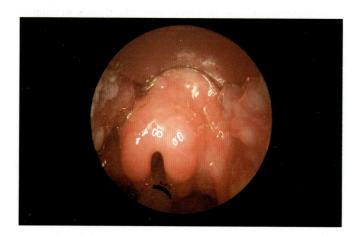

Figure 4.256

Acute epiglottitis: effect of intubation

Intubation provides an airway not only through the lumen of the tube but also on each side of the tube through chinks created by splinting the epiglottis outwards and forwards. Note the swelling in the valleculae and base of the tongue.

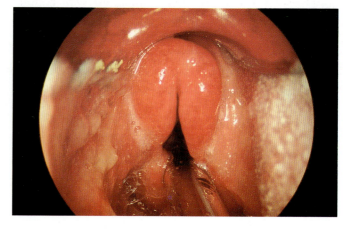

Figure 4.257

Acute epiglottitis after intubation

Ten-hour history of respiratory distress, quiet inspiratory stridor, muffled voice, painful swallowing and drooling of saliva. Endotracheal intubation is the treatment of choice to relieve the airway obstruction.

Dysplasia and neoplasia

Dysplasia is a histological term describing microscopic changes that indicate possible progression to malignancy. The characteristic cellular changes include atypical cells with large hyperchromatic nuclei and loss of cellular polarity. There is irregular stratification and increased mitosis. In moderate dysplasia the changes are confined to the basal layer but in severe dysplasia the changes extend towards the epithelial surface. In carcinoma in situ (intraepithelial carcinoma) the basal membrane is preserved.

These microscopic dysplastic changes cannot be differentiated by indirect or direct laryngoscopy. Large, multiple, carefully labelled biopsies of all suspicious areas are essential.

In invasive carcinoma nests or tongues of cells infiltrate the deeper tissues. Most malignant laryngeal tumours are squamous cell carcinomas: although they are more common in elderly males, the incidence in females is increasing. Squamous cell carcinomas of the larynx may be circumscribed, ulcerative, polypoid, nodular or exophytic. Some spread superficially on the surface of the mucosa while others infiltrate into deeper tissues. Suspicious endoscopic features include increased capillaries on the mucosal surface or on the periphery of a localized area, sometimes with contact haemorrhage, induration detected by palpation and partial or complete loss of vocal cord movement. Microlaryngoscopy, with telescopes for image magnification and detailed evaluation of all areas allows exact delineation of the surface changes and thus accurate

biopsies. When the lesion is uniform and clearly delineated a single representative biopsy may be taken, preferably from the edge so that it straddles the margin of the tumour and apparently nearby normal tissue. All biopsy samples should be generous, taken with forceps having jaws at least 3 mm in diameter. In other cases of suspected malignancy adequate, representative and multiple biopsies are important, where possible avoiding unnecessary violation of, or injury to, important anatomical structures such as the anterior commissure, vocalis muscle, vocal ligament or the vocal process of the arytenoid cartilage. For a large malignant tumour, multiple biopsies carefully labelled and mapped according to anatomical site are required for evaluation of the extent of the lesion. A small tumour, for example a suspected malignancy in the central part of the vocal fold, is better removed by excisional biopsy using cupped forceps and scissors rather than by destruction with the laser, as laser removal may totally destroy the tissue thereby precluding a microscopic diagnosis. Biopsy material for frozen section may be helpful when the necessity for further endoscopic or major extirpative surgery at the time of biopsy depends on the result.

In patients whose laryngeal mucosa shows premalignant epithelial dysplasia and cellular atypia, or in patients who have had radiation therapy for malignancy, repeated biopsies at short or long intervals may be required, the time for biopsy being indicated by changes in the voice and the appearance at indirect laryngoscopy.

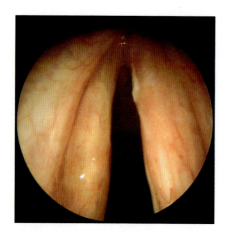

Figure 4.258

Leukoplakia

A small slightly raised area of leukoplakia at the anterior end of the right vocal fold. Histology demonstrated hyperkeratosis without atypia.

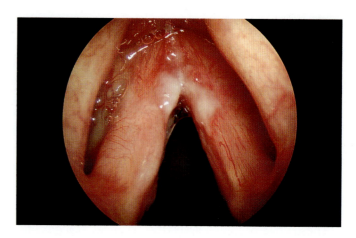

Figure 4.259

Leukoplakia

Leukoplakia at the anterior commissure and right and left vocal folds, photographed with a 30° telescope. Biopsies revealed hyperkeratosis with atypia. Regular follow-up is required.

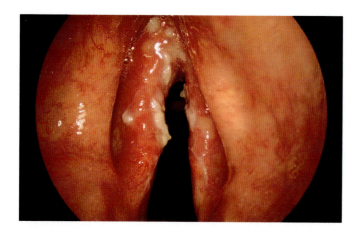

Figure 4.260

Severe dysplasia

Note the widespread abnormality of both vocal folds with multiple areas of irregular leukoplakia and erythroplasia. Malignancy was clinically suspected. However histologically severe hyperkeratosis and dysplasia were found.

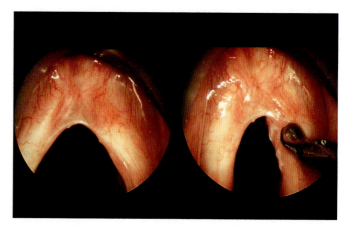

Figure 4.261

Severe dysplasia

Persistent recurring dysplasia for 12 years treated repeatedly by laser with the formation of an anterior glottic web. Photographs show the technique of 'rolling' the web to reveal the irregular patches of leukoplakia.

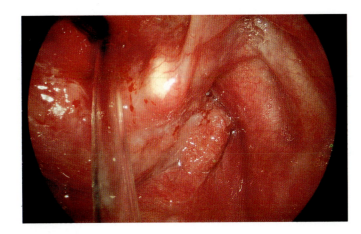

Figure 4.262

Carcinoma in situ

Multiple biopsies of this raised irregular lesion in the right piriform fossa showed carcinoma in situ but no invasive carcinoma.

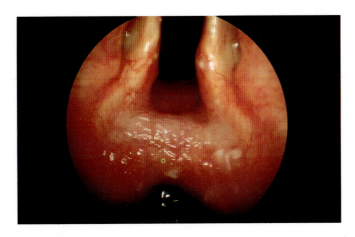

Figure 4.263

Interarytenoid pachydermia

Interarytenoid pachydermia with thickening of the squamous epithelium of the posterior glottic space. The cause is unknown and malignant changes may sometimes subsequently occur.

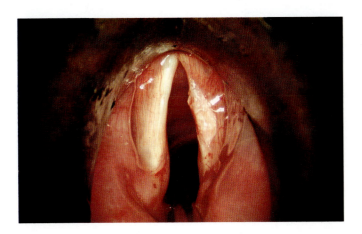

Figure 4.264

Squamous cell carcinoma

Infiltrating squamous cell carcinoma in the central third of the right vocal cord. Frozen section biopsy and laser excision with a margin of 2 mm. No recurrence 5 years later.

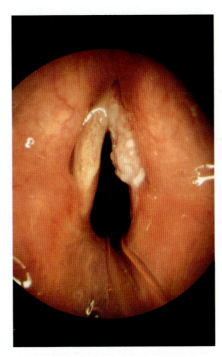

Figure 4.265

Squamous cell carcinoma

Infiltrating squamous cell carcinoma with an irregular surface and involving all of the membranous right vocal fold up to the anterior commissure. Endoscopic laser removal. Biopsies of the margin negative. No recurrence in 2 years.

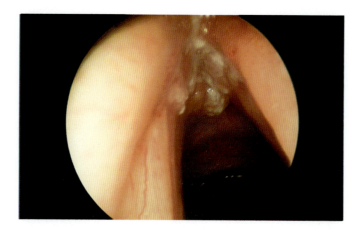

Figure 4.266
Squamous cell carcinoma

Infiltrating squamous cell carcinoma of the anterior commissure and subcommissure treated by anterior partial laryngectomy with recurrence within 8 months. Subsequently treated with radiotherapy.

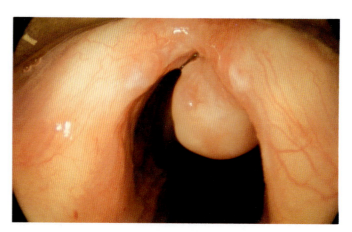

Figure 4.267
Spindle cell carcinoma

The large, rounded, polypoidal, firm mass arising from a pedicle under the anterior edge of the right vocal fold is a spindle cell carcinoma, which was treated with radiotherapy.

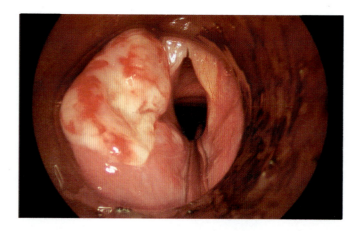

Figure 4.268
Squamous cell carcinoma

The irregular mass with haemorrhagic areas is an infiltrating squamous cell carcinoma of the left aryepiglottic fold and false cord. There was no left vocal cord movement. The lesion was treated by laryngectomy.

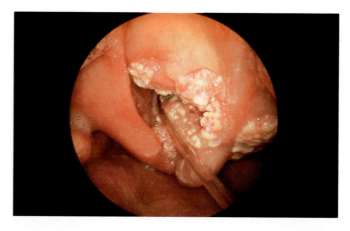

Figure 4.269
Squamous cell carcinoma

An infiltrating squamous cell carcinoma of the supraglottic larynx involving the tubercle of the epiglottis, false vocal cord and aryepiglottic fold and ulcerating into the medial aspect of the right piriform fossa. Treatment was by laryngectomy.

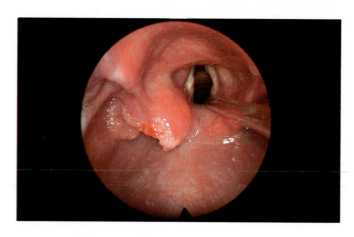

Figure 4.270
Squamous cell carcinoma

Infiltrating squamous cell carcinoma involving the anterior and lateral wall of the left piriform fossa and the upper aspect of the arytenoid. Good vocal cord movement was present, with no detectable regional lymph nodes and treatment was with radiotherapy.

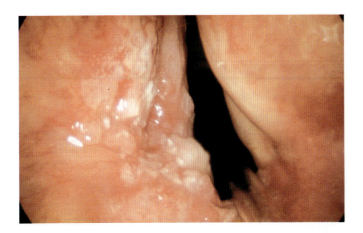

Figure 4.271

Verrucous carcinoma

Verrucous carcinoma of the posterior aspect of the left vocal cord, false cord and medial surface of the arytenoid. Repeated laser treatment achieved control.

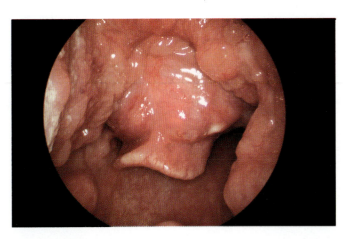

Figure 4.272

Squamous cell carcinoma

Squamous cell carcinoma in the pre-epiglottic space spreading to distend both valleculae and push the epiglottis posteriorly. The patient was being treated for papillomas in the larynx and was a heavy smoker.

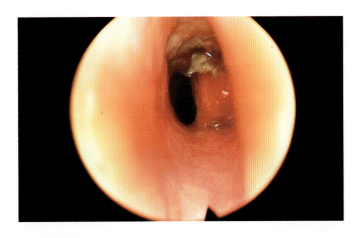

Figure 4.273

Carcinoma of the thyroid gland

Carcinoma of the thyroid gland ulcerating into the upper trachea, causing partial airway obstruction and intermittent bleeding.

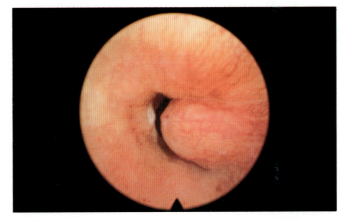

Figure 4.274

Adenoid cystic carcinoma of the trachea

Adenoid cystic carcinoma of the trachea with intact covering mucosa causing serious airway obstruction.

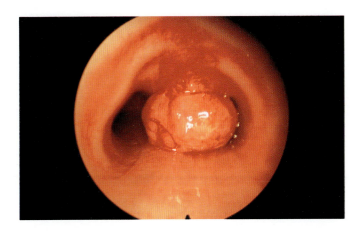

Figure 4.275

Tracheal tumour

This ectopic salivary gland tumour in the lower trachea caused almost total obstruction of the right main bronchus.

Foreign bodies

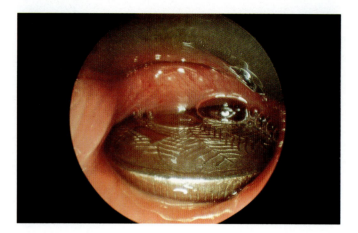

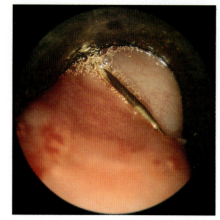

Figure 4.277

Ingested foreign body: brooch

Pin of a brooch in the upper oesophagus. The sharp point should be kept down during removal to minimize trauma.

Figure 4.276

Ingested foreign body: coin

This coin (Australian 10 cents) impacted in the upper oesophagus is shown immediately before removal using an open tube oesophagoscope under general anaesthetic. Sharp ingested foreign bodies such as fishbones may impact in the tonsil, base of tongue, laryngopharynx or postcricoid region. Drawing pins, badges and clasps usually impact in the upper oesophagus. Pieces of meat, vegetables, fruit and coins are held up in the oesophagus, usually the upper part. A plain radiograph will show a radio-opaque foreign body such as a coin or a piece of bone.

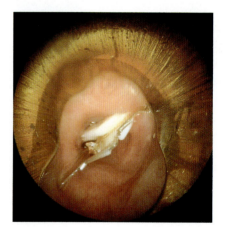

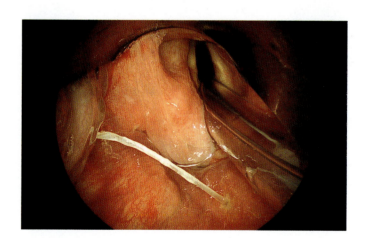

Figure 4.278

Ingested foreign body: star

Small, plastic, five-pointed star impacted in the upper oesophagus with some stagnant secretions and granulation tissue caused by the irritating points.

Figure 4.279

Ingested foreign body: fishbone

This large fishbone was impacted in the lateral pharyngeal wall, the sharp end medially in the posterior pharyngeal wall. Endotracheal intubation for anaesthesia allows safe removal.

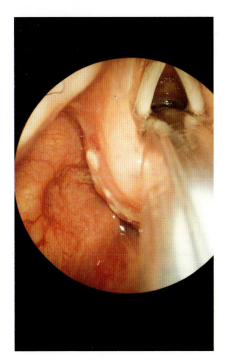

Figure 4.280

Site of foreign body impaction

Mucosal laceration in the left postcricoid region and lateral wall of the piriform fossa in a patient in whom a sharp foreign body had impacted and subsequently passed on before attempted endoscopic removal.

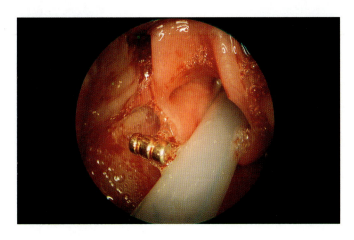

Figure 4.281

Ingested foreign body: ornamental pin

Upper aspect of an ornamental pin whose sharp end is downwards and resting in the postcricoid region.

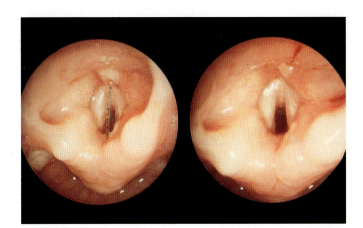

Figure 4.282

Foreign body in the larynx: glass

A foreign body in the larynx should be suspected when stridor, laryngospasm, husky voice, dyspnoea or inspiratory wheeze dominates the clinical picture. A piece of broken electric light bulb inhaled and impacted anteroposteriorly in the glottic opening in an 8-month-old baby, before and after removal.

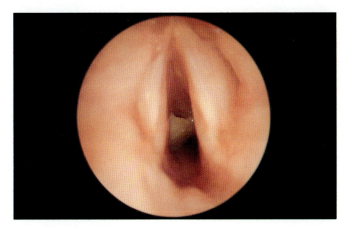

Figure 4.283

Impacted subglottic foreign body: nutshell

Note the nutshell firmly impacted in the subglottic space with surrounding oedema causing upper airway obstruction and presenting as 'atypical' croup. It may be safer to perform a tracheotomy to establish an airway before attempting the removal of a difficult laryngeal foreign body. Some inhaled foreign bodies impact in the larynx or subglottic region but most are inhaled into the tracheobronchial tree causing acute respiratory distress. If the patient is cyanosed and not improving, Heimlich's manoeuvre can be used to expel the foreign body from the airway. In most cases the acute respiratory distress will improve and after clinical and radiographic evaluation, bronchoscopy for removal under general anaesthesia must be undertaken.

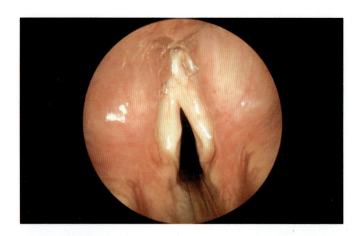

Figure 4.284

Foreign body extraction injury: chop bone

This man aged 22 years had an impacted chop bone removed from his larynx at the age of 2 years. He has had multiple operations in an attempt to correct the laryngeal scarring but his voice remains poor.

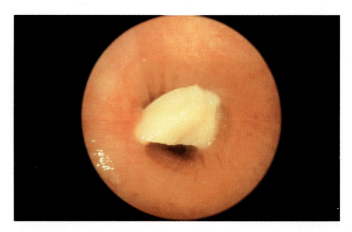

Figure 4.285

Inhaled foreign body: peanut

Peanut fragment impacted in the left main bronchus just prior to endoscopic removal under spontaneous respiration general anaesthesia. There is little surrounding reaction. The highest incidence of inhaled foreign body occurs during the second and third years of life. There is usually a history of a sudden coughing attack, choking, gagging, gasping, wheezing and cyanosis lasting minutes or hours.

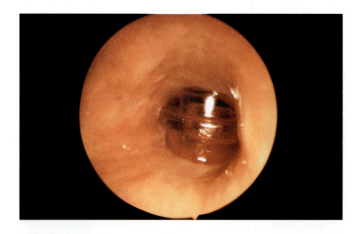

Figure 4.286

Inhaled foreign body: plastic object

Obstruction resulting from a foreign body in the main bronchus often produces a ball-valve obstruction with partial inspiratory air flow and bronchial constriction during expiration causing overdistention of the distal lung. A single negative chest radiograph is not sufficient to rule out the presence of a suspected inhaled foreign body. Note the round red plastic object impacted in the left main bronchus. A persistent wheeze could be heard at the bedside and by chest auscultation.

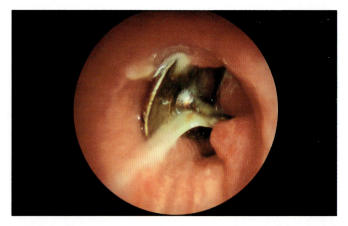

Figure 4.287

Inhaled foreign body: drawing pin

Drawing pin inhaled into the left main bronchus with some surrounding secretions; the point of the pin has provoked some proliferative granulation tissue.

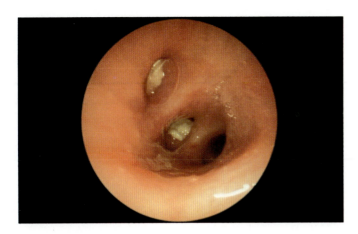

Figure 4.288

Inhaled foreign body: chicken meat

With delayed presentation there is chronic cough, wheeze and sometimes a diagnosis of 'unresolved pneumonia' with persistent changes in the chest radiograph. Clinical presentation may be days, weeks or months after the initial inhalation. Multiple small fragments of chicken in the left lower lobe segmental openings. A large piece of chicken meat has already been removed from the left main bronchus.

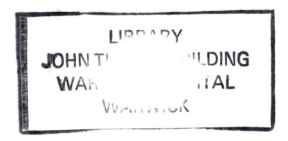
Rare and unusual laryngeal conditions

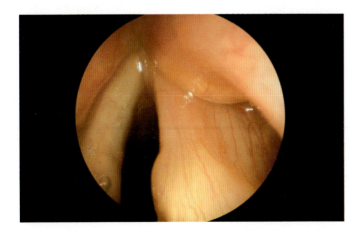

Figure 4.289

Lipoma

Note the smooth, round yellow lipoma protruding from the undersurface of the false cord into the anterior part of the right ventricle. Endoscopic technique using a 30° telescope.

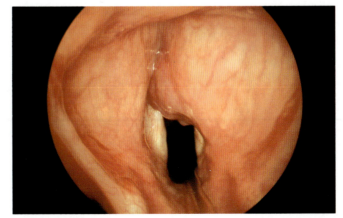

Figure 4.290

Amyloid

Large, round, but somewhat irregular, surface of a solitary mass of amyloid in the larynx of a young woman. Treated by local endoscopic removal.

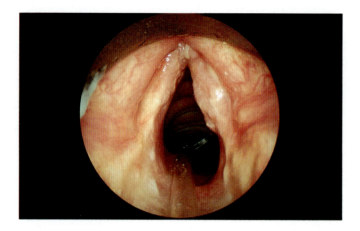

Figure 4.291

Amyloid

Amyloid infiltration in the vocal folds more on the right side than the left and causing severe dysphonia. Removal with carbon dioxide laser. There were no systemic manifestations.

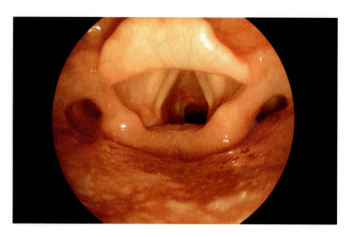

Figure 4.292

Idiopathic subglottic stenosis: indirect laryngoscopy

Indirect laryngoscopy appearance of idiopathic subglottic stenosis, an unusual condition that occurs only in females.

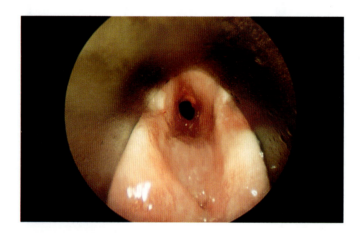

Figure 4.293

Idiopathic subglottic stenosis

Idiopathic subglottic stenosis in a 14-year-old girl, which was progressive for 2 years and then went into temporary remission before becoming active again.

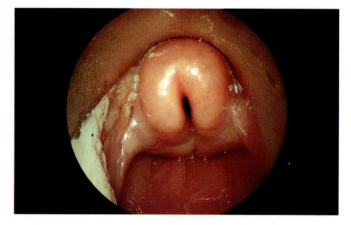

Figure 4.294

Sarcoid

Sarcoid in a 14-year-old boy, which presented as dyspnoea on exertion and some minor dysphagia. Painless, pale swelling of the epiglottis is characteristic of sarcoid in the larynx.

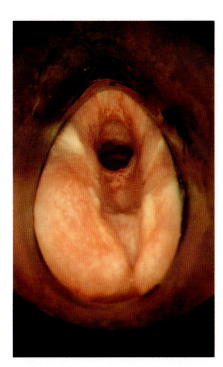

Figure 4.295

Wegener's granulomatosis

Wegener's granulomatosis in a 25-year-old woman whose pulmonary disease was diagnosed and treated 12 months previously. The acquired subglottic stenosis needed two laser treatments to restore an adequate airway.

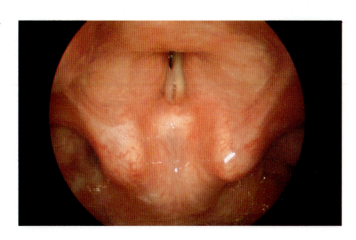

Figure 4.296

Rheumatoid arthritis

Severe rheumatoid arthritis causing chronic swelling in the posterior glottis, fixation of both cricoarytenoid joints and severe airway obstruction requiring a long-term tracheotomy.

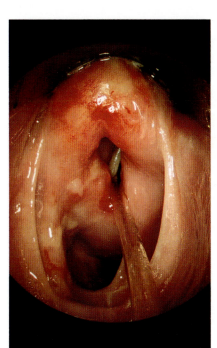

Figure 4.297

Pemphigoid

Pemphigoid during an active stage in a 45-year-old woman. The chronic fibrosis has caused scarring and thickening of the epiglottis and fibrous bands in the pharynx.

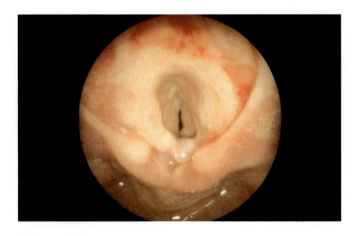

Figure 4.298

Epidermolysis bullosa

Epidermolysis bullosa in the active stage in a 7-year-old boy resulting in partial airway obstruction. See Figure 4.299.

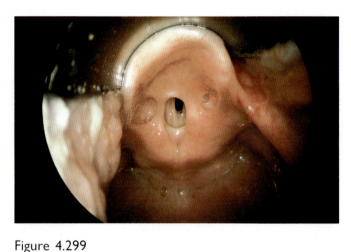

Figure 4.299

Epidermolysis bullosa

Epidermolysis bullosa in the chronic phase with supraglottic scarring and posterior glottic stenosis. This is the same patient as shown in Figure 4.298, 5 years later.

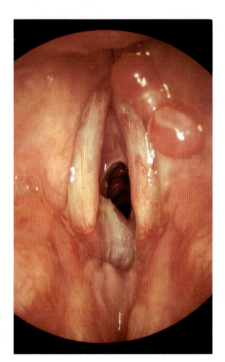

Figure 4.300

Plasma cell granuloma

A 60-year-old woman with three plasma cell granulomas on the right false cord, firm subglottic mass posteriorly on the left and a subglottic stenosis. The cause was unknown.

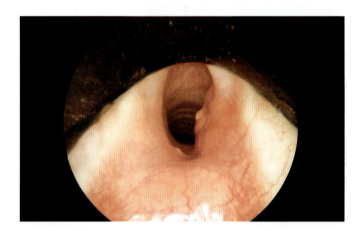

Figure 4.301

Subglottic granuloma

An idiopathic subglottic granuloma in an 11-year-old boy; the irregularity is from a previous biopsy.

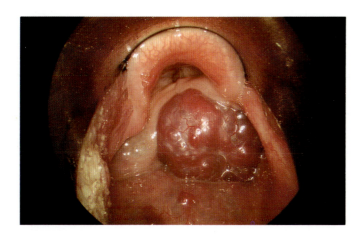

Figure 4.302

Haemangioma

A huge obstructing haemangioma in a 35-year-old woman, not controlled by radiotherapy. There was a rapid response to repeated intralesional injections of alcohol.

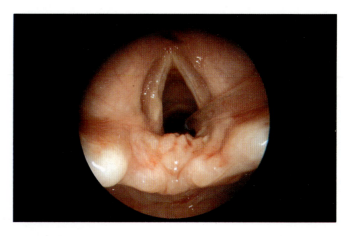

Figure 4.303

Pachyonychia congenita

Pachyonychia congenita in a 14-year-old boy with cutaneous manifestations. Note the proliferative mass in the posterior glottic space.

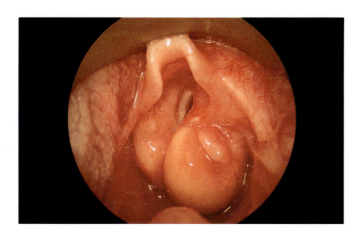

Figure 4.304

Xanthogranuloma

Benign juvenile xanthogranuloma in the larynx of an infant. Large rounded masses arising from arytenoid region. Glottic and subglottic narrowing required tracheotomy at 3 months of age.

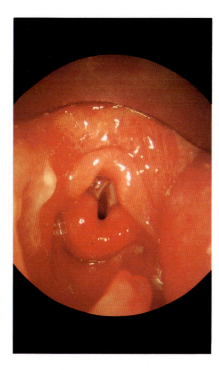

Figure 4.305

Congenital anomaly

Very rare congenital anomaly in a 12-hour-old infant with respiratory distress and inspiratory stridor. The epiglottis is rudimentary, almost absent. The arytenoids are large and the false cords hypoplastic.

5
The trachea

Bronchoscopy in adults usually relates to the diagnosis of intrabronchial tumours such as bronchogenic carcinoma, the investigation of chronic infection or segmental collapse and the clearance of secretions in intensive care patients. In children, bronchoscopy is necessary for removal of foreign bodies and in the investigation of congenital abnormalities.

Functional anatomy

The trachea begins at the lower border of the cricoid cartilage and passes down to bifurcate into the right and left main stem bronchi. It is a fibrous, muscular and cartilaginous tube lined internally by respiratory epithelium. The trachea is uniquely flexible and distensible, and can vary in length to adjust for diaphragmatic and respiratory movement, and extension and flexion of the vertebral column. It is supported by about 20 hyaline cartilage tracheal arches, C-shaped with the posterior open part closed by a sheet of fibroareolar connective tissue and transverse smooth muscle fibres. This trachealis muscle has two layers: an inner circular layer and an external longitudinal layer. Reduction of the tracheal lumen is caused by elongation of the trachea and by muscular contraction of the posterior transverse muscles. The elasticity of the tracheal cartilaginous arches passively dilates and widens the tracheal lumen during inspiration. The only complete cartilage ring in the respiratory tract is the cricoid cartilage, which is anatomically and functionally part of the larynx, not of the trachea. The respiratory mucosa is ciliated, pseudostratified columnar epithelium with a thin lamina propria; goblet mucous cells and some small subepithelial glands deliver secretions into the lumen. Scattered lymphoid aggregates are present within the lamina propria.

The tracheobronchial fluids are of great importance, working in conjunction with the respiratory cilia for mucociliary clearance, but there are other defence mechanisms such as immunological, proteolytic and phagocytic activities.

Tracheobronchoscopy

Endoscopic examination of the trachea and bronchial tree is performed commonly in both adults and children. Adult tracheobronchoscopy is performed mostly by physicians, internists, pulmonologists and critical care physicians, usually with a flexible bronchoscope and often under local anaesthetic. Tracheobronchoscopy in infants and children is performed by paediatric laryngologists, usually under general anaesthetic, using slim rigid rod lens telescopes for diagnostic examination (after suspension laryngoscopy has been achieved) or using rigid open tube bronchoscopes for procedures such as removal of a foreign body, suction clearance of secretions or biopsy.

Abnormalities of the cartilaginous tracheal arches are now more widely recognized. Tracheomalacia is a structural abnormality that allows collapse of the tracheal lumen or external compression by the innominate artery, a vascular ring or a mediastinal development cyst. The pathological changes in the trachea in tracheomalacia have been demonstrated clearly both in autopsy specimens and endoscopically. They consist of splayed, widened tracheal cartilages, widening of the posterior membranous wall and forward ballooning of the posterior membranous wall during expiration. Seen on a transverse section, the ratio of the length of tracheal cartilage to the width of the posterior membranous wall is normally about 4.5 : 1. The structural abnormality in tracheomalacia is often associated with a reduction of this ratio to 2 : 1, or in severe cases almost 1 : 1, so that the trachea becomes a flat tube with almost no anteroposterior lumen.

Injuries to the trachea caused by pressure from the cuff of an endotracheal tube during prolonged intubation and ventilation are now seldom seen with the use of high-volume, low-pressure cuffs, but unfortunately there has been no corresponding decrease in the incidence of laryngeal damage.

Radiological studies of the trachea include a plain anteroposterior chest radiograph, lateral views of the upper airway including the extrathoracic and intrathoracic trachea and a contrast oesophagogram. Narrowing or indentation of the normal air column in the trachea or compression or notching of the oesophageal outline will give useful information.

In infants, collapse, compression or stenosis of the trachea is suggested by a barking, seal-like cough, inspiratory and expiratory stridor, and cyanotic or apnoeic attacks. 'Dying spells' or reflex apnoea are common manifestations of tracheal compression caused by the innominate artery or as part of a wider abnormality in congenital tracheo-oesophageal fistula. Tracheomalacia occurs in adults, often in individuals who are considered to have 'intractable asthma' apparently resistant to standard treatment.

Endoscopic examination of the upper airways, principally of the trachea, is an essential part of the management of infants born with tracheo-oesophageal fistula and oesophageal atresia. Diagnostic indications include evaluation before operative repair (site of the tracheal aspect of the fistula, presence or absence of tracheomalacia, second or upper pouch fistula), diagnosis of an H-fistula, assessment of tracheomalacia, identification of recurrent, residual or second fistula, evaluation of the presence of associated anomaly, and evaluation of gastro-oesophageal reflux and oesophagitis or stenosis.

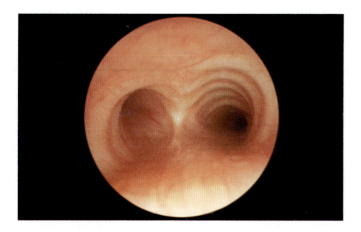

Figure 5.1

Normal trachea

The normal lower trachea, carina and openings of the right and left main bronchi in an adolescent. The diameter of the right main bronchus is usually about 50% greater than the diameter of the left main bronchus. Note the cartilaginous arches in the main bronchi.

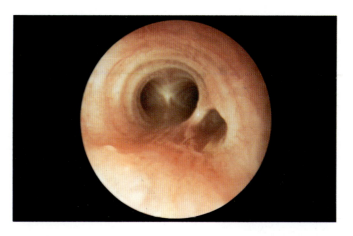

Figure 5.2

Right tracheal bronchus

A right tracheal bronchus in a 12-month-old child. This patient had a right upper lobe bronchus in the normal anatomical site. In other infants the right upper lobe bronchus originates from the lower trachea.

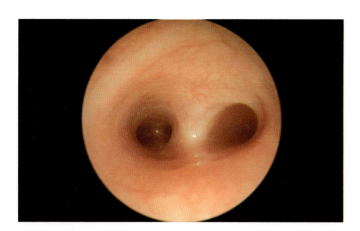

Figure 5.3

Congenital tracheal stenosis

The orifice seen on the left is the lower trachea and in the far distance there is a glimpse of the carina. The orifice on the right leads to a right tracheal bronchus.

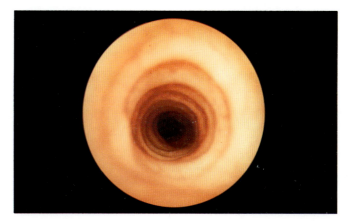

Figure 5.4

Congenital tracheal stenosis

Complete circular cartilaginous rings in the lower trachea. The orifice measures about 3.5 mm. There is often associated stenosis of the main bronchi with abnormal anatomy of the bronchi and the segmental openings.

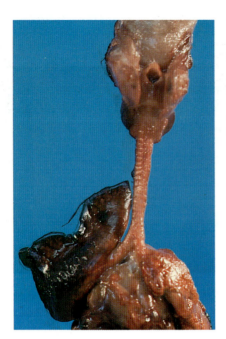

Figure 5.5

Congenital tracheal stenosis

Autopsy specimen of complete cartilaginous ring. There were multiple congenital anomalies. There was no vascular pulmonary sling in this patient, although it is a common association with congenital tracheal stenosis.

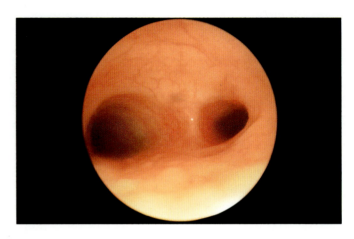

Figure 5.6

Congenital bronchial stenosis

There is a congenital stenosis of the right main bronchus, which has a lumen only about 50% that of the left main bronchus. Normally the diameter of the right main bronchus is about 50% greater than the left main bronchus.

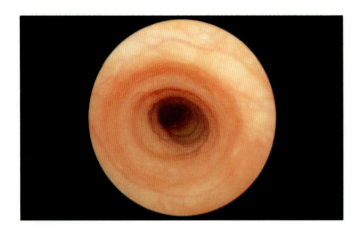

Figure 5.7

Congenital bronchial stenosis

Congenital stenosis of the right main bronchus with a normal trachea and left main bronchus. The cartilaginous rings in the bronchus are circular and complete.

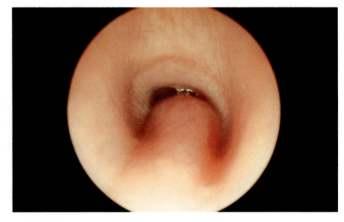

Figure 5.8

Congenital haemangioma

Haemangioma bulging the soft tissues of the posterior wall of the upper trachea in a 3-month-old infant. There was severe inspiratory and expiratory stridor. The appearance is sufficiently characteristic for an experienced observer to make a diagnosis without the need for biopsy.

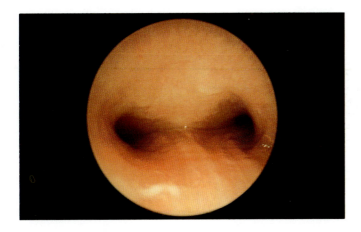

Figure 5.9

Congenital haemangioma

Congenital haemangioma external to the airways causing compression of the lower trachea and carina.

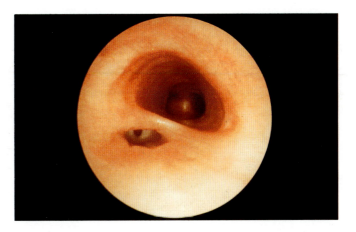

Figure 5.10

Congenital tracheo-oesophageal fistula

Tracheo-oesophageal fistula with a lower pouch fistula and an associated oesophageal atresia. The large opening of the fistula is located in the posterior wall of the trachea, towards the left of the midline.

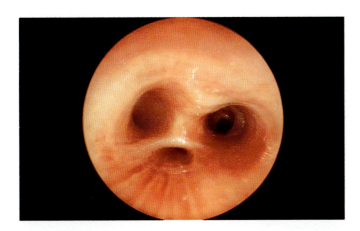

Figure 5.11

Congenital tracheo-oesophageal fistula

Congenital tracheo-oesophageal fistula with a large opening in the midline of the posterior wall just above the carina.

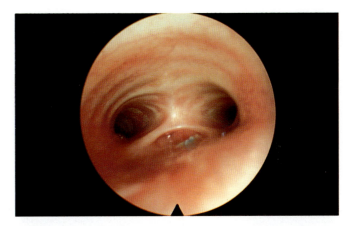

Figure 5.12

Repaired tracheo-oesophageal fistula in a 6-month-old child

This wide mouth of the residual pouch of the fistula is visible just above the carina. There is a small blue suture in it. In cases of repaired fistula, the residual pouch is invariably seen in the posterior tracheal wall as a diverticulum varying in length from a few millimetres to 15 mm.

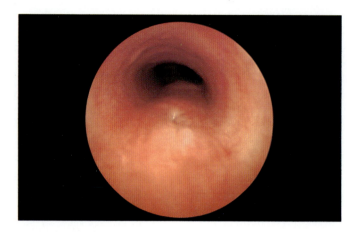

Figure 5.13

Congenital H-type tracheo-oesophageal fistula

There is a small tracheal opening in the midline of the posterior tracheal wall. It is usually in the upper third of the trachea.

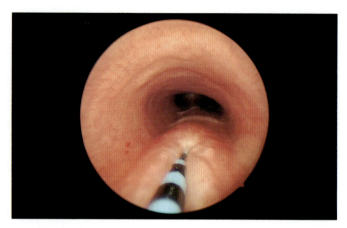

Figure 5.14

Congenital H-type tracheo-oesophageal fistula

Congenital H-type tracheo-oesophageal fistula with a 4 F catheter passed via the bronchoscope through the fistula and into the oesophagus. It remains in situ to help the surgeon identify the fistula at thoracotomy.

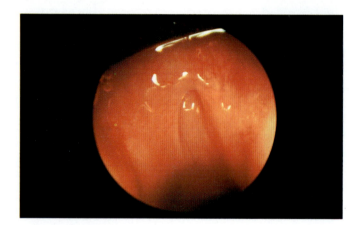

Figure 5.15

Oesophageal aspect of an H-type tracheo-oesophageal fistula

The characteristic appearance is of an inverted V-shaped orifice, which may be difficult to identify. A useful diagnostic test is to instil a few millilitres of saline into the upper oesophagus, apply positive pressure ventilation to the trachea through the endotracheal tube and, with an oesophagoscope in place, watch for bubbles of air.

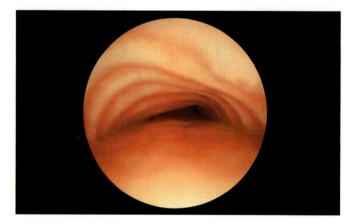

Figure 5.16

Severe tracheomalacia

Associated anomalies of the trachea and/or the oesophagus are common in patients with tracheo-oesophageal fistula and oesophageal atresia. These include congenital tracheal stenosis, tracheomalacia and sometimes congenital oesophageal stenosis. The tracheal cartilages have a half-circle shape rather than a normal horseshoe shape and the posterior membranes wall widens so that it bulges forward during expiration.

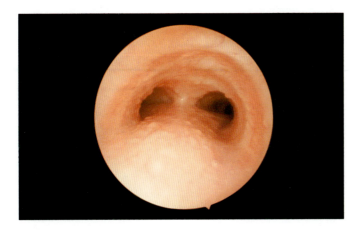

Figure 5.17

Mild tracheomalacia

Mild tracheomalacia with hypertrophy of multiple mucous glands in a child of 18 months.

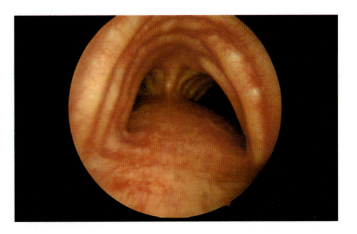

Figure 5.18

Mild tracheomalacia

Tracheomalacia in an adult. This is a congenital anomaly. The patient had been treated for unresponsive asthma. In tracheomalacia there is collapse, weakness and instability of the tracheal wall.

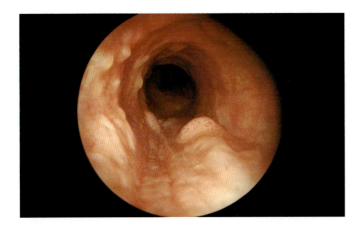

Figure 5.19

Recurrent respiratory papillomas in the trachea of an adult

Multiple sessile papillomas have spread over a wide area. In a patient with papillomas growing aggressively in the trachea or the bronchi, radiological study, including a CT scan, of the lungs may be necessary to detect parenchymatous spread with nodules or cystic spaces seen on the radiograph.

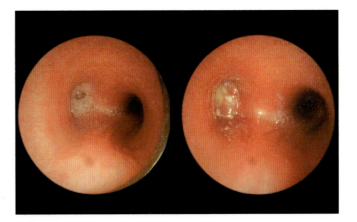

Figure 5.20

Tuberculosis

Changes due to primary tuberculosis after frothy mucus is sucked from the left main bronchus. The obstruction is caused by granulation tissue with areas of caseous material released by the ulceration of a caseating hilar lymph node.

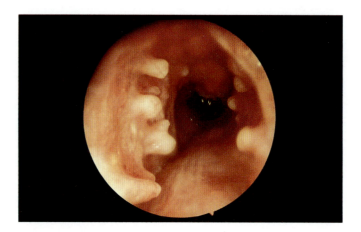

Figure 5.21

Tracheopathia osteoplastica

Tracheopathia osteoplastica is a rare finding, and is believed to be of degenerative nature and characterized by multiple osteocartilaginous nodules in the trachea and sometimes the bronchi. The osteocartilaginous nodules may be seen on a radiograph.

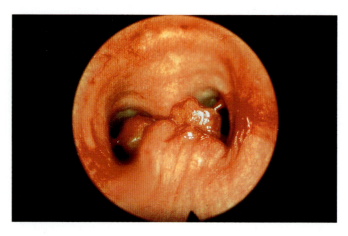

Figure 5.22

Bronchogenic carcinoma

Bronchogenic carcinoma invading the posterior wall of the trachea just above the carina and causing partial obstruction of airflow in both the right and left main bronchi. Palliative laser treatment was provided.

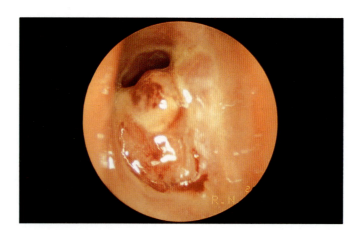

Figure 5.23

Thyroid carcinoma

Carcinoma of the thyroid gland has eroded the cartilaginous structures and ulcerated into the subglottic region causing severe airway obstruction and haemoptysis. Palliation with laser treatment was given.

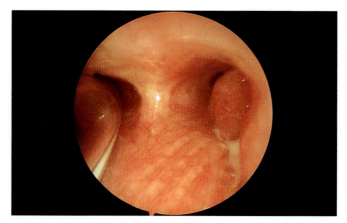

Figure 5.24

Adenoid cystic carcinoma

Adenoid cystic carcinoma on the lateral wall of the right main bronchus in a 16-year-old girl. Endoscopic biopsy was performed with an endotracheal tube administering one lung anaesthesia in the left main bronchus. There was little bleeding. A radical resection was performed subsequently; however, recurrence developed, which was likely due to insidious perineural spread.

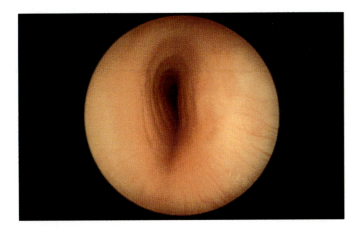

Figure 5.25

Mediastinal neuroblastoma

A mediastinal neuroblastoma causing side-to-side compression of the trachea in a baby only 1 month old. Most tracheal compression is anteroposterior.

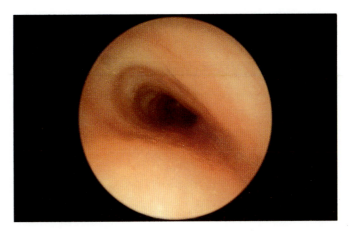

Figure 5.26

Innominate artery compression

Tracheal compression by the innominate artery occurs over a number of tracheal arches at the junction of the upper two-thirds and the lower third of the trachea. With innominate artery compression, and in contradistinction to other forms of tracheomalacia, a shorter segment of the lower trachea is involved and the associated findings of a wide posterior membranous wall with anterior bulging are not always present.

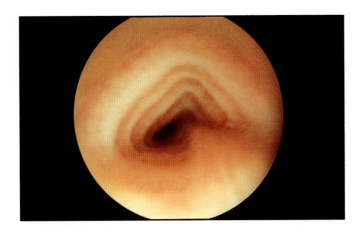

Figure 5.27

Double aortic arch

The narrow trachea appears almost triangular in appearance, the compression by a double aortic arch causing folding of the posterior membranous wall. Oesophagoscopy would show the posterior aortic arch passing behind the oesophagus at the junction of the upper third and the lower two-thirds.

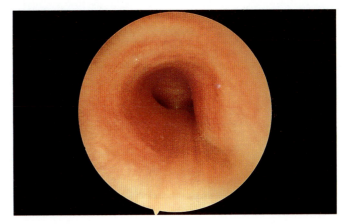

Figure 5.28

Double aortic arch

The vascular ring has markedly narrowed the lower trachea. In the distance the carina can be seen and there is some narrowing of the left main bronchus.

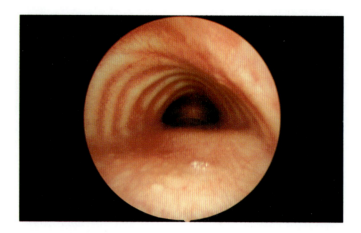

Figure 5.29

Pulmonary sling

A pulmonary sling is a vascular sling in which the left pulmonary artery passes between the trachea and the oesophagus. The degree of airway compression is usually not functionally significant.

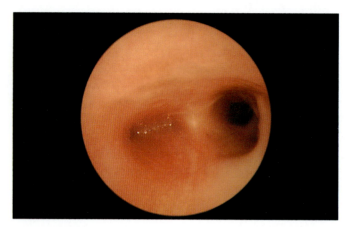

Figure 5.30

Pulmonary sling

A large single pulmonary artery causing compression of the left main bronchus with overdistension of the left lung. Proven with angiography.

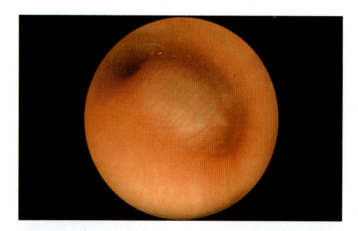

Figure 5.31

Duplication cyst of the trachea

A duplication cyst of the trachea in a baby a few weeks old with severe airway obstruction. Oesophagoscopy showed a rounded cystic mass from the right anterolateral wall. This rare duplication cyst of the trachea was removed at thoracotomy.

6

The head and neck

Many medical practitioners from numerous diverse specialty areas, including but not limited to general practitioners, general physicians, endocrine physicians and surgeons, general surgeons, plastic surgeons, oral surgeons, vascular surgeons and otorhinolaryngologists, may be called on to diagnose and treat diseases of the head and neck. To a large extent, which specialty treats which disease depends on a combination of historical, national and local factors. It is nevertheless important that all those individuals who manage neck disease have a good working knowledge of the diagnostic features and management of all those conditions that can occur in the neck.

Examination

A correct and reliable technique for examination of the structures contained in the neck is imperative if abnormalities are not to be missed. A systematic examination of the neck is required and each individual practitioner should develop a standard routine for examining all areas of the neck.

The neck should be fully exposed to below the levels of the clavicles to facilitate a thorough inspection. The initial inspection of the neck may reveal an obvious swelling, or the way in which the patient is 'holding' his or her head may suggest the presence of an inflammatory process. One technique of examination of the neck is described below.

The examination commences with an inspection of the neck from the front and from both sides. The practitioner then stands behind the seated patient. The patient is asked to relax and gently flex the neck while the examiner's fingers are placed simultaneously on each mastoid process. The fingers then palpate the preauricular area, the surface of the parotid gland, return under the pinna to the postauricular sulcus and move to the occiput before returning to the mastoid process.

The fingers now palpate down the anterior border of the trapezius to the clavicle, traverse the supraclavicular fossa and ascend the posterior border of the sternomastoid before returning to the mastoid process.

The fingers then move down the anterior border of the sternomastoid to the sternal notch and ascend in the midline. Care is required during this manoeuvre to avoid excessive and bilateral palpation over the carotid bulbs as this may occasionally produce syncope. As the fingers ascend in the midline, the thyroid gland is palpated and if the patient is asked to take a swallow at this time the movement of the thyroid gland can be assessed. The fingers progress in the midline to the point of the chin and palpate along the submental and submandibular triangles before returning to the mastoid process. If there is a palpable or described abnormality in the submental or submandibular regions then bimanual palpation with a gloved finger inserted into the mouth is mandatory.

If a significant external abnormality is found on examination of the neck then a thorough examination of the oral cavity, pharynx and larynx is generally required.

Assessment of neck lumps and neck nodes

The patient who develops a lump or swelling in the neck is a common clinical problem. The age of the patient is often a pointer to the nature of the swelling. Under the age of 20 years the lump is most likely to be inflammatory or congenital. Between the ages of 20 and 40 years the most common swellings are salivary, inflammatory or lymphoma. Beyond the age of 40 years a neck lump or swelling is metastatic malignant disease until proven otherwise. Inflammatory masses and salivary gland swellings are usually painful.

Midline neck masses

Most midline masses are solitary. Dermoid cysts are situated above the level of the hyoid bone, whereas thyroglossal cysts are identified below the hyoid bone. A thyroglossal cyst moves upwards when the patient is asked to protrude the tongue. A thyroid mass fails to move upwards on tongue protrusion but moves upwards when the patient swallows.

Posterior triangle masses

Masses in the posterior triangle of the neck typically arise from the lymph nodes. These lymph nodes may be enlarged as the result of a reactive process following a local infection or arise from specific infection such as Epstein–Barr virus infection (infectious mononucleosis), brucellosis, toxoplasmosis or cytomegalovirus infection, or enlarge as the result of neoplasia, either primary (lymphoma) or secondary (metastasis). One notable variation to these examples is the single bony hard cervical rib.

Supraclavicular masses

Supraclavicular masses are, unfortunately, often the result of metastatic lymph nodes from tumours either in the stomach or in the lung.

Salivary gland swellings

Submandibular gland swellings present beneath the angle of the mandible but do not extend below the level of the hyoid bone. A parotid tumour, when it is small, typically presents under the earlobe. Lateral protrusion of the earlobe is often an early sign of a parotid tumour. In this site the diagnosis of parotid tumour can be confused with an epidermoid cyst. The punctum of an epidermoid cyst should always be identified. Diffuse

parotid swellings can often be difficult to identify. Repeated clinical examination and the judicious use of fine-needle aspiration are useful in the management of a diffuse parotid swelling.

Vascular swellings

The identification of a painless pulsating mass at the level of the carotid bifurcation always raises the possibility of a carotid body tumour. Angiography, magnetic resonance imaging (MRI) and computerized scanning are all helpful in the diagnosis of lumps in this region.

Investigation of neck masses

In recent years the techniques to investigate neck masses have greatly increased. Computed tomography (CT) and MRI have become the preferred techniques to assess the size and anatomical extent of a neck lesion. The recent development of three-dimensional (3D) CT reconstruction promises to provide a very precise anatomical delineation of a neck lesion.

Ultrasound is very useful in determining whether a neck lesion is cystic or solid. Thyroid ultrasound combined with needle aspiration is an excellent technique in the management of thyroid gland cysts. Isotope scans are helpful in the diagnosis of a thyroid lump. A cold nodule on a thyroid isotope scan implies a cyst or a tumour.

Assessment of a suspected vascular lesion often requires angiography, which can now be combined with MRI or CT to give greater anatomical information.

Despite all the recent advances in imaging technology, the plain radiograph still has a definite place in the management of a number of conditions. Stones of the salivary glands can be easily identified on a plain radiograph. An elongated styloid process, cervical spine osteophytes and some ingested or inhaled foreign bodies will be well demonstrated on plain radiography.

Contrast studies such as the barium swallow are still the gold standard for the radiological assessment of swallowing disorders. Contrast studies of the parotid and submandibular glands (sialography) are widely practised. The information derived from sialography can be improved when combined with MRI and CT.

Fine-needle aspiration biopsy of a neck lump is one of the most useful diagnostic tests in the investigation of a neck mass. This investigation is required in most undiagnosed solid neck lumps. It is important that the local pathology laboratory and the investigating surgeon are aware of their own specificity and sensitivity in the fine-needle aspiration diagnosis of neck lumps. Fine-needle aspiration biopsy of a neck mass should nearly always be used prior to the need for an open biopsy.

Photography of neck disease

Lumps or swellings, unless exceptionally prominent, are sometimes difficult to demonstrate on a photograph. The creation of light and shadow is helpful in emphasizing an individual lesion.

Neck

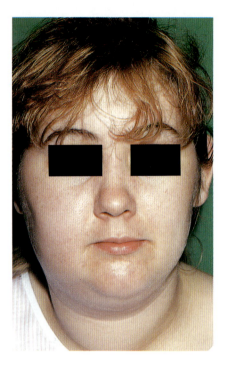

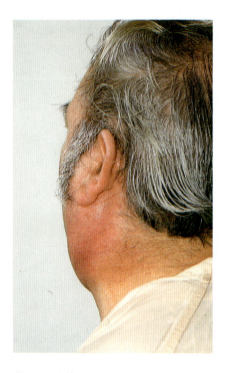

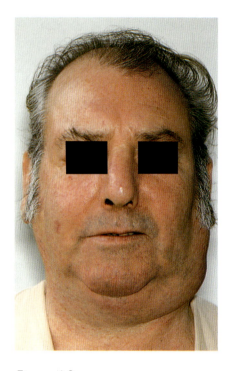

Figure 6.1
Parotitis (mumps)

The mumps virus is a member of the paramyxoma virus group. Mumps is the most common cause of acute parotitis. Swelling of one or both parotid glands is common, with the swelling being located characteristically below and in front of the ear. The swollen parotid gland may push the earlobe forward and laterally, and in severe cases it may even limit jaw movement. The swelling of one side may precede the other by as much as 4 days. This teenager has bilateral parotid swellings as a result of mumps.

Figure 6.2
Parotitis (bacterial)

Bacterial parotitis is most often due to a staphylococcal infection of the parotid gland in a dehydrated patient. This situation can arise in those patients with uncontrolled diabetes, renal failure or severe electrolyte disturbance. The gland becomes acutely swollen and tender and may, as shown in this case, progress to frank abscess formation. The skin overlying the gland has become red as the abscess develops.

Figure 6.3
Parotitis (bacterial)

This anterior view of the patient in Figure 6.2 shows the large parotid abscess which required surgical drainage.

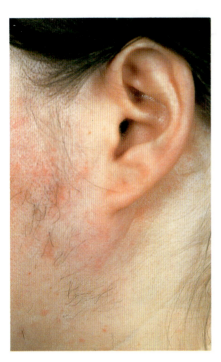

Figure 6.4
Parotid tumour (pleomorphic adenoma)

The pleomorphic adenoma or mixed cell tumour is the most common tumour of the parotid gland. Characteristically, a pleomorphic adenoma is a smooth, occasionally lobulated, firm tumour that presents under the earlobe. These tumours almost never present with pain nor do they produce a facial palsy. This illustration shows a pleomorphic adenoma pushing the earlobe laterally.

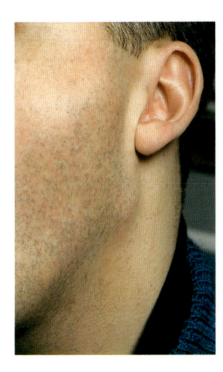

Figure 6.5
Parotid tumour (pleomorphic adenoma)

A parotid pleomorphic adenoma does not always present at the earlobe. There is potential clinical difficulty with the differential diagnosis of a lump in the area of the upper cervical lymph node chain, the posterior part of the submandibular triangle and the tail of the parotid. Fine-needle aspiration cytology can often be helpful in this diagnostic dilemma. In this illustration the swelling about 3 cm below the earlobe was shown to be a pleomorphic adenoma on fine-needle aspiration cytology. Surgery proved this to be a benign pleomorphic adenoma of the parotid gland.

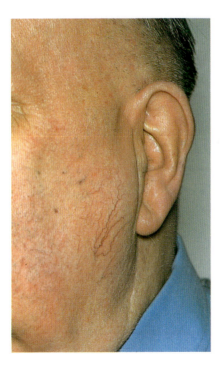

Figure 6.6
Parotid tumour (Warthin's)

Warthin's tumour (papillary cystadenoma lymphomatosum) is a monomorphic tumour and the second most common benign parotid tumour. It is a soft, fluctuant cystic tumour that typically affects elderly men and in 10% of cases is bilateral. The tumour is usually found in the tail of the parotid, although in this case the Warthin tumour involves most of the parotid gland.

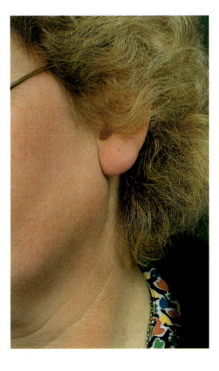

Figure 6.7
Parotid tumour (lymphoma)

Development of a rapidly swelling and uncomfortable mass in the parotid region is highly suspicious of malignancy. This woman had a rapidly enlarging mass in the parotid. Note how the earlobe is pushed laterally. Histology showed this mass to be a lymphoma. The absence of a facial palsy in association with rapidly expanding parotid tumour suggests the presence of a lymphomatous tumour.

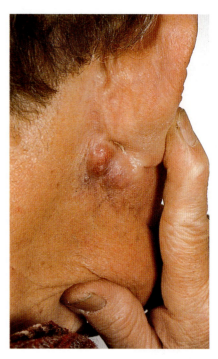

Figure 6.8
Parotid tumour (mucoepidermoid carcinoma)

This patient has a mass in the right parotid gland which is beginning to ulcerate through the skin below and behind the ear. Cutaneous breakthrough and subsequent ulceration can be a feature of a malignant parotid tumour. The histology showed a mucoepidermoid carcinoma.

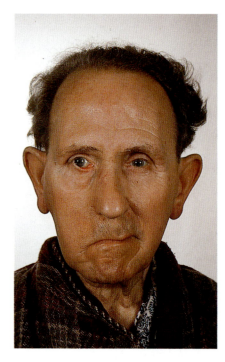

Figure 6.9
Parotid tumour (mucoepidermoid carcinoma)

This is the anterior view of the patient shown in Figure 6.8. Note the paralysis of the right side of the face, and the droop of the right hand corner of the mouth. A lateral tarsorrhaphy has been performed to protect the eye. A mucoepidermoid carcinoma of the right parotid, as shown in Figure 6.8, was the cause of the facial palsy.

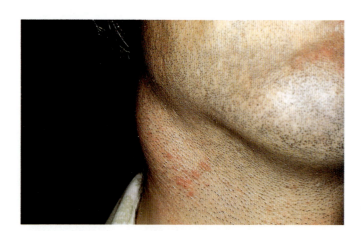

Figure 6.10
Branchial cyst (branchiogenic cyst)

A branchial cyst is a developmental cyst lined by stratified squamous epithelium interspersed with lymphoid tissue and containing a straw-coloured fluid. Cholesterol crystals can be found in the straw-coloured fluid. The cyst is smooth and fluctuant and is typically found at the anterior border of the sternomastoid, usually at the junction between the upper and middle third of the muscle. The young man in this illustration had a moderately large branchial cyst.

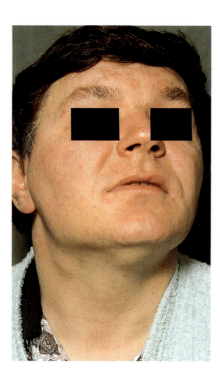

Figure 6.11
Branchial cyst (branchiogenic cyst)

This patient has a branchial cyst in its characteristic position. The swelling of the cyst can be seen below the angle of the mandible. The diagnosis was confirmed by fine-needle aspiration cytology.

Figure 6.12

Branchial fistula (first arch)

The exit to a first arch branchial fistula is visible anteroinferior to the earlobe. The tract of a first arch branchial fistula runs laterally from the junction of the cartilaginous and bony portions of the external auditory canal, passes between the branches of the facial nerve and exits onto the skin at a higher position than would normally be expected. The more usual site of exit of a first branchial fistula is anterior to the sternomastoid muscle at the level of the hyoid bone.

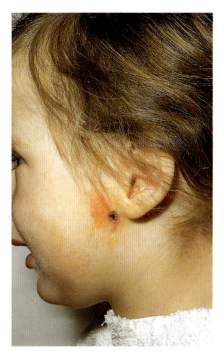

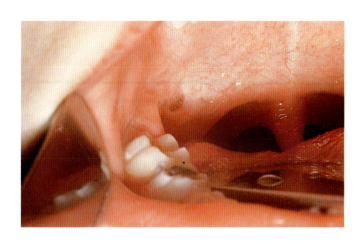

Figure 6.13

Branchial fistula (second arch)

The depression containing a number of bubbles located posteromedial to the retromolar trigone is the internal opening of a second arch branchial fistula in the supratonsillar region.

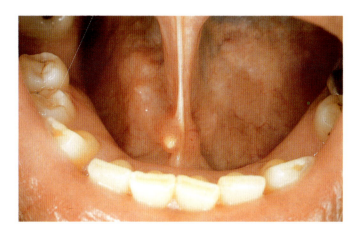

Figure 6.14

Impacted submandibular duct calculus

The cause of the acute swelling of this patient's left submandibular gland is the yellow calculus that has become impacted in the orifice of the submandibular duct. This type of stone can usually be removed by means of a small incision into the duct directly over the stone (sialolithotomy).

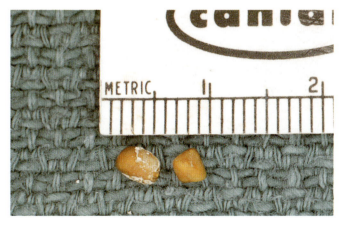

Figure 6.15

Submandibular duct calculi

These two characteristic yellow submandibular duct stones were removed by sialolithotomy.

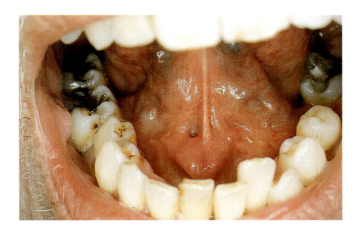

Figure 6.16
Submandibular duct fistula

A fistula has developed in this left submandibular duct at the site of a wide sialolithotomy performed for the removal of a large impacted calculus.

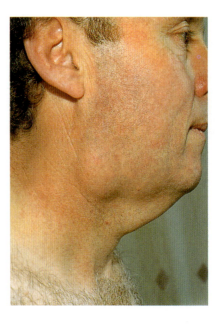

Figure 6.17
Submandibular swelling (lymphoma)

A swelling in the region of the submandibular triangle can be difficult to diagnose. Such a swelling may arise from structures within the submandibular triangle or from lesions that extend into the submandibular triangle either from the upper cervical lymph node chain or from the tail of the parotid. This swelling at the angle of the mandible was due to a lymphoma.

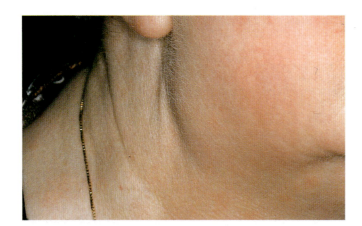

Figure 6.18
Submandibular swelling (chronic sialadenitis)

This woman developed a painful swelling of her submandibular gland whenever she ate. A fullness of the submandibular triangle can be seen in this illustration. The submandibular duct was obstructed by a stone.

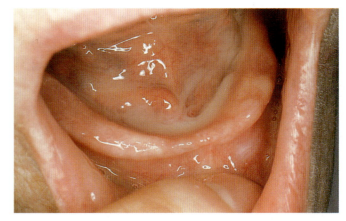

Figure 6.19
Acute on chronic submandibular sialadenitis

This patient with chronic submandibular gland sialadenitis and sialolithiasis developed a secondary acute bacterial sialadenitis. Note the purulent secretions that have been 'milked' from the gland.

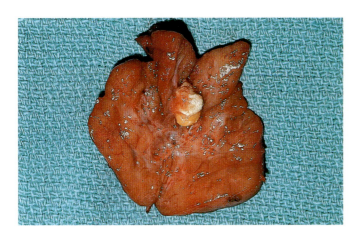

Figure 6.20
Chronic sialadenitis

This submandibular gland was removed for the relief of chronic sialadenitis. Note the large central calculus that was responsible for the recurrent infections.

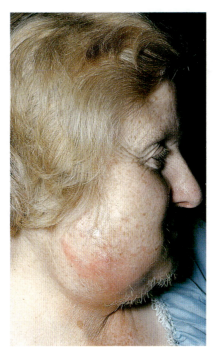

Figure 6.21
Submandibular gland abscess

This woman had a long-standing stone in her submandibular gland. A severe staphylococcal abscess developed within the gland resulting in this large fluctuant swelling overlying the angle of the jaw.

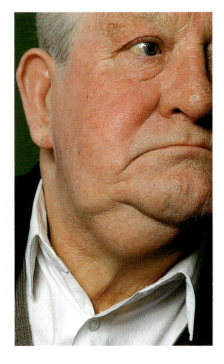

Figure 6.22
Metastatic squamous cell carcinoma

Squamous cell carcinoma of the aerodigestive tract that has spread to the lymph nodes of the neck can present in a number of ways. Some of these problems are shown in the following illustrations. This man presented with a firm 4 cm × 3 cm mass under the right side of his chin. These metastatic lymph nodes originated from a very small (<0.5 cm diameter) primary squamous cell carcinoma of the floor of the mouth.

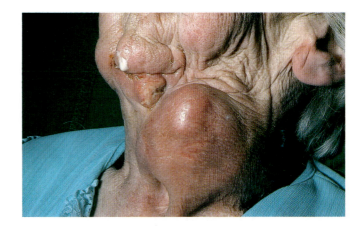

Figure 6.23
Metastatic squamous cell carcinoma

This woman has a squamous cell carcinoma of the floor of the mouth. There are masses of fixed lymph nodes and ulcerative tumour on the left side of the neck. The tumour was fixed to both the skin and the prevertebral tissue.

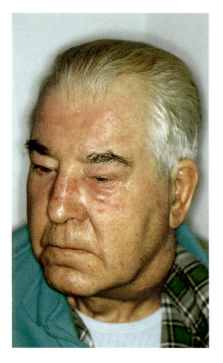

Figure 6.24

Metastatic squamous cell carcinoma

This man has metastatic squamous cell carcinoma in his submandibular triangle extending into the upper deep cervical lymph node chain. The visible swelling of this disease can be seen in the illustration. The tumour also obstructs the venous drainage of the left side of the face. Note the infraorbital and periorbital oedema.

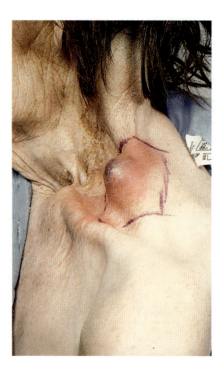

Figure 6.25

Metastatic squamous cell carcinoma

This patient presented with a red, painful, hard, nodular swelling in the supraclavicular fossa. This was metastatic squamous cell carcinoma arising from a laryngeal tumour. This man had paralysis of his brachial plexus as a result of these metastases.

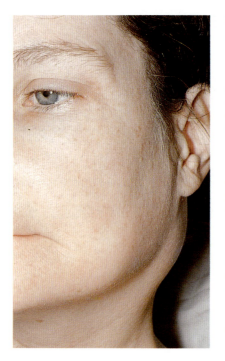

Figure 6.26

Metastatic squamous cell carcinoma

This woman presented with a large swelling of the left side of her neck. Fine-needle aspiration cytology demonstrated squamous cell carcinoma. The primary site for these metastatic nodes was the postnasal space. A Horner's syndrome due to interruption of the sympathetic chain is present in the left eye. Note the drooping upper eyelid and the constricted pupil.

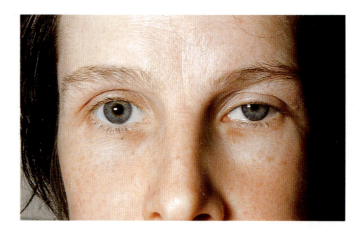

Figure 6.27

Metastatic squamous cell carcinoma

This illustration shows more clearly the left-sided Horner's syndrome of the patient shown in Figure 6.26.

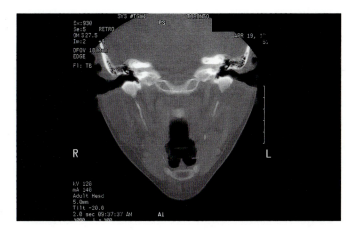
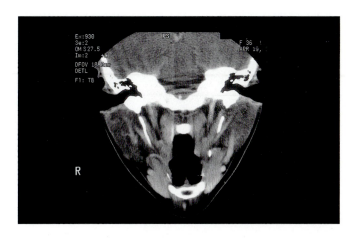

Figure 6.28

Eagle's syndrome (elongated styloid process)

This patient presented with recurrent stabbing pain in the region of the tonsillar fossae. The cause was ultimately discovered on CT, which revealed the presence of these grossly elongated styloid processes.

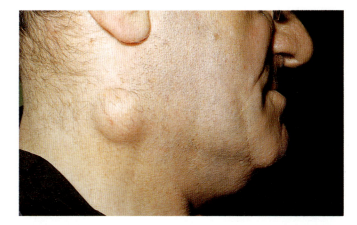

Figure 6.29

Sebaceous cyst

The large indentable, smooth subcutaneous mass with a central visible punctum sited at the angle of the jaw is a sebaceous cyst.

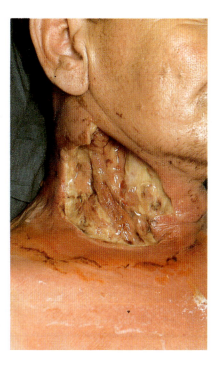

Figure 6.30

Necrotizing fasciitis

This man developed a rapidly spreading synergistic gangrene of the investing deep fascia of the neck. Wide débridement of the dead tissue was required combined with intensive antimicrobial therapy. A red line of demarcation can be seen surrounding the defect and further tissue débridement beyond this mark was required before the disease was contained. The sternomastoid muscle is visible in the centre of the neck defect.

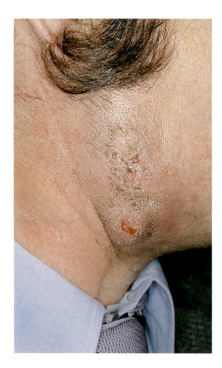

Figure 6.31

Cervicofacial actinomycosis

The chronic loculated area of suppuration at the angle of the jaw is due to actinomycosis. Note the multiple points of discharge overlying the brawny swelling. Sulphur granules were found in the pus.

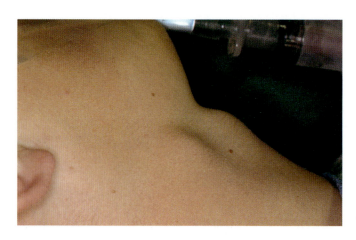

Figure 6.32

Tuberculous lymph node (scrofula)

This young man presented with a solitary lymph node lateral to his thyroid cartilage (the swelling closest to the photographer). The patient was otherwise well. Fine-needle aspiration cytology was unhelpful. Excision biopsy confirmed the diagnosis of tuberculosis. An atypical lymph node swelling in the neck of a young person should raise consideration of tuberculosis, lymphoma or HIV infection.

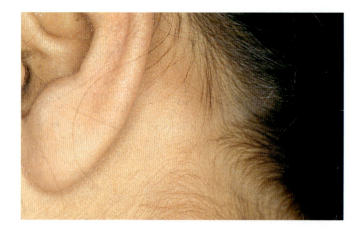

Figure 6.33

Tuberculosis (lymph node enlargement)

This 6-year-old girl with no systemic illness presented with a palpable lymph node behind the left ear overlying the mastoid bone, which had been present for 6 months, and unilateral tonsillar hypertrophy. Granulomatous changes of tuberculosis were found in the lymph node.

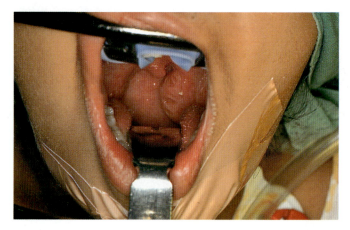

Figure 6.34

Tuberculosis (tonsillar enlargement)

This photograph shows the unilateral tonsillar enlargement of the young girl shown in Figure 6.33. The lymph node was on the same side as the tonsillar enlargement. Histology also revealed the granulomatous changes of tuberculosis within the tonsil.

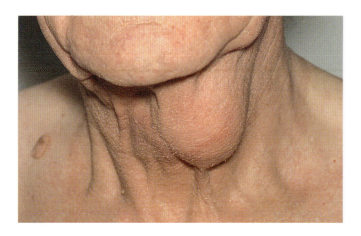

Figure 6.35
Lipoma of the neck

Lipomas can arise in any part of the neck and may be solitary or multiple. They are subcutaneous, slow growing and benign. This elderly woman has a large pendulous swelling on the left side of her neck. The swelling is a lipoma that had been present for 20 years.

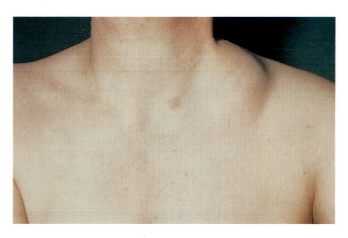

Figure 6.36
Lipoma of the neck

The soft rubbery swelling of this left supraclavicular fossa was a lipoma.

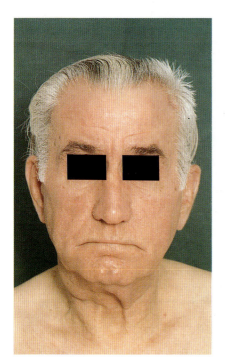

Figure 6.37
Laryngocele

This man has a compressible swelling of the right side of his neck. An increase in the air pressure within the pharynx increased the size of this laryngocele. The cystic swelling originated from the laryngeal ventricle.

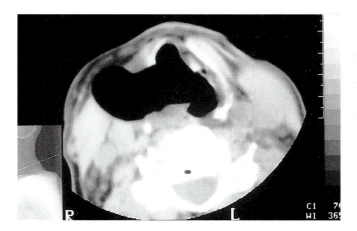

Figure 6.38
Laryngocele

This is an axial CT scan of the neck of the patient shown in Figure 6.37. A combined external and internal laryngocele can be seen.

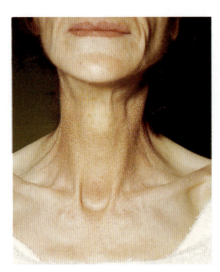

Figure 6.39
Pharyngeal pouch

The swelling visible on the left side of the neck of this thin and emaciated patient is a pharyngeal pouch or diverticulum. This pharyngeal pouch enlarged with eating and could be reduced by external compression.

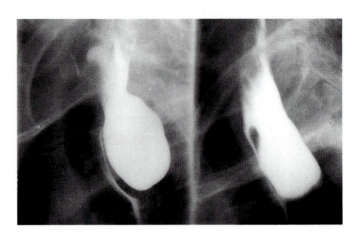

Figure 6.40
Pharyngeal pouch

This contrast radiograph shows the characteristic appearance of a pharyngeal pouch. The filling of the smooth pouch and the normal flow of barium down the oesophagus can be seen.

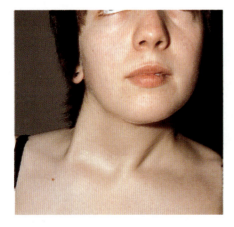

Figure 6.41
Torticollis

This torticollis in a young woman is the result of acute spasm in the right sternomastoid muscle, which developed from sleeping in an awkward position.

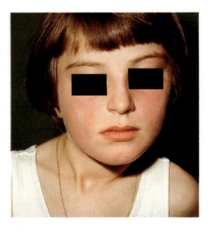

Figure 6.42
Torticollis

An inflammatory mass in the left side of the neck of this child gave rise to this torticollis. The child is pyrexial and both cheeks can be seen to be flushed. Intensive and prolonged antibiotic therapy resolved the torticollis.

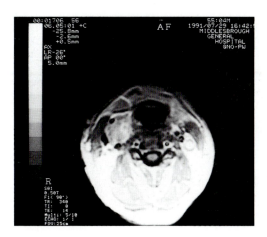

Figure 6.43

Carotid body tumour

This patient has a palpable, pulsatile swelling of the right side of the neck. This axial CT scan shows an enhancing mass on the right side of the neck. The internal and external carotid arteries are separated by the tumour. This is a carotid body tumour.

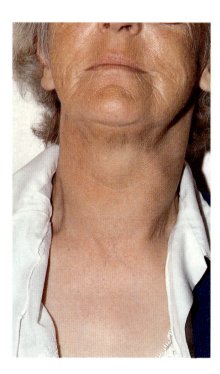

Figure 6.44

Goitre (Hashimoto's thyroiditis)

A goitre is a palpable or visible swelling of the thyroid gland. Hashimoto's thyroiditis is an autoimmune condition that is a common cause of bilateral and sometimes asymmetrical goitre. This woman has a smooth but asymmetrical swelling of her thyroid gland. The left lobe of the gland is considerably bigger than the right lobe.

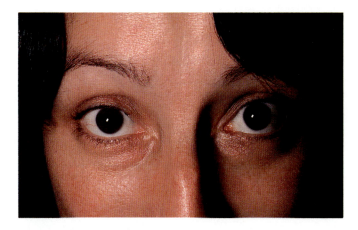

Figure 6.45

Endocrine orbitopathy (primary thyrotoxicosis)

This young woman with primary thyrotoxicosis (Graves' disease) demonstrates the clinical features of endocrine orbitopathy. Note a peculiar stare produced by retraction of the upper eyelid and the unnatural degree of separation between the margins of the two eyelids.

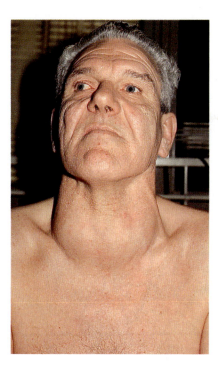

Figure 6.46

Goitre (multinodular thyroid)

This man has a massive multinodular goitre, which distorts his entire neck. He was euthyroid.

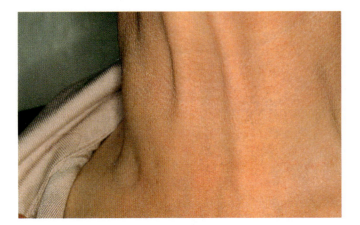

Figure 6.47

Goitre (papillary adenoma)

Loss of the profile of the strap muscles in the root of the neck can be a visible clue to a goitre. In this illustration there is a visible loss of the definition in the inferior portion of the right-sided strap muscles (sternohyoid). This loss of profile was due to a papillary adenoma affecting predominantly the right lobe of the thyroid gland.

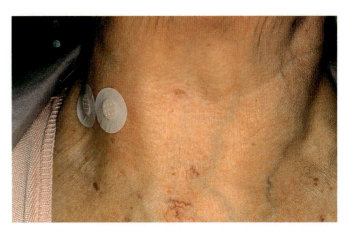

Figure 6.48

Goitre (with superior vena cava syndrome)

This 74-year-old woman presented with a very large goitre and a history of respiratory difficulty when she lay down. The goitre had extended into the superior mediastinum where it obstructed venous return from the head and neck. The large goitre can be seen in this illustration (particularly at the lateral aspects of the neck) with an associated dilatation of the cutaneous veins as a result of the superior mediastinal syndrome. The 'sticking plaster' covers the site of the fine-needle aspiration biopsy. This goitre was due to a very large multinodular goitre, which was successfully removed.

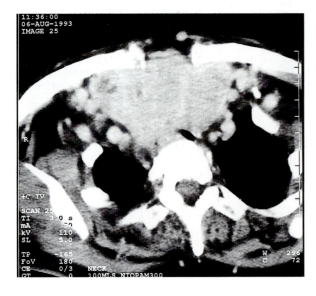

Figure 6.49

Goitre (with superior vena cava syndrome)

This axial CT scan demonstrates the extension of the multinodular goitre into the superior mediastinum of the patient shown in Figure 6.48.

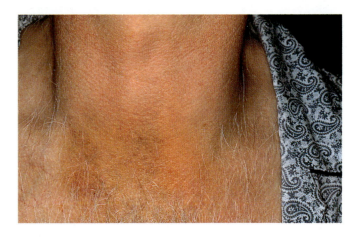

Figure 6.50

Goitre (spontaneous bleed)

This patient with a multinodular goitre was admitted to hospital as an emergency owing to progressive airway difficulty. Spontaneous bruising had occurred at the root of the neck heralding a bleed into the tissues of the neck rather than within the thyroid gland. Spontaneous bleeding within a multinodular goitre usually results in a painful swelling. The airway problem was treated by conservative therapy. Once the acute problem had settled, the multinodular goitre was removed and no further difficulties have arisen.

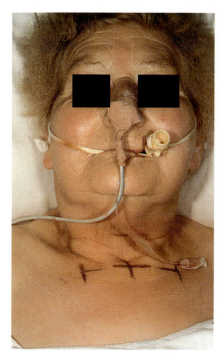

Figure 6.51

Thyroid lymphoma (respiratory obstruction)

This woman presented to an emergency department with airway obstruction. An emergency endotracheal tube was passed. It transpired that a thyroid lymphoma was the cause of her severe tracheal compression. External beam radiotherapy was planned and the patient was offered a temporary tracheostomy. She refused the tracheostomy and the endotracheal tube remained in place for the 4 weeks of treatment and a subsequent 2 weeks before successful extubation.

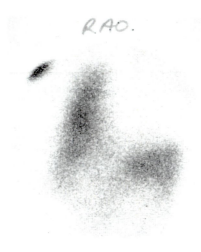

Figure 6.52

Thyroid scan (cold nodule)

Radioiodine thyroid scans are commonly used in the assessment of a thyroid swelling. Note the blank or 'cold area' of decreased iodine uptake in the left upper thyroid lobe, which suggests the presence of a solid malignant lesion or a cyst.

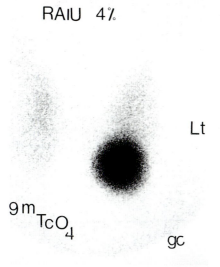

Figure 6.53

Thyroid scan (hot nodule)

This radioiodine thyroid scan shows an area of increased iodine uptake, i.e. a 'hot nodule'. This was an autonomous thyroid nodule of the left thyroid lobe.

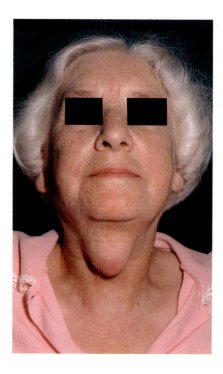

Figure 6.54

Thyroglossal cyst

The large midline neck swelling that moved upwards with swallowing and with protrusion of the tongue is a thyroglossal cyst.

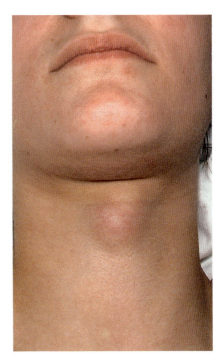

Figure 6.55
Thyroglossal cyst

This photograph shows the typical size of a thyroglossal cyst. There is often a slight discolouration of the skin over the smooth and firm cyst.

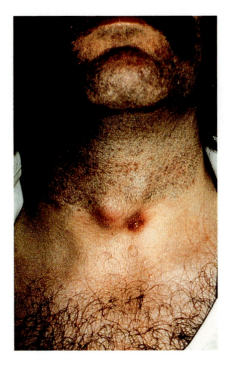

Figure 6.56
Thyroglossal sinus

A thyroglossal cyst may become infected. In this case, an infected thyroglossal cyst was incised and drained. A thyroglossal sinus resulted from that treatment. The discolouration medial to the prominence of the thyroid alae (Adam's apple) identifies the area of the sinus.

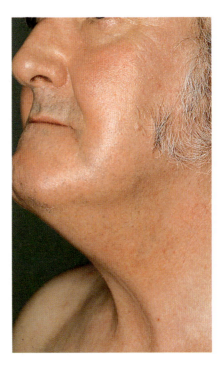

Figure 6.57
Dermoid cyst

The large swelling under the chin of this patient obliterated the angle between the chin and the neck. The palpable swelling was firm, circumscribed, approximately 3 cm × 3 cm and situated above the hyoid bone level. The excised specimen was a dermoid cyst.

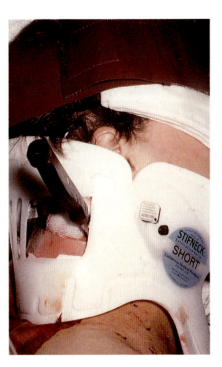

Figure 6.58
Neck trauma (knife injury to the neck)

This man was in an argument over the cost of the drug cocaine; a kitchen knife formed part of the negotiations. After the assault, the knife was stabilized by an extrication collar. Once radiological investigation had determined the position of the knife and confirmed the integrity and relative safety of the vascular structures in the neck, the knife was removed during surgical exploration.

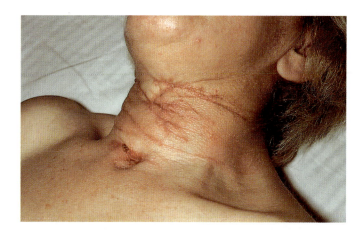

Figure 6.59

Neck trauma (suicide attempt with knife)

This man attempted suicide by multiple knife slashes to his own neck and wrists. The healing site of the emergency tracheostomy wound can be seen in addition to all the healing slash marks.

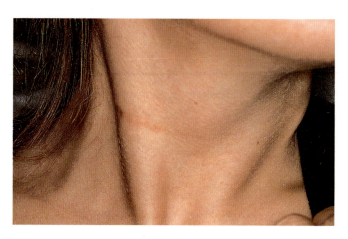

Figure 6.60

Neck trauma (strangulation)

This young woman was held down by the throat during an attempted rape. The assailant was right handed and the bruise caused by the thumb can be seen in the submandibular triangle. A circumferential bruise across the sternomastoid can be seen where the fingers encircled the throat.

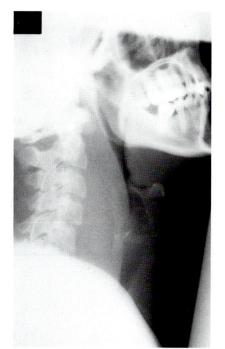

Figure 6.61

Neck trauma (kick from a horse)

This child received a kick on the side of the neck from a horse. An acute retropharyngeal swelling developed that resulted in airway difficulty. This lateral soft-tissue radiograph of the neck demonstrates the acute swelling.

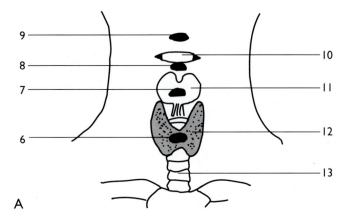

A

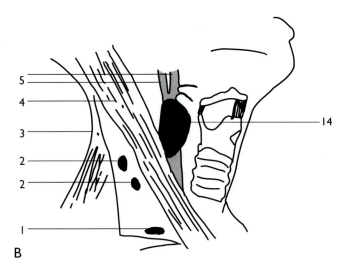

B

Figure 6.62

Assessment of neck lumps

A scheme for the diagnosis of lumps in the neck. A, Midline; B, lateral.

1 *Supraclavicular masses*
   Metastatic tumour (lung or stomach)
2 *Posterior masses*
   Lymphadenopathy from infectious mononucleosis, toxoplasmosis, brucellosis, lymphoma, metastatic tumour, tuberculosis
   Cervical rib
3 Trapezius
4 Sternomastoid
5 Carotid arteries
6 Thyroid nodule moves upward on swallowing
7 Chondroma
8 Thyroglossal cyst moves upward on swallowing and protruding the tongue
9 Dermoid cyst usually above hyoid bone
10 Hyoid bone
11 Thyroid cartilage
12 Thyroid gland
13 Trachea
14 *Lateral masses*
   Metastatic tumour
   Lymphoma
   Branchial cyst
   Laryngocele
   Carotid body tumour

Temporomandibular joint*

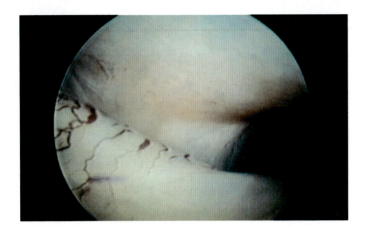

Figure 6.63

Temporomandibular joint arthroscopy

Arthroscopic view of the normal structures in the posterior aspect of the superior joint space of the temporomandibular joint (TMJ). The avascular disc is shown in the lower right. The vascularized synovium of the posterior attachment can be seen in the lower left. The rim of the glenoid fossa is shown above the disc and posterior attachment synovium.

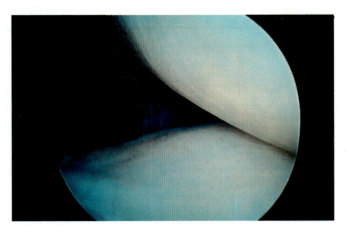

Figure 6.64

Temporomandibular joint arthroscopy

Normal arthroscopic anatomy showing the proper relationship between the disc (lower half of photograph) and the posterior slope of the articular eminence (upper right).

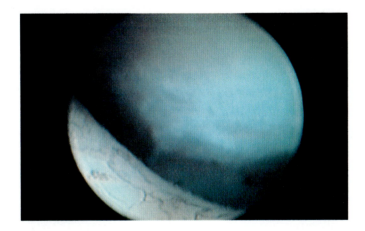

Figure 6.65

Anterior disc displacement

The posterior slope of the articular eminence (note the chondromalacia) is shown from 10 o'clock to 3 o'clock. The posterior attachment synovium is shown beneath the posterior slope of the articular eminence (from 5 o'clock to 9 o'clock). The disc which should normally be positioned beneath the posterior slope of the articular eminence (see Figure 6.64) is anteriorly displaced.

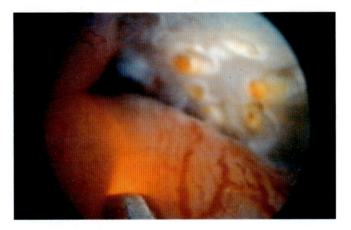

Figure 6.66

Synovitis in the posterior attachment synovium

The erythematous synovial tissue is shown in the lower half of the photograph. This arthroscopic finding is usually associated with significant TMJ pain preoperatively.

*   **The figures in this section are by courtesy of Dr Allen W. Tarro**

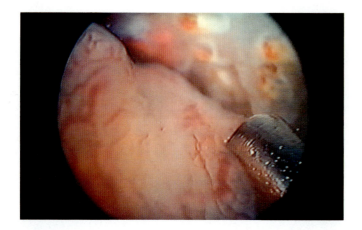

Figure 6.67

Treatment of synovitis with laser synovectomy using the holmium : YAG laser

The laser tip is shown in the lower right of the photograph. Note the decreased vascularity and erythematous appearance of the synovial tissue as compared with Figure 6.66.

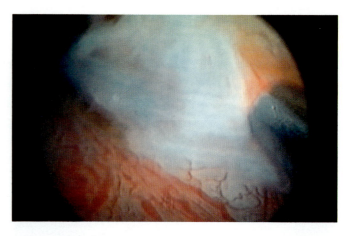

Figure 6.68

Stage 3 chondromalacia

Note the fibrillation of the articular cartilage shown on the posterior slope of the articular eminence, and the synovitis in the tissue below the articular eminence. The laser tip is shown on the right side of the photograph.

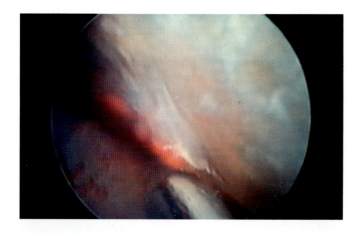

Figure 6.69

Laser resection

The holmium : YAG laser was used to remove most of the fibrillated tissue of the articular cartilage shown in Figure 6.68.

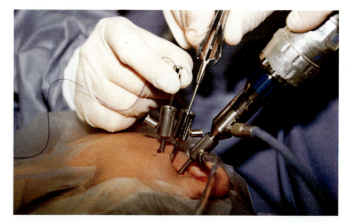

Figure 6.70

Multiport TMJ arthroscopy

A three-portal lateral approach is used in performing a TMJ disc suturing procedure. The suture is passed through the lumen of the needle used to pierce the disc (left cannula). The tissue graspers are used through the middle cannula to grasp the suture material that has been passed through the disc. The arthroscope is placed in the posterior (right) cannula to visualize the surgery in the joint.

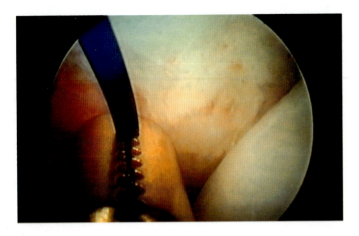

Figure 6.71

Multiport TMJ arthroscopy

Arthroscopic view of the tissue graspers securing the blue PDS suture material in the superior compartment of the TMJ. The disc is shown in the lower right of the photograph.

Select bibliography

Benjamin B, *Atlas of Paediatric Endoscopy: Upper Respiratory Tract and Oesophagus,* Oxford University Press: Oxford, 1981.

Benjamin B, *Diagnostic Laryngology: Adults and Children,* WB Saunders: Philadelphia, 1990.

Benjamin B, Art and science of laryngeal photography, *Annals of Otology, Rhinology and Laryngology* (1993) **102**: 271–82.

Benjamin B, Prolonged intubation injuries of the larynx: endoscopic diagnosis, classification and treatment, *Annals of Otology, Rhinology and Laryngology* (1993) (suppl 160) 102.

Bingham B, Hawke M, Kwok P, *Atlas of Clinical Otolaryngology,* Mosby YearBook: St Louis, 1992.

Hawke M, Telescopic otoscopy and photography of the tympanic membrane, *Journal of Otolaryngology* (1982) **11/1**: 35–9.

Hawke M, Endoscopic photography of the ear: an update, *Journal of Biological Photography* (1984) **52/2**: 19–23.

Hawke M, *Otitis Media: A Pocket Guide,* Decker Periodicals: Philadelphia, 1993.

Hawke M, Jahn AF, *Diseases of the Ear: Clinical and Pathological Aspects,* Gower Press: London, 1987.

Hawke M, Keene M, Alberti PW, *Clinical Otoscopy: An Introduction to Ear Diseases* (second edition), Churchill Livingstone: Edinburgh and London, 1990.

Hawthorn MR, Bingham BJ, *Synopsis of Operative ENT Surgery,* Butterworth: Oxford, 1992.

Hirano Minoru, Phonosurgical anatomy of the larynx. In: C Ford and D Bless (eds), *Assessment and Surgical Management of Voice Disorders,* Raven Press: New York, 1991: 25–41.

Kleinsasser O, *Tumours of the Larynx and Hypopharynx,* Georg Thieme Verlag: Stuttgart and New York, 1988.

Shankar L, Evans K, Stammberger H, Hawke M, *An Atlas of Imaging of the Paranasal Sinuses,* Martin Dunitz and JB Lippincott: London and Philadelphia, 1994.

Stammberger H, *Functional Endoscopic Sinus Surgery: The Messerklinger Technique,* BC Decker: Philadelphia, 1991.

Stammberger H, Hawke M, *Essentials of Functional Endoscopic Sinus Surgery,* Mosby YearBook: St Louis, 1993.

Index